PHARMACOLOGY
AN INTRODUCTORY TEXT

PHARMACOLOGY
AN INTRODUCTORY TEXT

MARY KAYE ASPERHEIM, M.D.

Private Practice, Charleston, South Carolina

Formerly Instructor of Pharmacology
St. Louis University School of Nursing
and Health Services
St. Louis, Missouri

EDITION

8

W.B. SAUNDERS COMPANY
A Division of Harcourt Brace & Company

Philadelphia London Toronto Montreal Sydney Tokyo

W.B. SAUNDERS COMPANY
A Division of Harcourt Brace & Company

The Curtis Center
Independence Square West
Philadelphia, Pennsylvania 19106

Library of Congress Cataloging-in-Publication Data

Asperheim, Mary Kaye.
Pharmacology: an introductory text / Mary Kaye Asperheim. — 8th ed.

p. cm.

Includes bibliographical references and index.

ISBN 0–7216–6038–X

1. Pharmacology.   2. Pharmaceutical arithmetic.   3. Nursing.   I. Title.
  [DNLM: 1. Pharmacology—nurses' instruction.   2. Drugs—nurses' instruction.
  QV 4 A839p   1996]

RM300.A8   1996

615′.1—dc20

DNLM/DLC   95–36451

Important Notice

In preparing this text, the author has made every effort to verify the drug selections and standard dosages presented herein. It is not intended as a source of specific or correct drug use or dosage for any patient. Because of changes in government regulations, research findings, and other information related to drug therapy and drug reactions, it is essential for the reader to check the information and instructions provided by the manufacturer for each drug and therapeutic agent. These may reflect changes in indications or dosage and/or contain relevant warnings and precautions. Attention to these details is particularly important when the recommended agent is a new and/or infrequently employed drug. Any discrepancies or errors should be brought to the attention of the publisher.

PHARMACOLOGY: AN INTRODUCTORY TEXT, Eighth Edition   ISBN 0–7216–6038–X

Last digit is the print number: 9   8   7   6   5   4   3   2   1

PREFACE TO THE EIGHTH EDITION

All categories of drugs have been reviewed and updated for the eighth edition.

Particular emphasis was placed on new categories of antibiotics and antihypertensive agents. Considerable expansion was made in the chapter on Geriatric Medication as well.

A new chapter on Drug Therapy in Home Health Care was added. The increasing number of patients that require skilled professional care outside the centralized hospital setting has resulted in many changes in drug therapy and has required new skills for those administering this care. The expanding roles of nurses and allied health professionals are covered, along with an overview of the drugs used in the home setting.

It is hoped that this text will continue to be useful as an overview of pharmacology for practical nurses and allied health care workers.

MARY KAYE ASPERHEIM FAVARO, M.D.

CONTENTS

UNIT 3
DRUG CLASSIFICATIONS 83

PHARMACOLOGY
AN INTRODUCTORY TEXT

U N I T

1

MATHEMATICS OF DOSAGE

U N I T   O B J E C T I V E S

■ 1. Write the basic Roman numerals for their Arabic equivalents.
■ 2. Read and write Roman numerals with 100 percent accuracy.
■ 3. Explain the meaning of a fraction and give an example of each type of fraction.
■ 4. Convert between improper fractions and whole or mixed numbers.
■ 5. Give the fundamental principles used in computing with fractions and give an example of each one.
■ 6. Demonstrate accurately the addition, subtraction, multiplication, and division of fractions and mixed numbers.
■ 7. Read and write decimals with 100 percent accuracy.
■ 8. Add, subtract, multiply, and divide decimals with 100 percent accuracy.
■ 9. Convert decimals to fractions with 100 percent accuracy.
■ 10. Convert common fractions to decimals with 100 percent accuracy.
■ 11. Convert percents to decimals, fractions to percents, percents to fractions, and decimals to percents.
■ 12. Use ratio-proportion technique with 100 percent accuracy.
■ 13. Convert temperature from the Fahrenheit scale to the centigrade scale and vice versa.

Roman Numerals

The system of Roman numerals uses letters to designate numbers. Their use is obviously restricted because mathematical procedures would become extremely complicated if the attempt were made to use these numerals in calculations. They are, however, retained in the apothecary system of measures used in writing prescriptions and dosages of drugs.

Basic Roman numerals are expressed as follows:

Roman Numeral	Arabic Number
I	1
V	5
X	10
L	50
C	100
D	500
M	1000

READING AND WRITING ROMAN NUMERALS

Procedure

1. When a Roman numeral precedes one of larger value, its value is subtracted from the larger. When a numeral follows one of larger value, its value is added to the larger.

Examples:

    a. IV = (5 − 1) = 4
    b. XI = (10 + 1) = 11
    c. LXI = (50 + 10 + 1) = 61

2. When two numerals of identical value are reported in sequence, their values are added. (Numerals may never be repeated more than three times in sequence.)

Examples:

    a. XXX = 30
    b. MMXXVII = 2028

3. When a numeral is placed between two numerals of greater value, the lesser is subtracted from the numeral following it.

Examples:

a. XIV = (10 + 5 − 1) = 14
b. XIX = (10 + 10 − 1) = 19
c. CXLIX = (100 + 50 − 10 + 10 − 1) = 149

EXERCISES

A. Express the following in Roman numerals:

1. 35
2. 89
3. 72
4. 55
5. 101

6. 92
7. 135
8. 1580
9. 341
10. 729

B. Express the following in Arabic numbers:

1. MCCXI
2. DCCXX
3. CLXVI
4. DXXIX
5. MMMVI

6. DCCC
7. LVI
8. LXXV
9. MMDCLXXIII
10. LXI

Fractions

A fraction indicates division and expresses the number of equal parts into which a whole is divided. If a whole is divided into a number of equal parts, then one or more parts of this number of equal parts is called a fraction.

Example: The fraction $\frac{3}{8}$ means 3 of 8 equal parts (Figure 2–1). This could also be written $3 \div 8$ because it indicates division into 8 equal parts.

The numbers 3 and 8 are called the "terms of the fraction." The lower number of a fraction is called the denominator, or the divisor, and tells into how many parts the unit is divided. The upper number of the fraction is called the numerator, or the dividend, and tells how many parts of the unit are taken.

KINDS OF FRACTIONS

Proper fraction. Sometimes called a common fraction, or just "fraction," this has a numerator that is smaller than the denominator and designates less than one whole unit.

Examples: $\frac{1}{3}, \frac{2}{5}, \frac{3}{17}$

Improper fraction. This is a fraction in which the numerator is larger than the denominator and designates more than one unit (Figure 2–2).

Example: $\frac{5}{4}$ or $1\frac{1}{4}$

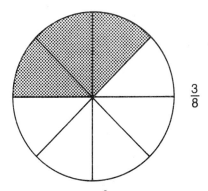

Figure 2–1. The fraction $\frac{3}{8}$ means 3 of 8 equal parts.

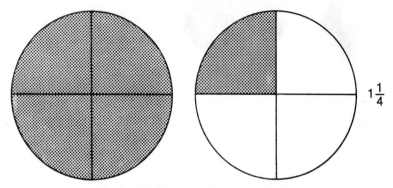

Figure 2–2. Example of improper fraction.

Mixed number. This consists of a whole number and a fraction.

Examples: $3\frac{3}{7}$, $4\frac{2}{3}$

Complex fraction. Both the numerator and the denominator (or just one of these) is in fraction form (Figure 2–3).

Examples: $\dfrac{\frac{2}{3}}{\frac{3}{8}}$, $\dfrac{4}{\frac{3}{7}}$

A fraction is said to be reduced to its lowest terms when the numerator and denominator cannot be divided exactly by the same number (except 1).

Example: $\frac{6}{8}$ This fraction is not reduced because both numerator and denominator can be divided by 2.

$$\frac{6\,(\div\,2)}{8\,(\div\,2)} = \frac{3}{4}$$ This is the reduced fraction.

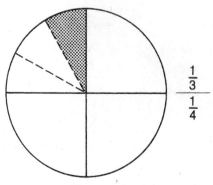

Figure 2–3. Example of complex fraction.

CONVERTING BETWEEN IMPROPER FRACTIONS AND WHOLE OR MIXED NUMBERS

Procedure for Changing an Improper Fraction into a Whole or Mixed Number

1. Divide the numerator by the denominator.
2. Write the remainder, if any, as a fraction reduced to the lowest terms.

Examples:

a. Change $\frac{8}{4}$ to a whole number.

$$8 \div 4 = 2$$

b. Change $\frac{16}{6}$ to a mixed number.

$$16 \div 6 = 2\frac{4}{6}, \text{ or reduced} = 2\frac{2}{3}$$

Procedure for Changing Mixed Numbers into Improper Fractions

1. Multiply the whole number by the denominator of the fraction.
2. Add this product to the numerator of the fraction.
3. Write the sum as numerator of the improper fraction; the denominator remains the same.

Examples:

a. Change $2\frac{3}{8}$ to an improper fraction.

$$2 \times 8 = 16, 16 + 3 = 19 \therefore \frac{19}{8}$$

b. Change $4\frac{2}{5}$ to an improper fraction.

$$4 \times 5 = 20, 20 + 2 = 22 \therefore \frac{22}{5}$$

c. Change $9\frac{1}{6}$ to an improper fraction.

$$9 \times 6 = 54, 54 + 1 = 55 \therefore \frac{55}{6}$$

EXERCISES

A. Change the following to whole or mixed numbers:

1. $\frac{12}{8} = 1\frac{4}{8} = 1\frac{1}{2}$ 2. $\frac{7}{5} = 1\frac{2}{5}$

3. $\dfrac{20}{10}$ 7. $\dfrac{79}{5}$

4. $\dfrac{12}{4}$ 8. $\dfrac{64}{9}$

5. $\dfrac{17}{9}$ 9. $\dfrac{26}{3}$

6. $\dfrac{25}{8}$ 10. $\dfrac{410}{100}$

B. Change the following to improper fractions:

1. $1\dfrac{1}{3}$ 6. $6\dfrac{4}{5}$

2. $4\dfrac{1}{2}$ 7. $2\dfrac{1}{8}$

3. $100\dfrac{3}{7}$ 8. $17\dfrac{1}{4}$

4. $9\dfrac{1}{8}$ 9. $80\dfrac{5}{12}$

5. $10\dfrac{4}{5}$ 10. $110\dfrac{1}{4}$

EQUIVALENT FRACTIONS

Equivalent fractions are fractions whose terms are different but that may be reduced to the same fraction. Equivalent fractions may be made by multiplying or dividing both terms of a fraction by the same number. Any number may be used, as long as the numerator and denominator are treated in the same way.

Examples:

a. $\dfrac{1(\times 2)}{8(\times 2)} = \dfrac{2}{16}$

b. $\dfrac{2(\times 32)}{3(\times 32)} = \dfrac{64}{96}$

c. $\dfrac{4(\div 2)}{6(\div 2)} = \dfrac{2}{3}$

Fractions may be changed to obtain a new fraction of any desired denominator by determining what number the present denominator must be multiplied by to give the desired denominator. Both numerator and denominator are then multiplied by this number.

Examples:

a. $\dfrac{1}{2} = \dfrac{?}{8}$

$8 \div 2 = 4$, so both numerator and denominator are multiplied by 4.

$$\dfrac{1}{2} \dfrac{(\times 4)}{(\times 4)} = \dfrac{4}{8}$$

b. $\dfrac{5}{9} = \dfrac{?}{72}$

$72 \div 9 = 8$, so both numerator and denominator are multiplied by 8.

$$\dfrac{5\ (\times\ 8)}{9\ (\times\ 8)} = \dfrac{40}{72}$$

EXERCISES

Change the following fractions to equivalent fractions having the specified denominator:

1. $\dfrac{1}{4} = \dfrac{?}{20}$ ___ ___

2. $\dfrac{6}{13} = \dfrac{?}{39}$ ___ ___

3. $\dfrac{6}{15} = \dfrac{?}{60}$ ___ ___

4. $\dfrac{7}{18} = \dfrac{?}{36}$ ___

5. $\dfrac{5}{4} = \dfrac{?}{32}$ ___

6. $\dfrac{8}{17} = \dfrac{?}{51}$ ___

7. $\dfrac{7}{9} = \dfrac{?}{63}$ ___

8. $\dfrac{9}{8} = \dfrac{?}{16}$ ___

9. $\dfrac{6}{7} = \dfrac{?}{21}$ ___

10. $\dfrac{63}{30} = \dfrac{?}{10}$ ___

FINDING THE LOWEST COMMON DENOMINATOR

Procedure

1. Find the lowest possible number that is divisible by all the denominators.
2. Change the fractions to equivalent fractions using this denominator.

Example: Find the lowest common denominator for the following:

a. $\dfrac{1}{3}$ and $\dfrac{2}{5}$ The lowest number divisible by 3 and 5 is 15, so this will be the new denominator.

$$\frac{1}{3} = \frac{?}{15} = \frac{5}{15}$$

$$\frac{2}{5} = \frac{?}{15} = \frac{6}{15}$$

b. $\frac{2}{3}$, $\frac{7}{8}$, and $\frac{1}{6}$ The lowest number divisible by 3, 8, and 6 is 24.

$$\frac{2}{3} = \frac{?}{24} = \frac{16}{24}$$

$$\frac{7}{8} = \frac{?}{24} = \frac{21}{24}$$

$$\frac{1}{6} = \frac{?}{24} = \frac{4}{24}$$

c. $\frac{2}{4}$ and $\frac{6}{8}$ The lowest common denominator is 8, so only the $\frac{2}{4}$ must be changed.

$$\frac{2}{4} = \frac{4}{8}$$

$$\frac{6}{8} = \frac{6}{8}$$

EXERCISES

Change the following to fractions having the lowest common denominator:

1. $\frac{7}{12}$ and $\frac{3}{6}$ ———

7. $\frac{2}{3}$, $\frac{1}{2}$, and $\frac{3}{4}$

2. $\frac{6}{7}$ and $\frac{2}{3}$ —

8. $\frac{3}{4}$, $\frac{5}{6}$, and $\frac{7}{8}$ - -

3. $\frac{1}{3}$ and $\frac{2}{9}$

9. $\frac{8}{9}$, $\frac{9}{10}$, and $\frac{1}{3}$

4. $\frac{2}{5}$ and $\frac{8}{20}$ —

10. $\frac{4}{15}$, $\frac{3}{5}$, and $\frac{4}{25}$

5. $\frac{1}{8}$ and $\frac{8}{24}$

11. $1\frac{1}{3}$, $\frac{3}{6}$, and $\frac{1}{4}$

6. $\frac{1}{4}$, $\frac{1}{5}$, and $\frac{1}{6}$

12. $\frac{3}{5}$, $\frac{4}{6}$, and $\frac{4}{10}$

ADDITION OF FRACTIONS AND MIXED NUMBERS

Procedure

1. If the fractions have the same denominator, add the numerators and write the sum over the common denominator and reduce to the lowest terms.

2. If the fractions have unlike denominators, first find their lowest common denominator; then add the numerators as mentioned.

3. To add mixed numbers, first add the fractions as mentioned and then add this to the sum of the whole numbers.

Examples:

a.
$$\frac{1}{5}$$
$$+\frac{2}{5}$$
$$\overline{\frac{3}{5}}$$

b.
$$\frac{3}{5} = \frac{9}{15}$$
$$+\frac{2}{3} = \frac{10}{15}$$
$$\overline{\frac{19}{15}} = 1\frac{4}{15}$$

c.
$$6\frac{1}{6} = 6\frac{8}{48}$$
$$+\ 9\frac{5}{8} = 9\frac{30}{48}$$
$$\overline{15\frac{38}{48}} = 15\frac{19}{24}$$

d.
$$1\frac{3}{8} = 1\frac{15}{40}$$
$$+9\frac{9}{10} = 9\frac{36}{40}$$
$$10\frac{51}{40}\left(\frac{51}{40} = 1\frac{11}{40}\right) = 11\frac{11}{40}$$

EXERCISES

Add the following numbers:

1. $\frac{1}{12}$, $\frac{2}{3}$, and $\frac{4}{9}$

2. $\frac{3}{5}$, $\frac{2}{3}$, and $\frac{4}{10}$

3. $2\frac{1}{3}$ and $4\frac{1}{8}$

4. $7\frac{1}{4}$, $6\frac{2}{8}$, and $4\frac{5}{6}$

5. $\frac{2}{3}$, $\frac{1}{2}$, and $\frac{1}{4}$

6. $3\frac{1}{2}$, $2\frac{3}{10}$, and $5\frac{2}{5}$

7. 5 and $\frac{7}{12}$

8. 2, $1\frac{4}{4}$, and $2\frac{5}{6}$

9. $24\frac{3}{8}$, $12\frac{6}{7}$, and $\frac{5}{14}$

10. $4\frac{1}{2}$, $2\frac{3}{8}$, and $3\frac{1}{4}$

SUBTRACTION OF FRACTIONS AND MIXED NUMBERS

Procedure

1. If the fractions have the same denominator, find the difference between the numerators and write it over the common denominator. Reduce to the lowest terms.

2. If the fractions have unlike denominators, first find the lowest common denominator, then proceed as mentioned.

3. To subtract mixed numbers, first subtract the fractions as mentioned and then find the difference between the whole numbers. If the fraction in the subtrahend (bottom number) is larger than the fraction in the minuend (top number), it is necessary to borrow from the whole number before subtracting the fractions.

Examples:

a. $\frac{4}{5} = \frac{8}{10}$

$-\frac{1}{2} = \frac{5}{10}$

$\frac{3}{10}$

b. $7\frac{16}{24} = 7\frac{16}{24}$

$-3\frac{1}{8} = 3\frac{3}{24}$

$4\frac{13}{24}$

c. $21\frac{7}{16} = 20\frac{16}{16} + \frac{7}{16} = 20\frac{23}{16}$

$-7\frac{12}{16}$

$-7\frac{12}{16}$

$13\frac{11}{16}$

EXERCISES

Subtract the following:

1. $\dfrac{8}{18} - \dfrac{3}{18}$ —— ——

2. $\dfrac{5}{7} - \dfrac{2}{3}$

3. $\dfrac{7}{8} - \dfrac{1}{4}$

4. $2\dfrac{4}{7} - 1\dfrac{1}{7}$

5. $4\dfrac{2}{8} - 2\dfrac{7}{8}$

6. $\dfrac{7}{15} - 3\dfrac{10}{15}$ ——————

7. $6 - 2\dfrac{2}{3}$

8. $25\dfrac{4}{5} - 11$

9. $20 - 16\dfrac{11}{12}$

10. $4\dfrac{2}{3} - 1\dfrac{1}{2}$

MULTIPLICATION OF FRACTIONS AND MIXED NUMBERS

Procedure

1. Change mixed numbers to improper fractions.
2. Cancel if possible by dividing any numerator and denominator by the largest number contained in each.
3. Multiply remaining numerators to find numerator of answer.
4. Multiply remaining denominators to find denominator of answer.

Examples:

a. $\dfrac{4}{5} \times \dfrac{15}{16} = \dfrac{\overset{1}{\cancel{4}}}{\underset{1}{\cancel{5}}} \times \dfrac{\overset{3}{\cancel{15}}}{\underset{4}{\cancel{16}}} = \dfrac{3}{4}$

b. $6 \times \dfrac{3}{8} = \dfrac{\overset{3}{\cancel{6}}}{1} \times \dfrac{3}{\underset{4}{\cancel{8}}} = \dfrac{9}{4} = 2\dfrac{1}{4}$

EXERCISES

Multiply the following:

1. $\dfrac{1}{3} \times \dfrac{1}{4}$ 6. $12 \times 2\dfrac{3}{4}$

2. $\dfrac{7}{8} \times \dfrac{5}{9}$ 7. $\dfrac{2}{3} \times 6$

3. $3\dfrac{1}{3} \times 1\dfrac{1}{5}$ 8. $\dfrac{4}{200} \times 1000$

4. $\dfrac{4}{5} \times 1\dfrac{8}{15}$ 9. $\dfrac{1}{3} \times \dfrac{4}{12} \times \dfrac{4}{6}$

5. $1\dfrac{1}{2} \times 2\dfrac{5}{6} \times 3\dfrac{1}{3}$ 10. $\dfrac{3}{4} \times \dfrac{4}{5} \times \dfrac{2}{15}$

DIVISION OF FRACTIONS AND MIXED NUMBERS

Procedure

1. Change mixed numbers to improper fractions.
2. Invert the divisor (the number after the division sign).
3. Follow the steps for multiplication of fractions.

Examples:

a. $\dfrac{2}{5} \div \dfrac{5}{8} = \dfrac{2}{5} \times \dfrac{8}{5} = \dfrac{16}{25}$

b. $8\dfrac{3}{4} \div 15 = \dfrac{\overset{7}{35}}{4} \times \dfrac{1}{\underset{3}{15}} = \dfrac{7}{12}$

EXERCISES

Divide the following:

1. $\dfrac{3}{5} \div \dfrac{7}{8}$ _____

2. $\dfrac{1}{12} \div \dfrac{1}{3}$ _____

3. $\dfrac{4}{6} \div \dfrac{6}{7}$ _____

4. $\dfrac{2}{3} \div 4$ _____

5. $3 \div \dfrac{1}{2}$ _____

6. $\dfrac{3}{4} \div \dfrac{4}{6}$ _____

7. $3\dfrac{1}{2} \div 1\dfrac{3}{4}$ _____

8. $1\dfrac{3}{4} \div 2$ _____

9. $1\dfrac{1}{2} \div 1\dfrac{1}{4}$ _____

10. $20\dfrac{1}{2} \div 50$ _____

RATIO

A ratio indicates the relationship of one quantity to another. It indicates division and may be expressed in fraction form.

Examples:

a. $\dfrac{3}{9}$ may be expressed as a ratio 3:9

b. 1:1000 may be expressed as a fraction $\dfrac{1}{1000}$

EXERCISES

Express the following ratios as fractions reduced to lowest terms:

1. 1:3 _____

2. 5:7 _____

3. 2:1000 _____

4. 7:63 _____

5. 42:83 _____

6. 2:17 $\frac{2}{17}$

7. 7:56 $\frac{7}{56} = \frac{1}{8}$

8. 1:11 $\frac{1}{11}$

9. 2:150 $\frac{2}{150} = \frac{1}{75}$

10. 4:9 $\frac{4}{9}$

Decimal Fractions

A decimal fraction is a fraction whose denominator is 10 or any multiple of 10, such as 100, 1000, 10,000, and so forth. However, it differs from a common fraction in that the denominator is not written but is expressed by the proper placement of the decimal point. Usually decimal fractions and mixed decimals are just called "decimals."

READING AND WRITING DECIMALS

Procedure

1. Observe the following scale. All whole numbers are to the left of the decimal point; all fractions are to the right.

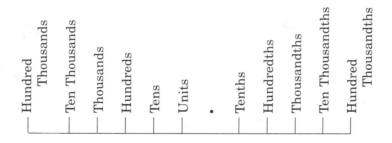

2. In reading a decimal fraction, read the number to the right of the decimal point and use the name that applies to the "place value" of the last figure.

Example: 0.257 = two hundred fifty-seven thousandths

3. In reading a mixed decimal, first read the whole number, then the decimal fraction. The word "and" shows the place of the decimal point.

Example: 327.006 = three hundred twenty-seven and six thousandths

EXERCISES

A. Read the following:

1. 0.03 _____

2. 0.089 _____

3. 23.5 _____

4. 5.21 _____

5. 0.0029 _____

6. 200.09 _____

7. 37.282 _____

8. 4256.353 _____

9. 256.01 _____

10. 0.0008 _____

B. Express the following as decimal fractions:

1. Four thousandths _____

2. Twenty-six hundredths _____

3. Five and three millionths _____

4. Seven hundredths _____

5. Three and one tenth _____

6. Eighty-eight thousandths _____

7. Two hundred thirty-three and fifty-seven millionths _____

8. Two and three tenths _____

9. Eight and four hundredths _____

10. Twenty-five and three one thousandths _____

ADDITION OF DECIMALS

Procedure

1. Write the decimals in a column, placing the decimal points directly under each other.

2. Add as in the addition of whole numbers.

3. Place the decimal point in the sum directly under the decimal points in the addends.

Examples:

a. 0.8 + 0.5 = 0.8
                0.5
                ———
                1.3

b. 3.27 + 0.06 + 2 = 3.27
                      0.06
                      2.00
                      ————
                      5.33

EXERCISES

Add the following:

1. 7.01 + 3.888

2. 26.78 + 6.28 + 16.53

3. 7.52 + 4.9

4. 0.72 + 0.81 + 5

5. 0.76 + 2 + 300

6. 0.81 + 0.973

7. 6 + 0.09

8. 0.8 + 6 + 0.245

9. 77.1 + 0.27 + 0.31

10. 0.3 + 0.37 + 1.8

SUBTRACTION OF DECIMALS

Procedure

1. The decimals should be written in columns, keeping the decimal points under each other.

2. Subtract as with whole numbers. (Zeros may be added after the decimal without changing the value.)

3. Place the decimal point in the remainder directly under the decimal point in the subtrahend and minuend.

Example: $0.6 - 0.524 =$ $\begin{array}{r} 0.600 \\ -0.524 \\ \hline 0.076 \end{array}$

EXERCISES

Subtract the following:

1. $1.65 - 1.004$

2. $0.21 - 0.17$

3. $64.28 - 23$

4. $756.824 - 28.127$

5. $0.07 - 0.052$

6. $10 - 6.78$

7. $5 - 0.3$

8. $36 - 1.5$

9. $3 - 0.163$

10. $109 - 3.29$

MULTIPLICATION OF DECIMALS

Procedure

1. Multiply as in the multiplication of whole numbers.
2. Find the total number of decimal places in the multiplier and multiplicand.
3. Starting from the right, point off in the product this total number of decimal places.
4. If the product contains fewer figures than the required decimal places, prefix as many zeros as necessary.

Example: $2.6 \times 0.0002 = $

$$
\begin{array}{r}
2.6 \\
\underline{0.0002} \\
0.00052
\end{array}
$$

EXERCISES

Multiply the following:

1. 4×0.8 _____   _____

2. 0.005×2.2 _____   .   _____

3. 3.15×0.03 _____   _____

4. 200×0.6 _____   _____

5. 59.38×0.015 _____   ____

6. 200×0.6 _____   _____

7. 0.003×0.03 _____   _____

8. 26.17×3.8 ____   _____

9. 100×1.2 _____   _____

10. 7.302×1.54 ___   _____

DIVISION OF DECIMALS

Procedure

1. If the divisor is a whole number, divide as in the division of whole numbers and place the decimal point in the quotient directly above the decimal point in the dividend.

2. If the divisor is a decimal, make it a whole number by moving the decimal point to the right of the last figure. Move the decimal point in the dividend the same number of places; proceed in division as in Step 1. (If the dividend contains fewer places than required, zeros may be added.)

$$
\begin{array}{r}
24.00 \\
625\overline{)15.000.00} \\
\end{array}
$$

Example: $15 \div 0.625 =$

$$
\begin{array}{r}
12\ 50 \\
\hline
2\ 500 \\
2\ 500 \\
\end{array}
$$

EXERCISES

Divide the following and carry to the third decimal place:

1. $300 \div 5.0$ _____

2. $14.03 \div 6$ _____

3. $69.4 \div 0.52$ _____

4. $24.78 \div 4$ _____

5. $48 \div 2.4$ _____

6. $0.2482 \div 0.068$ _____

7. $84 \div 4.2$ _____

8. $270.6 \div 32$ _____

9. $96.2 \div 28$ _____

10. $0.06128 \div 0.72$ _____

CHANGING DECIMALS TO FRACTIONS

Procedure

1. Express the decimal as it is written in fraction form.
2. Reduce to lowest terms.

Examples:

a. $0.375 = \dfrac{375}{1000} = \dfrac{3}{8}$

b. $0.40 = \dfrac{40}{100} = \dfrac{2}{5}$

c. $0.8 = \dfrac{8}{10} = \dfrac{4}{5}$

CHANGING COMMON FRACTIONS TO DECIMALS

Procedure

1. Divide the numerator by the denominator.
2. Place decimal point in proper position.

Examples:

a. $\dfrac{2}{5} = 5)\overline{2.00}^{\,0.4} = 0.04$

b. $\dfrac{19}{100} = 100)\overline{19.00}^{\,0.19} = 0.19$

c. $\dfrac{9}{7} = 7)\overline{9.000}^{\,1.29} = 1.29$

EXERCISES

A. Change the following to decimals.

1. $\dfrac{8}{10}$

2. $\dfrac{1}{6}$

3. $\dfrac{22}{100}$

4. $\dfrac{13}{15}$

5. $4\dfrac{2}{5}$

6. $7\frac{1}{8}$ _____ _____

7. $\frac{38}{54}$ _____ _____

8. $\frac{6754}{10000}$ _____ _____

9. $4\frac{23}{32}$ _____ _____

10. $\frac{94}{36}$ _____ _____

B. Change the following to fractions or mixed numbers:

1. 0.28 _____ _____

2. 5.07 _____ _____

3. 0.0022 _____ _____

4. 1.28 _____ _____

5. 3.04 _____ _____

6. 0.575 _____ _____

7. 0.76 _____ _____

8. 0.15325 _____ _____

9. 6.09 _____ _____

10. 0.01 _____ _____

4

Percentage

The term *percent,* and its symbol %, means hundredths. A percent number is a fraction whose numerator is expressed and whose denominator is understood to be 100. It can be changed to a decimal by moving the decimal point two places to the left to signify hundredths or to a fraction by expressing the denominator as 100.

Examples:

a. 5% means $\frac{5}{100}$ or 0.05

b. $\frac{1}{2}$% means $\frac{\frac{1}{2}}{100}$ or 0.005

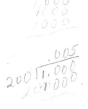

EXERCISES

Complete the following:

Fraction	Decimal	Percent
1. $\frac{1}{4}$	.25	25
2. $1\frac{1}{4}$	1.25	125
3. $\frac{3}{4}$	.75	75%
4. $\frac{1}{8}$ $\quad 8\overline{)1.0^{2}0}$ $\frac{125}{}$	.125	12.5 %
5. $\frac{56}{100}$	0.56	56 %
6. $\frac{6}{1000}$	.00.6	.6 %
7. $\frac{6}{100}$	.06	6%
8. $\frac{3}{4}$	0.75	75 %

25

9. $\frac{1}{5}$ .20   20%

10. $\frac{12}{100} = \frac{3}{25}$ .12   12%

11. $\frac{5}{100}$ 0.05   5%

12. $\frac{72}{100} = \frac{18}{25}$ .72   72%

FINDING PERCENT OF A NUMBER

Procedure

1. Change the percent to a decimal or common fraction.
2. Multiply the number by this decimal.

Examples:

    a. 23% of 64 = ?

$$64 \times 0.23 = 14.72$$

    b. 114% of 240 = ?

$$240 \times 1.14 = 273.6$$

EXERCISES

Find the following percents:

1. 6% of 300 $300 \times .06$ 18.00

2. $\frac{1}{2}$ % of 840 $840 \times .005 = 4.200$ 4.2

3. 5% of 15 $.05 \times 15$ .75

4. 8% of 2700   2700 .08 21600   216

5. 200% of 6.7   2.00 6.7 14.00   13.4

6. 0.2% of 10   .002 × 10   .02

7. 50% of 75 $\frac{50}{100} \times$ .50 37.50   37.5

8. 3% of 200   6

9. $\frac{1}{3}$ % of 360   360 00330 1080   1.08 1.20 1.080

$\frac{1}{3}$ 1,080

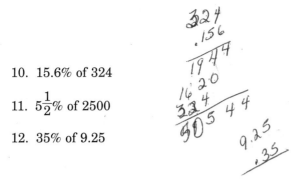

10. 15.6% of 324

11. $5\frac{1}{2}$% of 2500

12. 35% of 9.25

FINDING WHAT PERCENT ONE NUMBER IS OF ANOTHER

Procedure

1. Make a fraction of the two numbers using the number after the word "of" as the denominator.
2. Reduce the fraction to lowest terms.
3. Change the reduced fraction to a percent.

Examples:

a. 27 is what percent of 36?

$$\frac{27}{36} = \frac{3}{4} = 75\%$$

b. 9 is ? % of 20?

$$\frac{9}{20} = 0.45 = 45\%$$

EXERCISES

Find the following percents:

1. 2 is ? % of 20?

2. 10 is ? % of 25?

3. 15 is ? % of 85?

4. $2\frac{1}{2}$ is ? % of 8?

5. What % of 25 is 15?

6. 45 is ? % of 80?

7. $1\frac{1}{2}$ is ? % of $8\frac{1}{2}$?

8. What % of 25 is 50?

9. 60 is ? % of 15?

10. 3 is ? % of 15?

11. 240 is ? % of 1200?

12. What % of 15 is 30?

$\dfrac{50}{25} \times \overset{4}{100}$

$\dfrac{\overset{4}{60}}{15} \times 100$

$\dfrac{3}{15} \times \overset{20}{100}$

$\dfrac{\overset{2}{30}}{15} \times 100$

200 %

$15\overline{)60}$ 400 %

20 %

20 %

200 %

5

Proportion

A proportion shows the relationship between two equal ratios. A proportion may be expressed as:

$$8 : 16 : : 1 : 2$$
or
$$8 : 16 = 1 : 2$$

The first and fourth terms of a proportion are called the *extremes,* and the second and third terms are the *means*. In a proportion, the product of the means equals the product of the extremes.

It can be seen from the sample proportion above that the product of the extremes $(8 \times 2) = 16$; the product of the means $(16 \times 1) = 16$.

When one term of the proportion is unknown, it can easily be found.

Procedure

1. Multiply the means and the extremes, letting "x" signify the unknown term.
2. Divide the known product by the coefficient of "x" to solve for the unknown term.

Examples:

a. $3 : 5 = x : 10$

$$5x = 30$$
$$x = \frac{30}{5} = 6$$

b. $\frac{1}{2} : x = 1 : 8$

$$1x = 4\left(8 \times \frac{1}{2}\right)$$
$$x = \frac{4}{1} = 4$$

EXERCISES

Solve the following proportions for "x":

1. 2 : x :: 10 : 20   _____

2. 20 : x :: 30 : 600   _____

3. 10 : 15 :: x : 30   _____

4. x : 300 :: 2 : 60   _____

5. 6 : 3000 :: 10 : x   _____

6. 8 : 24 :: 16 : x   _____

7. 2.5 : x :: 50 : 60   _____

8. 3.4 : x :: 17 : 25   _____

9. 4 : 8 :: x : 72   _____

10. $3\frac{1}{2}$: 28 :: 6 : x   _____

11. 4 : 18 :: 20 : x   _____

12. 7 : 30 :: x : 60   _____

13. 4 : 7 :: x : 49   _____

14. x : 5.2 :: 1.6 : 8   _____

15. 20 : 100 :: 5 : x   _____

6

Fahrenheit and Centigrade

Two scales are commonly used to measure temperature: the Fahrenheit and centigrade scales. The inner tube of the thermometer contains mercury, which expands and rises in the tube as the heat increases, thus showing the temperatures on the scale (Figure 6–1).

The Fahrenheit scale is used on most clinical thermometers in the United States, but because some clinical thermometers do use the centigrade scale, the nurse should be able to convert from one scale to the other.

Five degrees on the centigrade scale correspond to nine degrees on the Fahrenheit scale, so the ratio is 5 : 9. Zero degrees centigrade corresponds to 32° Fahren-

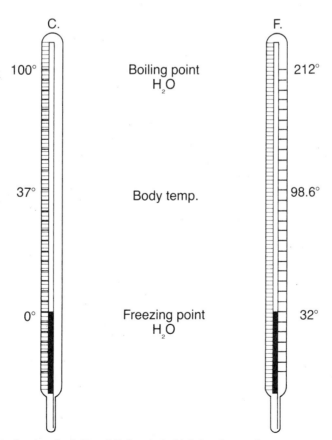

C.		F.
100°	Boiling point H_2O	212°
37°	Body temp.	98.6°
0°	Freezing point H_2O	32°

Figure 6–1. Centigrade *(left)* and Fahrenheit *(right)* scales used to measure temperature.

heit, so 32° must be subtracted from the Fahrenheit temperature in addition to considering the simple ratio.

Procedure for Converting Between Fahrenheit and Centigrade

1. Use the proportion formula C : F − 32 :: 5 : 9.
2. Substitute the known temperature in its proper place in the formula.
3. Solve for the unknown temperature as for the fourth term of a proportion.

Examples:

    a. Change 50° F to C

$$C : F - 32 :: 5 : 9$$
$$C : 50 - \underset{(18)}{32 :: 5 : 9}$$
$$9\,C = \frac{18 \times 5\,(90)}{90}$$
$$C = \frac{90}{9} = 10\,° \text{ on the centigrade scale}$$

    b. Change 75° C to F

$$C : F - 32 :: 5 : 9$$
$$75 : F - 32 :: 5 : 9$$
$$5(F - 32) = 675$$
$$5\,F - 160 = 675$$
$$5\,F = 835$$
$$F = 167° \text{ on the Fahrenheit scale}$$

EXERCISES

Convert the following:

1. 20° C = _____ ° F

2. 60° C = _____ ° F

3. 102° C = _____ ° F

4. 35° C = _____ ° F

5. 40° C = _____ ° F

6. 101° F = _____ ° C

7. 70° F = _____ ° C

8. 120° F = _____ ° C

9. 104° F = _____ ° C

10. 96.8° F = _____ ° C

Systems of Measurement

The systems of weights and measures commonly used in medicine are the metric and apothecary systems. Because both are used even in reference to a single drug or prescription, it is essential that the nurse become familiar with both systems and be able to convert from one to the other whenever necessary.

THE METRIC SYSTEM

The metric system is now being used exclusively in the *United States Pharmacopeia* and before long will probably be the only system used in drug dosage. Arabic numbers and decimals are used with this system.

The units used in the metric system are:

liter for volume	(fluids)
gram for weight	(solids)
meter for measure	(length)

These basic units are multiplied and divided always by a multiple of 10 to form the entire system. There are only a few equivalents that are used in medicine, however. These are:

Volume	Weight
1000 mL = 1 liter (L)	1000 mg = 1 gram (gm)
	1000 gm = 1 kilogram (kg)

A milliliter (mL) is equivalent to a cubic centimeter (cc), and for all practical purposes these units may be used interchangeably. Hence, 1000 cc = 1 L.

Procedure for Conversion Between Units of the Metric System

1. To change milligrams to grams, to change milliliters to liters, or to change grams to kilograms, divide by 1000.

2. To change liters to milliliters, grams to milligrams, or kilograms to grams, multiply by 1000.

Examples:

a. 64 mg = ? gm

$$1000 \text{ mg} : 1 \text{ gm} = 64 \text{ mg} : x \text{ gm}$$
$$1000 \text{ x} = 64$$
$$x = \frac{64}{1000} = 0.064 \text{ gm}$$

b. 325 mL = ? L

$$1000 \text{ mL} : 1 \text{ L} = 325 \text{ mL} : x \text{ L}$$
$$1000 \text{ x} = 325$$
$$x = \frac{325}{1000} = 0.325 \text{ L}$$

N.B. These rules may be used without use of the ratio and proportion method. The use of the proportion does serve to clarify the reasoning behind multiplying or dividing, however.

c. 3.5 L = ? mL

$$1000 \text{ mL} : 1 \text{ L} = x \text{ mL} : 3.5 \text{ L}$$
$$1 \text{ x} = 3500$$
$$x = 3500 \text{ mL}$$

EXERCISES

Change to equivalents within the metric system:

1. 1000 mg   =   _____ gm

2. 500 mg   =   _____ gm

3. 2000 mL   =   _____ L

4. 1500 mg   =   _____ gm

5. 0.1 L   =   _____ mL

6. 750 mg   =   _____ gm

7. 1 kg   =   _____ gm

8. 5 L   =   _____ mL

9. 4 mg   =   _____ gm

10. 100 gm   =   _____ kg

11. 0.25 L   =   _____ mL

12. 0.006 gm   =   _____ mg

13. 250 mg   =   _____ gm

14. 2.5 L   =   _____ mL

15. 0.05 gm   =   _____ mg

THE APOTHECARY SYSTEM

In this older system, Roman numerals and common fractions are used to designate units. The units of measure *precede* the numeral in correct form (e.g., the correct way to signify 20 grains would be "gr.xx"). A line is often written above the numerals, and a dot is placed above the numeral I to distinguish more clearly between two I's and a V or X hastily written. When using the apothecary system in calculations, however, the Arabic numbers are used.

Volume

60 minims (℥LX)	= 1 fluid dram (fl ʒ İ)
8 fluid drams	= 1 fluid ounce (fl ℥ İ)
16 fluid ounces	= 1 pint (O İ)

Weight

20 grains (gr. xx)	= 1 scruple (℈ İ)
3 scruples	= 1 dram (ʒ İ)
8 drams	= 1 ounce (℥ İ)
12 ounces	= 1 pound (lb İ)

The weight of one grain is based on the average weight of a grain of wheat.

A minim is roughly equivalent to one drop. However, for extremely accurate procedures, each dropper must be exactly calibrated because there is a great variety in the sizes of drops, depending on the dropper, the viscosity of the liquid, and so forth.

When speaking of fluid measures, sometimes the prefix "fl" is used (e.g., fl dram instead of only dram when designating a liquid). Either is correct, however.

Procedure for Conversion Within the Apothecary System

The proportion method is the simplest for these conversions.

1. Write the equivalent between the terms to be converted as the first two terms of the proportion.

2. Being careful to keep the units in the last two terms in the same order as they occur in the first, write the known quantity and the unknown equivalent as the third and fourth terms of the proportion.

Examples:

a. 6 drams = ? ounces

$$8 \text{ drams} : 1 \text{ ounce} = 6 \text{ drams} : x \text{ ounces}$$
$$8x = 6$$
$$x = \frac{6}{8} = \frac{3}{4} \text{ ounce}$$

b. 2 drams = ? minims

$$60 \text{ minims} : 1 \text{ dram} = x \text{ minims} : 2 \text{ drams}$$
$$1x = 120$$
$$x = 120 \text{ minims}$$

EXERCISES

Change to equivalents within the apothecary system:

1. 4 ounces   =   _____ pint

2. 40 drams   =   _____ ounces

3. 30 pounds   =   _____ ounces

4. $\frac{1}{2}$ ounce   =   _____ drams

5. 16 drams   =   _____ ounces

6. 120 minims   =   _____ drams

7. 12 fluid ounces =   _____ pint

8. 240 minims   =   _____ drams

9. 3 drams   =   _____ minims

10. 960 minims   =   _____ ounces

Household Measurements

Household measurements may be used to measure approximately the amount required. These include glasses, cups, tablespoons, teaspoons, and medicine droppers. Household measurements are not accurate and should be avoided in the administration of medication. The American standard teaspoon has been established by the American Standards Association as containing approximately 5 mL, and this measurement is accepted in the *United States Pharmacopeia*.

Drops and minims are said to be equivalent, but when a certain number of minims is ordered, the dose should always be measured in minims.

Some approximate equivalents to household measurements are as follows:

$$1 \text{ teaspoon } = 1 \text{ fluid dram } = 5 \text{ mL}$$
$$1 \text{ tablespoon } = \frac{1}{2} \text{ fluid ounce } = 4 \text{ fluid drams } = 15 \text{ mL}$$
$$2 \text{ tablespoons } = 1 \text{ fluid ounce } = 30 \text{ mL}$$

EXERCISES

Change to approximate equivalents in household measurements:

1. 10 mL   = _____ teaspoons

2. 120 mL   = _____ tablespoons

3. 2 ounces   = _____ teaspoons

4. 60 mL   = _____ ounces

5. 20 tablespoons = _____ ounces

6. $\frac{1}{2}$ fluid ounce = _____ tablespoons

7. 60 mL   = _____ teaspoons

8. 6 teaspoons   = _____ fluid ounces

9. 12 ounces   = _____ teaspoons

10. 16 tablespoons = _____ fluid ounces

CONVERSION BETWEEN THE METRIC AND APOTHECARY SYSTEMS

Some essential equivalents must be learned to convert between the metric and the apothecary systems (Table 7–1). The proportion method of conversion is the easiest way to carry out these conversions. The same procedure is used here as when carrying out operations within the apothecary system.

Table 7-1. METRIC DOSES WITH APPROXIMATE APOTHECARY EQUIVALENTS*

These *approximate* dose equivalents represent the quantities usually prescribed, under identical conditions, by physicians trained, respectively, in the metric and in the apothecary system of weights and measures. In labeling dosage forms in both the metric and the apothecary systems, if one is the approximate equivalent of the other, the approximate figure shall be enclosed in parentheses.

When prepared dosage forms such as tablets, capsules, pills, etc., are prescribed in the metric system, the pharmacist may dispense the corresponding *approximate* equivalent in the apothecary system, and vice versa, as indicated in the following table.

Caution—For the conversion of specific quantities in a prescription that requires compounding or in converting a pharmaceutical formula from one system of weights or measures to the other, *exact* equivalents must be used.

Liquid Measure		Liquid Measure	
Metric	Approx. Apothecary Equivalent	Metric	Approx. Apothecary Equivalent
1000 mL	1 quart	3.00 mL	45 minims
750 mL	1 1/2 pints	2.00 mL	30 minims
500 mL	1 pint	1.00 mL	15 minims
250 mL	8 fluid ounces	0.75 mL	12 minims
200 mL	7 fluid ounces	0.60 mL	10 minims
100 mL	3 1/2 fluid ounces	0.50 mL	8 minims
50 mL	1 3/4 fluid ounces	0.30 mL	5 minims
30 mL	1 fluid ounce	0.25 mL	4 minims
15 mL	4 fluid drams	0.20 mL	3 minims
10 mL	2 1/2 fluid drams	0.10 mL	1 1/2 minims
8 mL	2 fluid drams	0.06 mL	1 minim
5 mL	1 1/4 fluid drams	0.05 mL	3/4 minim
4 mL	1 fluid dram	0.03 mL	1/2 minim

Weight		Weight	
Metric	Approx. Apothecary Equivalent	Metric	Approx. Apothecary Equivalent
30.00 gm	1 ounce	30.00 mg	1/2 grain
15.00 gm	4 drams	25.00 mg	3/8 grain
10.00 gm	2 1/2 drams	20.00 mg	1/3 grain
7.50 gm	2 drams	15.00 mg	1/4 grain
6.00 gm	90 grains	12.00 mg	1/5 grain
5.00 gm	75 grains	10.00 mg	1/6 grain
4.00 gm	60 grains (1 dram)	8.00 mg	1/8 grain
3.00 gm	45 grains	6.00 mg	1/10 grain
2.00 gm	30 grains (1/2 dram)	5.00 mg	1/12 grain
1.50 gm	22 grains	4.00 mg	1/15 grain
1.00 gm	15 grains	3.00 mg	1/20 grain
0.75 gm	12 grains	2.00 mg	1/30 grain
0.60 gm	10 grains	1.50 mg	1/40 grain
0.50 gm	7 1/2 grains	1.20 mg	1/50 grain
0.40 gm	6 grains	1.00 mg	1/60 grain
0.30 gm	5 grains	0.80 mg	1/80 grain
0.25 gm	4 grains	0.60 mg	1/100 grain
0.20 gm	3 grains	0.50 mg	1/120 grain
0.15 gm	2 1/2 grains	0.40 mg	1/150 grain
0.12 gm	2 grains	0.30 mg	1/200 grain
0.10 gm	1 1/2 grains	0.25 mg	1/250 grain
75.00 mg	1 1/4 grains	0.20 mg	1/300 grain
60.00 mg	1 grains	0.15 mg	1/400 grain
50.00 mg	3/4 grain	0.12 mg	1/500 grain
40.00 mg	2/3 grain	0.10 mg	1/600 grain

Note—A milliliter (mL) is the approximate equivalent of a cubic centimeter (cc).

*Adopted by the latest *Pharmacopeia, National Formulary* and *New and Nonofficial Remedies* and approved by the U.S. Food and Drug Administration.

$$60 \text{ mg} = 1 \text{ grain}$$
$$1 \text{ gm} = 15 \text{ grains}$$
$$30 \text{ gm} = 1 \text{ ounce}$$
$$2.2 \text{ lb} = 1 \text{ kg}$$

$$1 \text{ mL} = 15 \text{ minims}$$
$$30 \text{ mL} = 1 \text{ fluid ounce}$$
$$500 \text{ mL} = 1 \text{ pint}$$
$$1000 \text{ mL} = 1 \text{ quart}$$

$$1 \text{ teaspoonful} = 1 \text{ dram} = 4 \text{ or } 5 \text{ mL}$$
$$1 \text{ tablespoonful} = \frac{1}{2} \text{ ounce} = 4 \text{ drams} = 15 \text{ mL}$$
$$1 \text{ teacupful} = 6 \text{ ounces} = 180 \text{ mL}$$
$$1 \text{ glassful} = 8 \text{ ounces} = 240 \text{ mL}$$

Examples:

a. 45 gm = ? ounces
$$30 \text{ gm} : 1 \text{ ounce} = 45 \text{ gm} : x \text{ ounces}$$
$$30 \, x = 45$$
$$x = \frac{45}{30} = 1\frac{1}{2} \text{ ounces}$$

b. 150 lb = ? kg
$$2.2 \text{ lb} : 1 \text{ kg} = 150 \text{ lb} : x \text{ kg}$$
$$2.2 \, x = 150$$
$$x = \frac{150}{2.2} = 68.2 \text{ lb}$$

EXERCISES

A. Explain the procedure for conversion from one system of measurement to another.

B. Convert to apothecary equivalent:

1. 2 gm
2. 24 mL
3. 30 mg
4. 300 mg
5. 0.6 gm
6. 500 mL
7. 0.3 gm
8. 0.065 gm
9. 4 mL
10. 100 mg

C. Convert to metric equivalent:

1. gr XV
2. 6 fluid ounces
3. 30 minims
4. 8 drams
5. 4 ounces
6. gr $\dfrac{1}{8}$
7. 60 drops
8. 10 fluid drams
9. 11 lb
10. your weight

ADDITIONAL EXERCISES

Convert the following:

1. 0.5 L = _____ mL

2. 4 mL = _____ minims

3. gr $\frac{1}{4}$ = _____ mg

4. 0.1 gm = _____ mg

5. 500 mL = _____ pint

6. $\frac{1}{2}$ = _____ ml

7. $\frac{1}{2}$ ounce = _____ drams

8. 30 drops = _____ teaspoons

9. 1500 mg = _____ gm

10. gr 90 = _____ gm

11. 5 tablespoons = _____ mL

12. 5 tablespoons = _____ ounces

13. gr $\frac{1}{8}$ = _____ mg

14. 10 mL = _____ teaspoons

15. 10 mL = _____ minims

16. $2\frac{1}{2}$ quarts = _____ mL

17. 0.6 gm = _____ grains

18. 3 kg = _____ lb

19. 165 lb = _____ kg

20. 3 pints = _____ quart

Dosage for Children

Children are not able to tolerate adult doses of drugs. There are several formulas for graduating dosage according to age and weight. The recommended dosage per kilogram or pound of body weight is more accurate than calculating dosage according to age. Other factors besides age and weight enter into dosage for children. For this reason, some physicians use the "body surface area" method to estimate the dosage for children. Charts are available to determine the body surface area in square meters according to height and weight.

Nurses must be able to determine dosage and recognize the safe amount of drug to be administered to an infant or child. It is important to become familiar with the method or methods used by the employing physician or institution.

The following three formulas are useful in calculating dosage for infants and children:

Young's rule:

$$\frac{\text{Age of child}}{\text{Age of child} + 12} \times \text{average adult dose} = \text{child's dose.}$$

Young's rule is not valid after 12 years of age. If the child is small enough to warrant a reduced dose after 12 years of age, the reduction should be calculated on the basis of Clark's rule.

Clark's rule:

$$\frac{\text{Weight of child}}{150} \times \text{average adult dose} = \text{child's dose.}$$

Fried's rule, which is sometimes used in calculating dosages for infants less than 2 years old, used the formula

$$\frac{\text{Age in months}}{150} \times \text{average adult dose} = \text{child's dose.}$$

Any unit of measure may be used in these formulas. The answer will be in the same units as used. If another unit is desired, conversion may be carried out as previously illustrated.

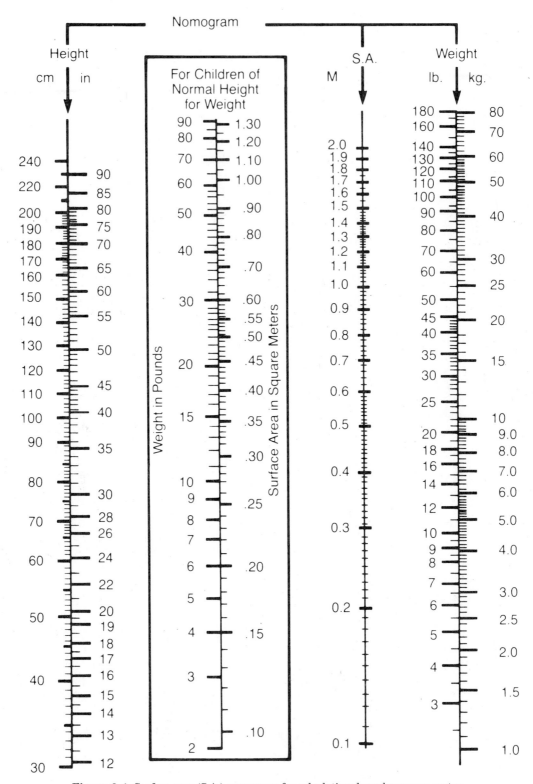

Figure 8–1. Surface area (S.A.) nomogram for calculating doses by square meter.

Examples:

    a. Find the dose of phenobarbital for a 4-year-old child (adult dose: 30 mg).

$$\frac{4}{4 + 12} \times 30 \text{ mg} = 7.5 \text{ mg}$$

    b. Find the dose of cortisone for a 30-lb infant (adult dose: 100 mg).

$$\frac{30}{150} \times 100 \text{ mg} = 20 \text{ mg}$$

Surface Area Nomogram

The surface area nomogram is used for calculating pediatric doses by square meter of body surface (Figure 8–1). The center enclosed box gives the square meters by weight in pounds only for children of normal height and weight. For children who are slender or obese, a straight line that connects the height and weight on the two outside scales can be used to read the square meters of body surface.

EXERCISES

Calculate the following children's doses:

1. If the adult dose of codeine sulfate is 30 mg, what is the dose for a 3-year-old child? _____

2. The adult dose of Dilantin suspension is 125 mg/5 mL. How much would you use when 75 mg is ordered for a child? _____

3. The adult dose of Achromycin is 250 mg. What is the dose for an 8-year-old child? _____

4. The vial is labeled Demerol 100 mg/cc. The order is for 60 mg. How much will be given? _____

5. The adult dose of phenobarbital is 30 mg. How much would you administer this drug to a 30-lb child? _____

6. The pediatrician has ordered Tylenol elixir 2 cc. The bottle is labeled 120 mg/5 cc. How much will be given? _____

7. The adult dosage of procaine penicillin is 300,000 U once daily. Calculate the dosage for a 6-year-old child using Young's rule. _____

8. If each milliliter of procaine penicillin supplies 300,000 U, how many minims would you give this 6-year-old child? _____

9. Gantrisin suspension is available in a dose of 500 mg/5 mL. How much is needed for a 100-mg dose? _____

10. The adult dose of a drug is 50 to 100 mg. What is the dose for a 6-month-old infant using the minimum dose? _____

11. a. Calculate the dose of Seconal for a child weighing 50 lb. The adult dose is gr 1 1/2. _____
    b. What is the metric equivalent? _____

12. Keflex pediatric drops are available in a dose of 100 mg/mL. The order is for 60 mg. How much will be given? _____

13. The adult dose of Ritalin is 15 mg. What is the dose for a 30-lb child? _____

14. The adult dose of paregoric is 10 mL. How much would be given to a 20-lb infant? _____

15. Ampicillin oral suspension 250 mg/mL is available. Calculate the amount to be given for the following dosages:
    a. 150 mg _____   b. 100 mg _____
    c. 125 mg _____   d. 375 mg _____

16. The dose of azathioprine is 125 mg per squared meter per day. Find the total daily dose for a 44-lb child of average height and weight. _____

17. Find the total daily dose of azathioprine for a child who is 40 inches tall and overweight at 60 lb. _____

9

Dosage of Drugs Standardized in Units

INSULIN DOSAGE

Insulin and many other drugs that are obtained from animal sources are standardized in units based on their strengths rather than on weight measures such as milligrams and grams. The reason for this is that the strength of these animal drugs varies greatly, depending on the sources, conditions, and manner in which they are obtained. Many of the hormones (e.g., insulin) are too complex to be completely purified to obtain the exact weight of the drug per unit volume.

Insulin is supplied in 10-cc vials labeled in the number of units per cubic centimeter; thus, U 100 insulin means there are 100 units per cubic centimeter. In the past, insulin was administered in U 40 and U 80 dosage forms. Today, however, the U 100 form has almost totally replaced the weaker strengths. The smaller volume required per dose decreases local reactions at the injection site, and mathematical calculations when a fraction of a cubic centimeter is required are obviously simplified.

The simplest and most accurate way to measure insulin is within an insulin syringe. The syringe is calibrated in units, and the desired dose may be read directly on the syringe. A typical insulin syringe has calibrations on one side for use with U 40 insulin and calibrations on the other side for use with U 80 insulin. Similarly, a 100-U syringe has calibrations for use with U 100 insulin. In Figure 9–1, 35 units are shown drawn up on the 100-U syringe.

If an insulin syringe is not available, a tuberculin syringe may be used and the unit dosage converted to the equivalent number of minims or cubic centimeters, using the proportion method.

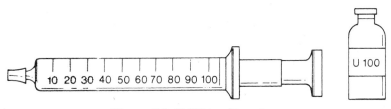

Figure 9–1. U 100 insulin syringe.

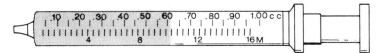

Figure 9–2. Tuberculin syringe.

Example: Give 25 units of insulin, using U 40 insulin.

$$40 \text{ units}: 1 \text{ cc} = 25 \text{ units}: x \text{ cc}$$
$$40 \text{ x} = 25$$
$$x = \frac{25}{40} = \frac{5}{8} \text{ cc} = 0.625 \text{ cc}$$

The problem could be worked to use the minim scale.

$$40 \text{ units}: 16 \text{ minims} = 25 \text{ units}: x \text{ minims}$$
$$40 \text{ x} = 400$$
$$x = 10 \text{ minims}$$

Figure 9–2 shows a tuberculin syringe with 10 minims drawn up.

HEPARIN DOSAGE

Like insulin, heparin is derived from animal sources, in this case porcine intestinal mucosa, and is standardized for its activity as an anticoagulant.

Heparin is supplied in unit dose or multiple dose vials and in strengths ranging from 1000 to 20,000 units per milliliter. There is often no set dose for the use of heparin; the individual's requirements are obtained from blood clotting studies done every 4 hours. Blood clotting time is generally maintained at twice the normal clotting rate to provide a safe yet effective way to decrease the formation of blood clots in the body.

Heparin is often given intravenously to produce a rapid effect and then is given in deep subcutaneous injection in larger and more infrequent doses.

ANTIBIOTIC DOSAGE

Many antibiotics are still standardized in units. These may be prepared for injection in the form of a liquid containing a specified number of units per cubic centimeter. The entire amount in the vial may be ordered, but sometimes only part of the contents is used. It is, therefore, important to *always read the label carefully*. Antibiotics are also available in the form of a dry powder in a vial that must first be diluted with water or another diluent. The powder should be diluted so that the desired dose is in 1 or 2 cc if the dose is to be given intramuscularly. If it is to be given intravenously, a larger amount of diluent may be used.

When the dose is less than 1 mL, the milliliter amount can be converted to minims. Use 15 minims when the denominator of the fraction can be divided into 15. Use 16 minims when the denominator of the fraction can be divided into 16.

Procedure for Preparing the Desired Concentration of Antibiotic

1. Using the proportion method, state the desired concentration as the first two terms of the proportion.

2. The total number of units in the vial is the third term. The unknown volume of diluent, represented by "x," is the fourth term.

Examples:

a. Dilute a vial containing 600,000 units of penicillin so that each cubic centimeter contains 50,000 U.

$$50,000 \text{ U}: 1 \text{ cc} = 600,000 \text{ U}: x \text{ cc}$$
$$50,000 \text{ x} = 600,000$$
$$= \frac{600,000}{50,000} = 12 \text{ cc of diluent}$$

b. The physician orders 100,000 units of penicillin. How can this be given from a vial containing 1,000,000 units in powder form?

$$100,000 \text{ U}: 1 \text{ cc} = 1,000,000 \text{ U}: x \text{ cc}$$
$$100,000 \text{ x} = 1,000,000$$
$$x = 10 \text{ cc}$$

EXERCISES

A. Using a tuberculin syringe, how many minims of insulin would be given for the following doses?

1. 25 units of U 80   _____

2. 75 units of U 80   _____

3. 75 units of U 100   _____

4. 20 units of U 40   _____

5. 20 units of U 80   _____

6. 20 units of U 100   _____

7. 30 units of U 100   _____

8. 15 units of U 100   _____

9. 60 units of U 100   _____

10. 35 units of U 100 _____

11. 25 units of U 100 _____

12. 12 units of U 40 _____

13. 80 units of U 80 _____

14. 80 units of U 100 _____

15. 50 units of U 100 _____

B. Calculate the following antibiotic dosages:

1. The vial contains 600,000 U. How much sterile distilled water would be added to give a 150,000-unit dose? _____

2. A vial contains 5,000,000 U of penicillin in powder form. The order is 500,000 U every 6 hours. How much diluent will be used? _____

3. The drug is supplied in 1-gm vials. The manufacturer's directions indicate that 5 mL of diluent is to be added. How much drug will be contained in 1 mL? _____

4. The order is for 250 mg of streptomycin. How much diluent will be added to the vial that contains 5 gm of streptomycin? _____

5. The vial of Bicillin contains 600,000 U/cc. The order is for 200,000 U. How much will be given? _____

6. The order is for Garamycin 60 mg IM tid. Garamycin is available in 2-cc vials containing 40 mg/cc. How many cubic centimeters will be necessary to give one dose? How many minims? _____

7. The order reads Keflin 500 mg every 4 hours IM for 5 days. The ampules on hand contain 1 gm. How many ampules will be needed to give the required doses? _____

8. The order is for 500 mg IM. The label on the vial reads 0.5 gm/mL. How much will you give? _____

9. The 2-mL vial of Lincocin reads 300 mg/cc. The order is for 200 mg IM. How much will you give? _____

10. Lincocin 450 mg IM is ordered. How much will you give using a vial labeled 300 mg/cc? _____

BASIC PHARMACOLOGY

U N I T   O B J E C T I V E S

■ 1. Understand the principles of drug administration.
■ 2. Know common abbreviations related to route of administration and frequency of dosage.
■ 3. Demonstrate accuracy in converting from one system of measurement to another.
■ 4. Identify drugs according to clinical use.
■ 5. Recognize symptoms of untoward reactions.
■ 6. Possess a foundation and interest for further study of pharmacology.

10

Introduction to Pharmacology

Objectives for the Student

BE

ABLE

TO
- 1. Name four sources of drugs and give an example of each.
- 2. Give the definition of terms as assigned.
- 3. List the responsibilities of the nurse for drug administration.
- 4. Prepare your own objectives for this course.

The administration of medications is one of a nurse's most important responsibilities. As a member of the professional team engaged in caring for the sick, it is most important that the nurse apply him- or herself diligently in acquiring all possible knowledge of medicines, their use or abuse, correct dosage, methods of administration, symptoms of overdosage, and abnormal reactions that may arise in the treatment of various conditions. This knowledge is obviously an indispensable aid in giving the best possible patient care.

The attitude of the nurse toward drug administration is important to the effectiveness of the drug. Ideally, the body functions best when given adequate food, rest, relaxation, and freedom from undue emotional stress. However, because of physical or mental abnormalities, it is necessary at times to resort to drugs to produce a near-normal state of body function. At best, drugs are *crutches,* and undue dependence on

them can be *very dangerous.* Used intelligently, they are a life-saving boon; used unwisely, they can produce irreparable harm. The nurse who combines diligent and intelligent observation with moral integrity and plain *common sense* in administering drugs will undoubtedly make many lasting contributions to the profession and to the patients for whom she or he cares.

Pharmacology has undergone tremendous changes during the past few decades. Many new agents on the market today were totally unheard of a generation ago, and scarcely a day goes by that literature is not received on new agents or medicines and new techniques and theories of drug administration. The newest advancements are always a source of interest and intrigue to the beginning student, but it is only by applying him- or herself first of all to the task of obtaining a well-rounded background in drug therapy that the student will begin to appreciate these new "miracles of the modern age."

The information presented in this manual attempts to lay the foundation for this well-rounded background, but, as in all other areas of nursing, the responsibility for making this knowledge one's own rests with the students themselves. A true dedication to the profession only places the student in the starting position of a lifelong pursuit—a pursuit that, though admittedly arduous, promises the unfailing reward of continuous new horizons and that casts new light on the great task entrusted to the nurse in every service to the sick.

DEFINITIONS

Pharmacology: a broad term that includes the study of drugs and their actions in the body.

Pharmacy: the art of preparing, compounding, and dispensing drugs for medicinal use.

Toxicology: the science that deals with poisons: their detection and the symptoms, diagnosis, and treatment of conditions caused by them.

Drug: any substance used as medicine (e.g., used to diagnose, cure, mitigate, treat, or prevent disease).

Drugs include the following:

Chemical substances: agents that may be made synthetically (e.g., sulfonamides, aspirin, sodium bicarbonate).

Plant parts or products: crude drugs that may be obtained from any part of various plants and used medicinally. Leaves, bark, fruit, roots, rhizomes, resin, and other parts may be used (e.g., ergot, digitalis, opium).

Animal products: glandular products are the chief medicinals currently obtained from animal sources (e.g., thyroid hormone, insulin).

Certain food substances: substances that under some conditions serve both as foods and as medicinal substances (i.e., vitamins and minerals in various foods).

Addition: the combined effect of two drugs, which is equal to the sum of the effects of each drug taken alone.

Adverse or untoward effect: an action different from the planned effect.

Allergic reaction: a reaction that develops after the individual has taken the drug a few times.

Antagonism: the combined effect of two drugs that is less than the effect of either drug taken alone.

Depression: a decrease in activity of cells caused by the action of a drug.

Diagnostic: refers to the art or act of determining the nature of a patient's disease.

Idiosyncrasy: abnormal sensitivity to a drug.

Palliative: an agent or measure that relieves symptoms.

Potentiation: an effect that occurs when a drug increases or prolongs the action of another drug, the total effect being greater than the sum of the effects of each used alone.

Prophylactic: an agent or measure used to prevent disease.

Side effect: an unpredictable effect that is not related to the main action of the drug.

Stimulation: an increase in the activity of cells produced by drugs.

Synergism: the joint action of agents in which their combined effect is more intense or longer in duration than the sum of their individual effects.

Therapeutic: refers to treatment of disease.

Tolerance: increasing resistance to the usual effects of an established dosage of a drug as a result of continued use.

Drug Legislation and Standards

Objectives for the Student

BE

ABLE

TO

■ 1. Identify drugs according to the current schedule of the Controlled Substances Act.
■ 2. List Official Drug Standards.
■ 3. Use the *Physicians' Desk Reference* to identify a selected list of drugs according to generic and proprietary names.

AMERICAN DRUG LEGISLATION

Drug legislation in the United States underwent major revisions as of May 1, 1971, when the Controlled Substances Act became effective. This law requires that every person who manufactures, dispenses, prescribes, or administers any controlled substance be registered annually with the Attorney General; this registration function is the responsibility of the Bureau of Narcotics and Dangerous Drugs (BNDD).

Legislation and controls were revised to establish five schedules of controlled substances. Drugs in the original schedules are subject to revision on an annual basis on notification by the BNDD, and many changes have been made within the schedules since the legislation first went into effect.

Complete listings of the drugs in each sched-

ule are available from district BNDD offices. Only a few examples of the more well-known drugs in each schedule are included here.

Schedule I

1. The drug or other substance has a high potential for abuse.
2. The drug or other substance has *no* currently accepted medicinal use in treatment in the United States.
3. There is a lack of accepted safety for use of the drug or other substance under medical supervision.

Drugs Included:

1. Opiates: ketobemidone, allylprodine.
2. Opium derivatives: heroin.

3. Hallucinogens: lysergic acid diethylamide (LSD), marijuana, mescaline, peyote.

Schedule II

1. The drug or other substance has a high potential for abuse.

2. The drug or other substance has a currently accepted medical use in treatment in the United States or a currently accepted medical use with severe restrictions.

3. Abuse of the drug or other substance may lead to severe psychological or physical dependence.

Drugs Included:

1. Opium and any derivative of opium (e.g., raw opium, morphine, codeine, ethylmorphine, hydrocodone, metopon, thebaine).

2. Coca leaves and derivatives, e.g., cocaine.

3. Opiates: anileridine, dihydrocodeine, diphenoxylate, levomethorphan, methadone, meperidine, oxycodone.

4. Stimulants: methamphetamine, amphetamine, phenmetrazine, methylphenidate.

5. Depressants: amobarbital, secobarbital, pentobarbital, methaqualone.

Schedule III

1. The drug or other substance has a potential for abuse less than the drugs in Schedule I or II.

2. The drug or other substance has a currently accepted medical use in treatment in the United States.

3. Abuse of the drug or other substance may lead to moderate or low physical dependence or high psychological dependence.

Drugs Included:

1. Phendimetrazine, phentermine, diethylpropion, glutethimide, methyprylon, nalorphine.

2. Combinations of amobarbital, secobarbital, or pentobarbital with other active ingredients.

3. Compounds containing limited concentrations of codeine, dihydrocodeinone, ethylmor-

phine, opium, or morphine with one or more active non-narcotic ingredients in recognized therapeutic amounts.

Schedule IV

1. The drug or other substance has a low potential for abuse relative to the drugs or other substances in Schedule III.

2. The drug or other substance has a currently accepted medical use in treatment in the United States.

3. Abuse of the drug or other substance may lead to limited physical or psychological dependence relative to the drugs in Schedule III.

Drugs Included:

1. Chloral hydrate, chloral betaine, ethchlorvynol, meprobamate, paraldehyde, phenobarbital, chlordiazepoxide, diazepam, propoxyphene, flurazepam, chlorazepate, pemoline, pentazocine, oxazepam.

Schedule V

1. The drug or other substance has a low potential for abuse relative to the drugs in Schedule IV.

2. The drug or other substance has a currently accepted medical use in treatment in the United States.

3. Abuse of the drug or other substance may lead to limited physical or psychological dependence relative to the drugs in Schedule IV.

Drugs Included:

1. Compounds containing limited amounts of codeine, dihydrocodeine, ethylmorphine, opium, or diphenoxylate in combination with other non-narcotic active ingredients. (In all cases the allowable concentration of these agents is lower than those compounds included in Schedule III.)

2. Diphenoxylate and atropine preparations (e.g., Lomotil).

AMERICAN DRUG STANDARDS

The United States Pharmacopoeia/National Formulary (USP). Formerly two standards, the *Pharmacopoeia* and the *National Formulary* have been combined into one official volume to provide standards for drug quality and strength. Before official standards, drugs, particularly from plant sources, could vary in strength from being ineffective to providing almost a fatal dose, depending on the quality of the plant, the soil, and the growing conditions. The *Pharmacopoeia* includes a list of approved drugs and defines them with respect to source, chemistry, physical properties, tests for identity, method of assay, storage, and dosage and provides directions for compounding and general use. It is revised periodically by an appointed committee to include new drugs and exclude those no longer in general use.

New Drugs. In 1965 the American Medical Association (AMA) began publishing this annual text, which lists drugs whether or not they have been approved for official standards. It is organized according to therapeutic uses for the drugs, and the information is based on evaluation by the Council on Drugs. The inclusion does not imply acceptance by the AMA.

Additional Sources of Drug Information

Physicians' Desk Reference (PDR). Revised annually and readily supplied to all hospitals and physicians, this reference source is probably the most widely used. It is not intended as an official standard. Each manufacturer supplies information for inclusion, usually by trade name, and gives the accepted uses, side effects, and doses for commercially available pharmaceutical agents.

Drug Information. This annual publication by the American Hospital Formulary Service contains useful and current information on drugs.

BRITISH AND CANADIAN DRUG STANDARDS

British Pharmacopoeia (BP). Similar in content to the *United States Pharmacopoeia/ National Formulary,* this text sets the standards for drugs that are official in the United Kingdom and its dominions and colonies. It is published by the British Pharmacopoeia Commission under the direction of the General Medical Council.

British Pharmaceutical Codex (BPC). A text similar to the *British Pharmacopoeia,* this is published by the Pharmaceutical Society of Great Britain and gives official drug information and standards.

Canadian Formulary (CF). Published by the Canadian Pharmaceutical Association, this text is recognized by the Canadian Food and Drug Act and contains formulas for many Canadian pharmaceutical preparations. It has some drugs not included in the *British Pharmacopoeia.*

INTERNATIONAL DRUG STANDARDS

Pharmacopoeia Internationalis (IP). The World Health Organization was originally responsible for the publication of this text in an attempt to standardize drugs for many European nations. The nomenclature of drugs is in Latin; all doses are in the metric system.

CANADIAN DRUG LEGISLATION

Canadian Food and Drug Act

The Food and Drug Act, passed in 1941, empowers the Governor-in-Council to prescribe drug standards and limit variation in any food or drug.

Schedule A. This schedule contains a list of diseases or disorders for which a cure may not be advertised. It includes diseases such as gangrene, influenza, and appendicitis.

Schedule B. This schedule contains lists of official drug standard texts, such as the *United States Pharmacopoeia,* the *British Pharmacopoeia,* and other previously mentioned Canadian volumes.

Schedule C. This schedule contains a list of drugs derived from animal tissues, such as liver extract and insulin, for which special standards of quality and purity apply.

Schedule D. This schedule contains a list of drugs obtained from microorganisms, such as antibiotics, and their requirements for manufacture.

Schedule E. This schedule contains a list of sensitivity discs or tablets and their standards.

Schedule F. Thalidomide is the only drug currently in this schedule; its sale is prohibited. Also included in this schedule is a regulation noting drugs that must be dispensed by prescription only.

Schedule G. A list of controlled drugs with strict prescribing regulations is included in this schedule. It includes amphetamines, barbiturates, benzphetamine, butorphanol, chlorphentermine, diethylpropion, methamphetamine, methaqualone, methylphenidate, pentazocine, phendimetrazine, phenmetrazine, phentermine, and thiobarbituric acid.

Schedule H. This schedule contains a list of hallucinogenic drugs that are restricted, allowing no practitioner to prescribe them, including LSD, psilocin, and harmaline.

Canadian Narcotic Control Act and Regulations

This act defines who may prescribe a narcotic drug, such as physicians, dentists, research personnel, and their agents, and places conditions on the recipient of a narcotic prescription, requiring disclosure of all previous narcotics received within the last 30 days.

In addition, the act describes procedures for record keeping and dispensing by pharmacists. Hospital regulations are also outlined.

Methadone is covered individually in this act, which sets requirements for authorized practitioners who prescribe and dispense this drug.

PROPRIETARY (TRADE) NAMES

Most pharmaceutical houses market their drugs primarily under trade names rather than under generic names. Today there is a great multiplicity of trade names under which a single drug may be sold. The practice of using these brand names is often confusing to the nurse and sometimes even to the physician, to say nothing of the inconvenience to the pharmacist who must stock four or five different brands of the same drug. Currently, there is a trend to return to the use of official or generic names on prescriptions. Many hospital pharmacies provide the nursing divisions with a formulary that lists the official or generic names for the commercial products stocked in the pharmacy.

When a specific trade name is ordered by a physician, however, it must be dispensed by the pharmacist. No other brand, even if the product is exactly the same as the one ordered, may be substituted without the physician's knowledge and consent.

Review Questions

1. Why is it necessary to have governmental control over narcotics?

2. Name some drugs that have a high potential for abuse.

3. Name some drugs that have a high potential for abuse but are used in treatment in this country with restrictions.

4. Investigate the facilities for treatment of drug abuse in your community.

5. Locate the sources of poison information in your community, county, and state.

6. Discuss the difference between the generic name and the trade name of a medication.

Pharmaceutical Preparations

Objectives for the Student

B E

A B L E

T O

■ 1. Name all of the various pharmaceutical preparations.
■ 2. Distinguish between an elixir and a tincture and give an example of each.
■ 3. Discuss the advantage of administering a capsule instead of a pill.
■ 4. Distinguish between a lotion and a liniment and give an example of each.

Because of the various properties of the different drugs and their many uses, it is necessary to have different ways of preparing them for patient use. Listed here are the more common pharmaceutical preparations.

Solutions: aqueous liquid preparations containing one or more substances completely dissolved. Every solution has two parts: the *solute* (the dissolved substance) and the *solvent* (the substance, usually a liquid, in which the solute is dissolved).

Waters: saturated solutions of volatile oils (e.g., peppermint water, camphor water).

Syrups: aqueous solutions of a sugar. These may or may not have medicinal substances added (e.g., simple syrup, ipecac syrup).

Spirits: alcoholic solutions of volatile substances. These are also known as essences (e.g., essence of peppermint, camphor spirit).

Elixirs: solutions containing alcohol, sugar, and water. They may or may not be aromatic and may or may not have active medicinals. Most frequently they are used as flavoring agents or solvents (e.g., terpin hydrate elixir, phenobarbital elixir).

Tinctures: alcoholic or hydroalcoholic solutions prepared from drugs (e.g., iodine tincture, digitalis tincture).

Fluidextract: alcoholic liquid extract of a drug made by percolation so that 1 cc of the fluidextract contains 1 gm of the drug. Only vegetable drugs are used (e.g., glycyrrhiza fluidextract).

Emulsions: suspensions of fat globules in water (or water globules in fat) with an emulsifying agent (e.g., Haley's MO, Petrogalar). (Homogenized milk is also an emulsion.)

Liniment: a mixture of drugs with oil, soap, water, or alcohol intended for external application with rubbing (e.g., camphor liniment, chloroform liniment).

Lotions: aqueous preparations containing suspended materials intended for soothing, local application. Most are patted on rather than rubbed (e.g., calamine lotion, Caladryl lotion).

Powders: single-dose quantities of a drug or mixture of drugs in powdered form wrapped separately in powder papers (e.g., Seidlitz powder).

Tablets: single-dose units made by compressing powdered drugs in a suitable mold (e.g., aspirin tablets). Special forms of tablets include *sublingual* tablets (to be held under the tongue until dissolved) and *enteric-coated* tablets (with a coating that prevents their absorption until they reach the intestinal tract).

Long-acting or sustained-release dosage forms: active pharmaceutical agents are either layered in tablet form for release over several hours or placed in pellets within a capsule. The pellets are of varying size and disintegrate over a period of 1 to 8 hours.

Pills: single-dose units made by mixing the powdered drug with a liquid such as syrup and rolling it into a round or oval shape. These are largely replaced by other dosage forms today (e.g., Hinkle's pills).

Capsules: powdered drugs within a gelatin container. Liquids may be placed in soft gelatin capsules (e.g., cod liver oil capsules, Benadryl capsules).

Suppositories: mixtures of drugs with some firm base such as cocoa butter, which can then be molded into shape for insertion into a body orifice. Rectal, vaginal, and urethral suppositories are the most common types (e.g., Furacin vaginal suppositories, Dulcolax suppositories, but nasal or otic suppositories may be made).

Ointments: mixtures of drugs with a fatty base for external application, usually by rubbing (e.g., zinc oxide ointment, Ben-Gay ointment).

Gels: aqueous suspensions of insoluble drugs in hydrated form. Aluminum hydroxide gel, USP, is an example.

Aerosols: active pharmaceutical agents in a pressurized container.

Troches or lozenges: flat, round, or rectangular preparations that are held in the mouth until dissolved.

Review Questions

1. Explain the difference between the following:
   a. a capsule and a tablet.
   b. a sustained-release capsule and a tablet.
   c. an elixir and a tincture.

2. Give three common types of suppositories.

3. Name five pharmaceutical preparations that are used for local application.

4. How does an ointment differ from a lotion?

5. What precautions do you consider important in the use of agents for external use?

Special Assignment: If laboratory work is not included in the course, a visit to the hospital pharmacy to observe the various pharmaceutical preparations will enhance the learning situation at this time.

Introduction to Dosage

Objectives for the Student

- 1. Interpret a medication order with 100 percent accuracy.
- 2. Interpret a prescription with 100 percent accuracy.
- 3. Use accepted abbreviations with 100 percent accuracy.
- 4. List the factors influencing dosage.
- 5. Demonstrate beginning skill in transcribing orders.

Dosage is the amount of a medicine or agent prescribed for a given patient or condition. *Dose* is the measured portion of medicine to be taken at one time. Factors influencing dosage are as follows:

Age: The age of a patient will affect his or her response to drugs. Children and elderly persons require less than the usual adult dose.

Sex: The sex of a patient sometimes affects the response to drugs. Women are more susceptible to the action of certain drugs and are usually given smaller doses. The administration of medication to women in the early weeks of pregnancy may cause damage to the fetus. During the third trimester there is the possibility of premature labor caused by drugs that may stimulate muscular contractions.

Condition of the patient: Smaller doses are indicated when resistance in the patient is lowered. Impaired kidney and liver function may cause drugs to accumulate to toxic levels.

Psychological factors: A person's personality often plays an important part in his or her response to certain drugs.

Environmental factors: The setting in which drugs are given and the attitude of the nurse who is administering the medication may influence the effects of drugs.

Temperature: Heat and cold also affect the response to drugs. It may be necessary to decrease the dosage of certain drugs during hot weather.

Method of administration: Generally, larger doses are ordered when a medication is given by mouth or by rectum and smaller doses when the parenteral route is used.

Genetic factors: Drug idiosyncrasy is an abnormal susceptibility of some individuals that causes them to react differently to a drug than most people. This intolerance to small amounts of some drugs is thought to be due to genetic factors.

Body weight: The dosage of certain potent drugs is often calculated on the basis of the ratio of milligrams of the drug to pounds or kilograms of the patient's body weight. The more a person weighs the more dilute the drug will become, and a smaller amount will accumulate in the tissues. On the other hand, the less a person weighs the greater the accumulation in the tissues, and a more powerful drug effect is produced.

THE PRESCRIPTION

The prescription is probably as old as the written history of humankind. The first real literature dealing with pharmacy was a scroll called the Ebers Papyrus, which included methods of conjuring away diseases as well as lists of medicinal agents and methods of compounding.

A prescription is an order written by a physician to be filled by a pharmacist indicating the medication needed by the patient and containing all the necessary directions for the pharmacist and the patient (Figure 13–1). The prescription consists of several parts:

1. The date and the patient's name and address.
2. The inscription, which states the name and quantities of ingredients.
3. The subscription, which gives directions to the pharmacist.
4. The signa (Sig), which gives directions to the patient.
5. The signature, address, and registry number of the physician if they are not printed on the prescription blank.

Parts of an Order

A physician or dentist writes orders for the administration of drugs. A nurse who administers drugs must be familiar with the Nursing Practice Act of the state in which she is licensed to practice and with the policies of the employing agency.

A complete drug order consists of the name of the drug, the dosage, when the drug is to be given, how it is to be given, how many times it is to be given, the date of the order, and the signature of the physician who wrote the order.

Antibiotics and narcotics are examples of drugs that have an automatic stop policy. A new order is required for the drug to be continued

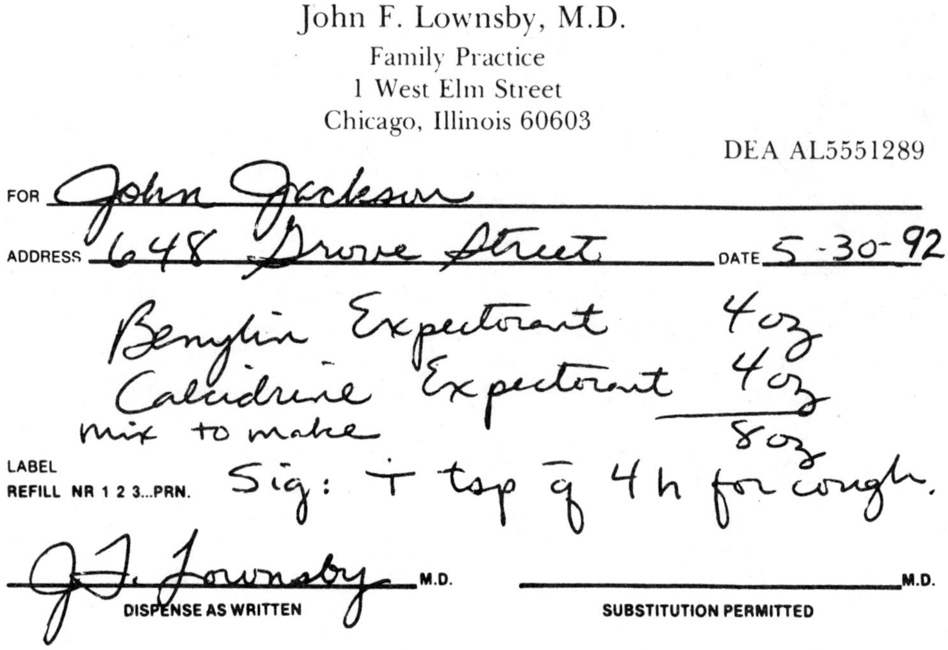

John F. Lownsby, M.D.
Family Practice
1 West Elm Street
Chicago, Illinois 60603

DEA AL5551289

FOR John Jackson

ADDRESS 648 Grove Street   DATE 5-30-92

Benylin Expectorant   4 oz
Calcidrine Expectorant   4 oz
mix to make   8 oz

LABEL
REFILL NR 1 2 3...PRN.   Sig: ⊤ tsp q̄ 4 h for cough.

J. F. Lownsby M.D.
DISPENSE AS WRITTEN

_____ M.D.
SUBSTITUTION PERMITTED

Figure 13–1. A sample prescription.

Table 13-1. COMMON PRESCRIPTION ABBREVIATIONS

Abbreviation	Meaning	Abbreviation	Meaning
aa	of each	pc	after meals
ac	before meals	po	by mouth
ad lib	as much as desired	prn	as needed
bid	twice a day	q	every
c	with	qd	every day
caps	a capsule	qh	every hour
cc	cubic centimeter	q2h	every 2 hours
elix	elixir	q3h	every 3 hours
et	and	qid	4 times a day
fldext	fluidextract	qod	every other day
gm	gram	qs.	quantity sufficient
gr	grain	Rx	take
gtt	a drop	s̄	without
hs	at bedtime	ss	one half
HT	hypodermic tablet	SC	subcutaneously
IM	intramuscularly	Sig	label
IV	intravenously	sp frumenti	whiskey
L	liter	stat	immediately
μg	microgram	syr	syrup
ml	milliliter	tab	tablet
od	once daily	tid	3 times a day
od	right eye	tr	tincture
os	left eye	U	unit
ou	both eyes		

after a specified time that has been established by the institution.

ABBREVIATIONS

To administer medications safely, it is necessary to become thoroughly familiar with accepted abbreviations. The amount of a drug to be given may be written in either the metric or apothecary system. In the metric system the quantity of the drug is written in Arabic and decimal numbers before the metric measure. Some examples are: 100 mg, 2500 mL, 0.5 gm, 2 L. In the apothecary system both the Arabic and Roman numerals are used. The measure is usually written before the amount of drug to be given, such as gr 10, gr ¼, gr IV. The abbreviation ss is often used to stand for ½.

When Roman numerals are used, the I is expressed as i. Some examples are: gr ii, gr viiss.

There are various ways to write drug orders using Roman numerals. Some examples are: gr x, gr ix, gr xv, gr iss.

The list of abbreviations in Table 13–1 includes those most often found in prescriptions and physicians' orders.

EXERCISES

1. Write the meaning of the following abbreviations:

h _____

qd _____

ac   _____

mg   _____

qid   _____

qod   _____

hs   _____

stat   _____

bid   _____

2. Interpret the following orders:
   a. Milk of magnesia 30 mL qod.
   b. Penicillin VK 500 mg q 4h po.
   c. Orinase 250 mg ac daily.
   d. Tylenol tabs ii stat and q 4h prn.

3. Differentiate an order for codeine gr ½ q 4h prn from one for codeine sulfate gr ½ q 4h.

4. Write the following dosages using the metric system of measurement and accepted abbreviations:
   a. Erythromycin two hundred fifty milligrams every six hours.
   b. Phenobarbital grains one and one half at bedtime.
   c. Demerol fifty milligrams intramuscularly every four to six hours as needed for pain in operative site.
   d. N.P.H. Insulin fifteen units subcutaneously every morning before breakfast.
   e. Fluidextract of cascara fifteen milliliters at bedtime as needed.

Administration of Medications

Objectives for the Student

BE ABLE TO

■ 1. Differentiate between local and systemic effects and give four examples of each.
■ 2. Name the four methods of administering drugs.
■ 3. Define the term *parenteral* and give examples of types of parenteral methods of administering drugs.
■ 4. List advantages and disadvantages of giving drugs by the parenteral route.
■ 5. List guidelines for safe administration of drugs.
■ 6. Identify reasons for errors in medication administration.
■ 7. Use common abbreviations with 100 percent accuracy.
■ 8. Demonstrate beginning skill in pouring medications.
■ 9. Calibrate the rate of flow of intravenous solutions.

Safety is the paramount concern in drug administration. The following are guidelines to be used in the promotion of safe medication administration.

GUIDELINES FOR SAFETY IN DRUG ADMINISTRATION

1. Know the policies of the hospital or agency.
2. Give only those medications for which the physician has written and signed the order.
3. Check with the head nurse or physician when in doubt about any medication.
4. Make certain that the data on the medicine card or Kardex correspond exactly with the label on the patient's medicine.
5. Always have another person, for example, the head nurse or pharmacist, check calculations.
6. Do not converse during drug administration unless seeking help. Remember that attentiveness is the most important aspect of safety.

7. Keep the medication cabinet or drug cart locked at all times when not in use.
8. Do not give keys to the medication cabinet or drug cart to an unauthorized person.

Six

Five Rights for Correct Drug Administration

1. Right patient
2. Right time and frequency of administration
3. Right dose
4. Right route of administration
5. Right drug
6. Right documentation

METHODS OF DRUG ADMINISTRATION

The methods by which drugs are administered modify their effect on the body. Certain drugs are suited to only one method of administration, whereas others may be given in a number of ways, depending on the preparation used and the reason for which the medication is given. As a general rule we are concerned with two types of drug administration: local (intended for an effect limited to the site of application) and systemic (intended for a general effect in which the drug is absorbed into the blood and carried to one or more tissues in the body).

Administration for Local Effects

A local effect is obtained when the drug is applied in the immediate area. Occasionally undesired absorption may be obtained from a local site, and an untoward or toxic effect may result. Boric acid, methyl salicylate, and hexachlorophene have been shown to exert harmful effects systemically when applied to large or denuded areas particularly.

Application to the Skin. Intact skin, with the exception of a newborn's skin, is generally impermeable to most agents. Ointments containing anti-inflammatory or antibiotic agents are useful for their local effects. Care should be taken not to apply topical agents to denuded areas without knowledge of the physician, because undesired absorption may occur.

Application to the Mucous Membrane. The application of drugs to the various mucous membranes of the body may be made for local or systemic effects. The mucous membranes in the mouth, eye, nose, vagina, and rectum are constantly bathed in watery solutions and are generally more permeable than skin.

Suppositories. Suppositories may be inserted in the rectum for local effects, such as Dulcolax for its local action to promote a laxative effect, or in the form of soluble bases to gain a systemic effect (i.e., antinauseants, pain-relieving agents, or drugs such as aspirin for antipyretic effect). Vaginal suppositories are generally for treatment of local infections, although some systemic absorption may occur.

Enemas. Enemas are most commonly used to promote a laxative effect; however, some oil-based retention enemas may contain drugs intended for systemic effects.

Intranasal Preparations. Intranasal preparations may be used to treat systemic conditions such as asthma or to exert a local effect in decreasing nasal congestion. Care should be taken that the nasal passages are free from exudate before administering a nasal preparation, and the tip of the spray bottle should be protected from contamination. Nasal spray nozzles should be cleaned after each use.

Ophthalmic Preparations. Care should be taken to keep eye preparations from contamination. The eye dropper bottle or ointment tube should never touch the membranes of the eye. These preparations generally have an expiration date to guarantee their sterility; this should be checked before using any ophthalmic preparation.

Ear Preparations. Absolute sterile technique is not necessary for ear preparations. With the patient lying down, the ear drops should be instilled into the ear canal after first gently pulling the external ear to straighten the ear canal. The patient should remain in a recumbent position for a few minutes after instillation of the drops to ensure their effect.

Administration for Systemic Effects

To obtain systemic effects from a drug, it must first be absorbed into the blood and carried to the tissue or organ on which it acts. To produce these effects, drugs may be administered orally, sublingually, rectally, parenterally, by inhalation, or in some cases even by topical administration.

Oral Administration. Although the most popular method from the standpoint of patient acceptability and convenience, oral administration has the disadvantage of being slower in onset of action than parenteral administration; this method should not be used if a very rapid effect is desired. Some drugs, such as insulin, are not effective when given orally, because they are destroyed by the juices in the gastrointestinal tract.

Drugs given orally may be administered as tablets, capsules, pills, or liquids. Taste is an important factor from the patient's viewpoint. Many drugs that have disagreeable tastes may be disguised by giving them in a large amount of fluid, such as fruit juices or effervescent drinks, or in syrups or emulsions. Fluids that have an unpleasant taste should be given cold, often with ice, and followed by a drink of water.

Food delays or reduces the absorption of many drugs, including aspirin and some forms of penicillin. Other drugs are better absorbed and less irritating to the stomach when taken with food. Examples of drugs better taken with food are iron products and some forms of erythromycin.

Reduced absorption may occur if certain drugs are given with certain food products. For example, tetracycline was given with milk for a time to reduce gastric irritation. It was later found that the tetracycline was severely disabled and rendered much less effective because the calcium, magnesium, and mineral supplements bound with the tetracycline, thus reducing the amount of the drug available to the body.

When taking oral medications the patient should be advised as follows:

1. Read all directions, warnings, and interactions about the drug. These are generally clearly printed on over-the-counter preparations. Over-the-counter preparations are drugs too and should not be ignored as a cause of possible side effects with prescription drugs.

2. Take medications generally with a full glass of water to enable the drug to be dissolved and begin working faster.

3. Medications should never be combined with alcohol. Some cough syrups contain alcohol in sufficient amounts to be noted.

4. Do not mix medications in hot drinks. The hot temperature can destroy some drugs, and the tannic acid in hot tea can reduce the absorption of certain medications.

5. Do not mix medications in food unless specifically ordered.

6. Vitamin and mineral supplements have substances that can interfere with drug absorption. These should be noted as over-the-counter drugs.

Procedure for Pouring and Administering Oral Medications

1. Wash hands.
2. Identify the patient by checking his or her arm band. If the arm band is missing and there is any question as to the patient's ability to respond correctly to his or her name, ask a reliable staff member to identify the patient.
3. Compare the drug label with the medicine card or the Kardex when taking the container from its location, before pouring, and before returning the container to its location.
4. Pour pills, tablets, and capsules into lid of bottle before placing in medicine cup. Avoid touching them with fingers.
5. When pouring liquids, pour away from the label. Wipe neck of bottle with damp paper towel or tissue before replacing cap.
6. Hold medicine glass, graduate, or minim glass at eye level and place thumb on glass at desired volume.
7. When giving more than one medication to a patient, the following order should be used: Give tablets and capsules followed by water or other liquid; then give liquids diluted with water as required. Cough medicine is given undiluted and is not followed by liquids. Sublingual and buccal tablets are given last.

NAME *Jane Kingsby*

ROOM   338-1

MEDICATION *Danthusin*

R   604871

DOSAGE   0.5 Gm.

TIME   9-1-5-9

Figure 14–1. A sample medicine card.

8. Remain with patient until all medication has been swallowed.
9. Record on Kardex or medicine sheet only after medication has been given.
10. Report and record medication ordered but not given.

A medicine card similar to the one illustrated in Figure 14–1 is usually made out for each medication a patient receives. Each hospital has its own slightly modified form. Many hospitals and long-term care facilities transcribe medication orders to a Kardex.

Many drugs commonly used are available in unit-dose packages. A unit-dose package contains the amount of drug for a single dose in the proper form for administration by the prescribed route. Tablets, capsules, and liquid medications can be prepared in single-dose packages. All unit-dose packages are labeled with the generic name, trade name, precautions, expiration date, if appropriate, and instructions for storing.

Packaging of drugs provides for medication safety because it is not necessary to calculate dosages. Strip packages provide for ease of counting narcotics, because all doses in the strip are numbered. This package also prevents contamination caused by pouring tablets into the hands when counting.

Liquid medications may be measured in a graduate, minim glass, or medicine glass, depending on the volume desired and the amount of accuracy required (Figure 14–2). Very small

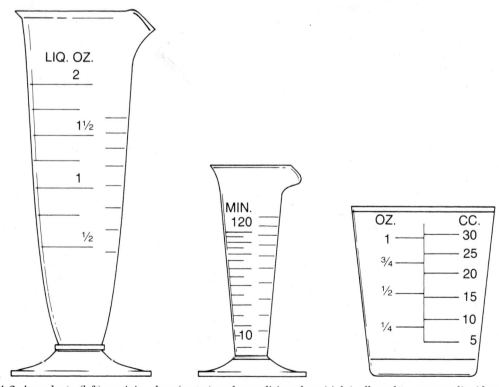

Figure 14–2. A graduate *(left)*, a minim glass *(center)*, and a medicine glass *(right)*, all used to measure liquid medication.

or exact volumes should not be measured in a medicine glass.

Sublingual Administration. The procedure for giving sublingual medications follows that for oral administration of drugs. However, the medication is not swallowed; it is placed under the patient's tongue, where it must be retained until it is dissolved or absorbed. The number of drugs that may be administered in this way is limited.

Parenteral Administration. The term *parenteral* refers to all the ways in which drugs are administered with a needle. Although this is undoubtedly the most efficient method of drug administration, because it avoids all the variables of topical and gastrointestinal absorption, it can also be the most hazardous. Untoward effects may be rapid and even fatal.

Whenever the skin is broken, it is possible for infections to develop; thus, strict aseptic technique must be used. Injections may cause nerve damage if placed incorrectly, and the accidental penetration of blood vessels may cause hematoma formation or the incorrect placement of a drug intended for intramuscular use directly into a blood vessel.

Medications intended for use by injection are supplied in the form of ampules or vials, as illustrated in Figure 14–3. Ampules are designed for use only once, and the unused portion must be discarded. Ampules should be used whenever a drug is administered intravenously. Rubber-stoppered vials are used for multiple withdrawals of drugs. If any sign of precipitation, color change, or cloudiness develops within the vial, it should be discarded.

Some parenteral drugs are supplied within the ampule as a powder that must first be diluted by the nurse before administration. Directions for reconstitution are enclosed with the package literature, advising dilution with sterile saline or water, and should be strictly observed.

Prefilled disposable syringes for all medications to be given subcutaneously, intramuscularly, and intravenously are available (Figure 14–4). Some of the advantages of prefilled disposable syringes are the following:

1. Sterility is ensured.

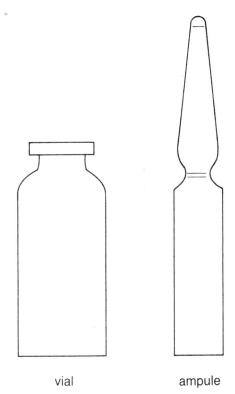

vial   ampule

Figure 14–3. Injected medications are supplied in vials *(left)* and ampules *(right)*.

2. Accuracy is ensured.
3. There is less trauma to tissue caused by blunt needles.
4. They are immediately available.

These unit doses of disposable syringes are the most convenient but also the most costly forms of parenteral medications.

Intradermal Injection. This form of injection is used exclusively for skin testing. The needle is inserted at an angle almost parallel to the skin surface. When correctly placed, a small bubble will be raised in the skin surface where the intradermal material is deposited. The inner surface of the arm or the back is generally chosen for skin testing (Figure 14–5).

Subcutaneous Injection. In subcutaneous injection, the solution is placed beneath the skin into the fat or connective tissue just underlying the dermis layer. A 25-gauge needle is generally used, with the length from ⅜ to ⅝ inch, depending on the thickness of the patient's subcutaneous tissue. A 45-degree angle is generally

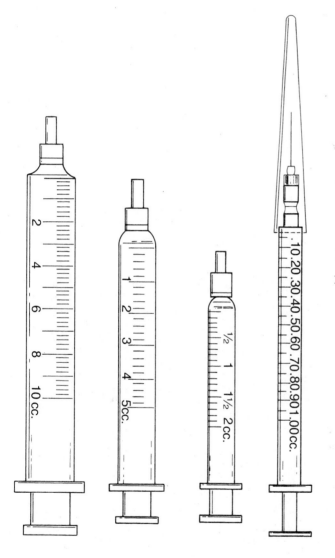

Figure 14–4. Prefilled disposable syringes.

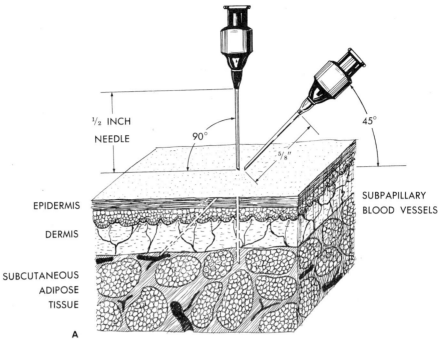

EPIDERMIS

DERMIS

SUBCUTANEOUS
ADIPOSE
TISSUE

SUBPAPILLARY
BLOOD VESSELS

½ INCH
NEEDLE

90°

5/8"

45°

A

Figure 14–5. Three types of injections. *A,* Subcutaneous; *B,* intradermal; *C,* intramuscular. (Reprinted with permission from Asperheim, M.K.: Pharmacologic Basis of Patient Care, 5th ed. Philadelphia, W.B. Saunders Co., 1985.)

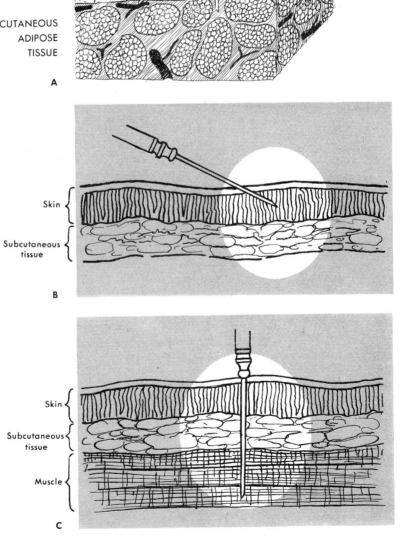

Skin

Subcutaneous
tissue

B

Skin

Subcutaneous
tissue

Muscle

C

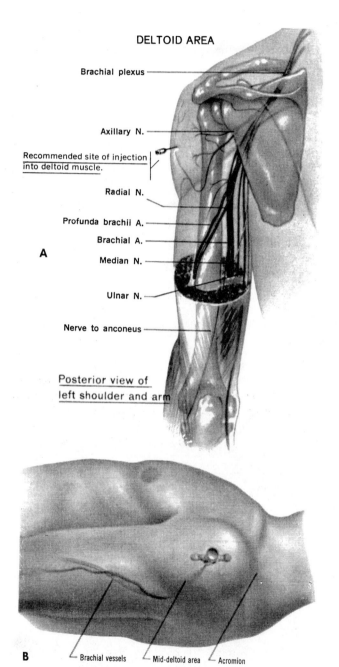

DELTOID AREA

Brachial plexus

Axillary N.

Recommended site of injection into deltoid muscle.

Radial N.

Profunda brachii A.

Brachial A.

Median N.

Ulnar N.

Nerve to anconeus

A

Posterior view of left shoulder and arm

B

Brachial vessels   Mid-deltoid area   Acromion

Figure 14–6. *A* and *B,* Two views of the deltoid site for intramuscular injection. (Reprinted with permission from Asperheim, M.K.: Pharmacologic Basis of Patient Care, 5th ed. Philadelphia, W.B. Saunders Co., 1985.)

VASTUS LATERALIS

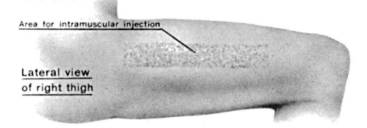

Area for intramuscular injection

Lateral view
of right thigh

Figure 14–7. Vastus lateralis site for intramuscular injection in adults. (Reprinted with permission from Asperheim, M.K.: Pharmacologic Basis of Patient Care, 5th ed. Philadelphia, W.B. Saunders Co., 1985.)

used, although with a short needle a 90-degree angle may be used as well (see Figure 14–5).

After careful cleansing with alcohol or other anti-infective, the skin is gently pinched and lifted from the muscle. The skin is released before the medication is injected. Before injection, the needle is aspirated to make sure a blood vessel has not been entered, then the material is deposited. Generally amounts injected subcutaneously are less than 2 mL.

Intramuscular Injection. For intramuscular injection (IM) a 1- to 3-inch needle is used. The gauge of the needle generally is based on the viscosity of the material injected. A 21-gauge needle is often used for penicillin injections, but a smaller gauge is chosen for solutions of other drugs.

There are several sites that may be used for intramuscular injections, including the deltoid muscle in the upper arm (Figure 14–6), the vastus lateralis in the lateral thigh (Figure 14–7),

and the gluteus maximus in the buttocks (Figure 14–8). Sites should be rotated if repeated administration of IM medications is ordered.

When giving intramuscular injections to children, a smaller-length needle is chosen. With infants often a ⅜ inch is used. The vastus lateralis in the anterolateral thigh is the preferred site for infants and young children because the gluteal muscles are not well developed. The needle is inserted in an anteroposterior position after the muscle is firmly grasped and the child firmly restrained (Figures 14–9 and 14–10).

Care should be taken to aspirate the syringe before the medication is delivered.

Intravenous Administration. The intravenous (IV) route is used when the most rapid onset of drug action is desired. The medication is injected directly into a vein as a preparation either administered directly from an ampule especially constituted for IV use or diluted in a bottle of fluids for more gradual administration.

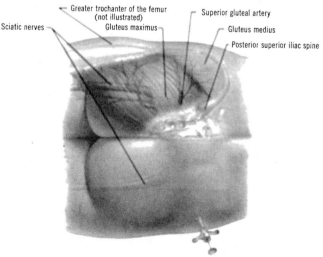

Greater trochanter of the femur
(not illustrated)
Sciatic nerves
Gluteus maximus
Superior gluteal artery
Gluteus medius
Posterior superior iliac spine

Figure 14–8. Intramuscular injection in the gluteal area. (Reprinted with permission from Asperheim, M.K.: Pharmacologic Basis of Patient Care, 5th ed. Philadelphia, W.B. Saunders Co., 1985.)

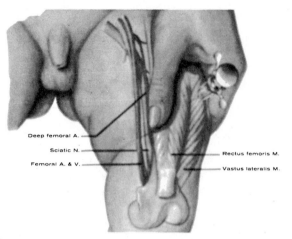

Deep femoral A.
Sciatic N.
Femoral A. & V.

Rectus femoris M.
Vastus lateralis M.

Figure 14–9. Vastus lateralis site for intramuscular injection in children.

Any surface vein may be used, or a cutdown is employed to utilize the subclavian vein or deeper extremity veins.

Just as the intended effect of the drug takes place within a few seconds in many cases, the untoward effects may occur with the same rapidity. For this reason the direct supervision of a physician is often necessary.

The IV route can be used when drugs are too irritating to be injected into the subcutaneous or intramuscular sites, because the intima of the blood vessels is ordinarily quite resistant to the effect of these agents. Care should be taken to prevent extravasation of these agents; sloughing of local tissues can result.

The IV route is also used to administer fluids, electrolytes, dextrose or other sugars, and proteins. Care should be taken to avoid incom-

VENTROGLUTEAL SITE

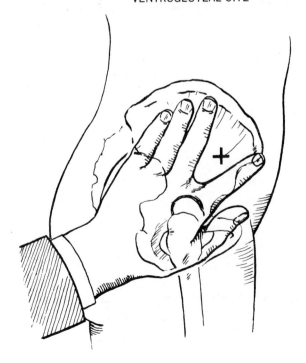

Figure 14–10. Ventrogluteal site. The injection is made between the index and middle fingers, which are spread as far as possible to form a V. (Reprinted with permission from Asperheim, M.K.: Pharmacologic Basis of Patient Care, 5th ed. Philadelphia, W.B. Saunders Co., 1985.)

patibilities when mixing drugs in various IV solutions. If cloudiness, discoloration, or precipitates occur when a drug is mixed, the solution should not be used.

The rate of flow of the IV solution is monitored by maintaining the proper number of drops per minute. The number of drops per minute varies with the caliber of the IV set used and should be carefully checked by the nurse in each instance. Calibrations may vary from 10 to 60 drops/mL.

Calibrating the Rate of Intravenous Solutions. IV bottles are supplied in 250-, 500-, and 1000-mL sizes. The order may read for a specified solution to be given at stated intervals (e.g., 150 mL per hour for 8 hours), or a specified amount may be administered continuously (e.g., 500 mL is to run for a 6-hour period). In every case the proper number of drops per minute is determined by the calibration of the particular IV set used.

Example

1000 mL of 5% dextrose in water is ordered to be given over an 8-hour period. The equipment is calibrated so that 15 drops = 1 mL. What should be the rate of flow in drops per minute?

First: Determine the number of milliliters per hour.

$$\frac{1000 \text{ mL}}{8 \text{ hr}} = 125 \text{ mL/hr}$$

Second: Determine the number of milliliters per minute.

$$\frac{125 \text{ mL/h}}{60 \text{ (min/hr)}} = 2.1 \text{ (or 2 mL/min)}$$

Third: Convert the milliliter per minute to the drops required.

$$1 \text{ mL} = 15 \text{ drops}$$

Therefore, 2 mL = 30 drops per minute.

Example

How long will it take for 250 mL of IV solution to be delivered if it is flowing at 30 drops per minute? This set is calibrated at 60 drops/mL.

First: Convert drops to milliliters. If 60 drops = 1 mL, 30 drops = 0.5 mL/min.

Second: Determine how many minutes it will take for this amount of fluid to be absorbed.

$$\frac{250 \text{ mL}}{0.5 \text{ mL/min}} = 500 \text{ min}$$

Third: Convert minutes to hours.

$$\frac{500 \text{ min}}{60 \text{ min/hr}} = 8.3 \text{ hr}$$

Intra-Arterial Injection. In special cases, most notably in the administration of antineoplastic agents, the drug is injected directly into an artery leading to the affected tissue or organ. A special administration set is used for this purpose. Intra-arterial administration can deliver high doses of a drug to a restricted area of the body, thus eliminating some of the systemic side effects of the agent. Presently, patients can be discharged with intra-arterial medications prepared for self-administration over extended periods of time.

Review Questions

1. Discuss the methods used to apply medication to mucous membranes of the nose, throat, eyes, urinary tract, and vagina.

2. Name the methods used to administer drugs to obtain systemic effects.

3. Define the term *parenteral.*

4. What advantage does oral administration of drugs have over parenteral administration?

5. Give an example of each of the following methods of injection:
   a. intradermal
   b. subcutaneous
   c. intramuscular
   d. intravenous

6. What are some habits that you should develop to administer medications safely?

7. Discuss the correct procedure for pouring and measuring 15 mL of milk of magnesia, using a bottle that contains 8 oz of the drug.

8. Without the use of a reference, prepare a list of common abbreviations used in writing medication orders.

Additional learning opportunities:

1. If the course in pharmacology does not correlate with the basic nursing course, it is recommended that equipment for pouring the various forms of oral medications be provided for examination.

2. Practice transcribing orders by various methods.

Vitamins, Minerals, and General Nutrition

Objectives for the Student

B E

A B L E

T O

■ 1. List the characteristics of vitamins.
■ 2. State the function of vitamins in the body.
■ 3. State the function of minerals in the body.
■ 4. Identify fat-soluble vitamins.
■ 5. Identify water-soluble vitamins.
■ 6. Give an example of a source of each vitamin.
■ 7. Identify symptoms of specific vitamin deficiencies.
■ 8. Identify symptoms of specific mineral deficiencies.
■ 9. Identify the components of a healthy diet.

At the lowest scale of life, primitive microorganisms are able to synthesize most of the nutrients they need and demand few ready-made raw materials from their environment.

Some of this ability to synthesize requirements is lost, however, in higher plants and animals, because they have many highly specialized cells and organs that depend entirely on other cells for their nourishment. Humans depend on other organisms to supply many vital constituents of their food; this is particularly true of one class of compounds that is required in minute amounts—the vitamins.

It has been known for some time that deficiencies in diet cause diseases. It was noticed by the British that sailors on long voyages, away from fresh fruits and vegetables, developed a disease known as scurvy, which was characterized by loosening of the teeth, bleeding gums, irritability, and fatigue. It was found that if citrus fruits were part of the diet this disease could be prevented. (Citrus fruits are notably rich in vitamin C.) One of the fruits frequently used was the lime; hence, the word "limey" was often applied to the English sailor.

Unfavorable symptoms are also noted when

an overdose of vitamins (especially the fat-soluble vitamins) is consumed. Actual toxicity may be produced. Polar bear liver, because of the extremely high concentration of stored oil-soluble vitamins, will produce toxicity of this type if it is consumed by humans.

Hypervitaminosis: the disease that develops because of an overdose of vitamins.

Avitaminosis: the disease that develops because of a lack of vitamins.

NOMENCLATURE OF VITAMINS

The duplication and confusion apparent in the naming of vitamins are understandable only in the historical context of the development of our knowledge of vitamins. Successive letters of the alphabet were assigned to new vitamins as they were characterized and isolated, and some letters were assigned out of order. Vitamin K, for example, refers to the Scandinavian word "Koagulation," because of the part this vitamin plays in the clotting mechanism of blood. Vitamin H refers to the German word "Haut," which means skin.

It soon became evident that the original vitamin B was not a single vitamin at all but actually a group of vitamins; therefore, subscript numbers were added, giving us vitamins B_1, B_2, and others. There are currently many numbers missing in the series, because some of the fractions separated were subsequently found to be identical.

CHARACTERISTICS OF VITAMINS

Vitamins are

- Organic in nature;
- Required in very small amounts;
- Required preformed in the diet or synthesized by intestinal flora;
- Necessary for normal growth and maintenance;
- Sensitive to light, heat, and oxidation and must be stored in a cool place in dark bottles;
- Necessary for enzyme systems.

General vitamin-deficiency symptoms include tiredness, aches, pains, and a general "poor feeling." The general populace has far too many symptoms of this type, however, to blame them on vitamin deficiencies exclusively. An adequate diet is the best answer for the prevention of vitamin deficiencies.

FAT-SOLUBLE VITAMINS

Vitamin A

Source: fish liver oils (especially cod liver), dairy products, and vegetables such as carrots and spinach.

Deficiency symptoms: night blindness, nerve degeneration of the spinal cord and peripheral nerves, skin lesions.

Minimum daily requirement (MDR): 5000 units.

Commercial products: Stabil-A, Aquasol A.

Vitamin D

Source: fish liver oils (especially cod and halibut), ultraviolet radiation (sunshine), dairy products.

Deficiency symptoms: If the deficiency occurs in childhood, the condition is known as rickets and is characterized by an abnormally large abdominal region, soft skull, and deformed arms and legs; if the deficiency occurs in later life, it is known as osteomalacia and is characterized by softening of the bones.

Activity: This vitamin enables the body to deposit calcium and phosphorus in the bones. An overdose leads to low calcium concentration in the blood, tetany, and eventual death.

MDR: 400 units.

Commercial products: Drisdol, Dical-D.

Vitamin K

Source: alfalfa, synthesized by intestinal flora.

Deficiency symptoms: hemorrhagic tendency.

Activity: This vitamin is required for the formation of prothrombin in the liver, which is needed for blood to clot normally.

MDR: not known exactly because it is manufactured by intestinal flora.

Commercial products: Synkayvite, Hykinone (water-soluble synthetic form of the vitamin), Mephyton (vitamin K).

Vitamin E

Source: wheat-germ oil.

Deficiency symptoms: Its function in humans is not known. A deficiency in rats causes sterility; in guinea pigs muscular dystrophy is produced.

MDR: unknown.

Commercial products: Eprolin, Epsilan-M.

WATER-SOLUBLE VITAMINS

These vitamins may be subdivided into two general groups: those concerned with the release of energy from food (e.g., thiamine, riboflavin) and those concerned with the formation of red blood cells (e.g., folic acid, vitamin B_{12}).

Thiamine (Vitamin B_1)

Source: widely distributed in nature, especially in yeast, liver, and lean meat.

Deficiency symptoms: The condition is known as beriberi and is characterized by inflammation of the peripheral nerves, paralysis, mixed sensations of heat and cold, congestive heart failure, and edema.

MDR: 2 mg.

Commercial products: sold merely as thiamine hydrochloride.

Riboflavin (Vitamin B_2)

Source: liver, kidney, milk.

Deficiency symptoms: vascularization of the cornea followed by ulcerations, dermatitis, and lip lesions.

MDR: 2 mg.

Commercial products: sold merely as riboflavin.

Nicotinamide (Niacinamide) and Nicotinic Acid (Niacin)

Source: liver, yeast, peanuts.

Deficiency symptoms: The condition produced is known as pellagra. The symptoms are insomnia, appetite loss, irritability, dizziness, and morbid fears, followed by subsequent lesions of the mucous membranes and dermatoses, especially on areas of the chest and neck exposed to the sun.

MDR: 15 mg.

Commercial products: sold merely as nicotinamide.

Side effect: A facial flush occurs quite often when nicotinic acid is administered, but the flush is not commonly seen when nicotinamide is used.

Pyridoxine (Vitamin B_6)

Source: liver, yeast, milk, meats, molasses.

Deficiency symptoms: skin lesions, hypochromic anemia, and convulsions in some instances.

MDR: 2 mg.

Commercial products: sold merely as pyridoxine.

Pantothenic Acid

Source: meat, vegetables, cereals, legumes, eggs, milk.

Deficiency symptoms: deficiency symptoms as an isolated deficiency have not been described; occurs in overall deficiency states.

MDR: not described. Therapeutic preparations have no known use. It is used empirically to treat many neurologic and metabolic disorders in combination.

Folic Acid

Source: green leafy vegetables, liver, yeast.

Deficiency symptoms: macrocytic anemia. The red blood cells do not mature properly and are larger than normal. This increased size reduces the amount of total surface area; consequently, less oxygen is transported to the tissues.

MDR: no dose determined; 0.25 mg is recommended.

Commercial products: Folvite.

Vitamin B$_{12}$

Source: animal tissue, especially liver.

Deficiency symptoms: pernicious anemia. Vitamin B$_{12}$ is known as the extrinsic factor for the production of red blood cells. For effective utilization of this vitamin from the gastrointestinal system, the intrinsic factor must be in the stomach of the individual. If it is not, the vitamin is not absorbed. In most cases of demonstrated deficiency of this vitamin, it is actually this intrinsic factor that is at fault, because vitamin B$_{12}$ is so widely distributed in nature that it would be rather unlikely that the individual has a dietary inadequacy. In a deficiency, then, vitamin B$_{12}$ is ordinarily administered parenterally to circumvent this intrinsic factor needed for absorption from the oral route.

MDR: 2 µg.

Commercial products: Coplex, Rubramin.

Ascorbic Acid or Cevitamic Acid (Vitamin C)

Source: green vegetables, berries, fruits. Because this vitamin is rapidly destroyed by air, the fruits must be fresh. Canning and cooking destroy the vitamin.

Deficiency symptoms: scurvy, characterized by gingivitis, loose teeth, slow healing of wounds, and petechial hemorrhages.

MDR: 30 to 125 mg.

Commercial products: sold as ascorbic acid.

Multiple Vitamin Preparations

It is well recognized that when one vitamin deficiency exists, there is invariably a dietary deficiency in several other vitamins as well. Thus, most commonly a multiple vitamin supplement is prescribed. There are many multivitamin supplements available. A few of the more common brands are: Allbee with C, Becotin-T, Dayalets, Lederplex, MVI, Multicebrin, Optilets, Stresscaps, Theragran, ViDaylin, and Vigran.

The multivitamins available for over-the-counter purchasing generally have a lower vitamin content, particularly in the oil-soluble vitamins, than those available by prescription only.

MINERALS

There are many minerals, or essential elements, necessary for normal body functions. Most of these are required in trace amounts only and are found so freely in the environment, the soil, plants used for food, and seafood that they rarely, if ever, need to be discussed in terms of a deficiency leading to ill health.

Trace elements are used by the body as components of enzymes and in some cases as catalysts necessary for proper enzymatic function. Copper, cobalt, fluorine, manganese, and zinc are a few of the trace elements known to be essential.

Other minerals perform a more dynamic function in the body and must be ingested regularly in some form, since they are either excreted daily in urine or feces or are depleted in the process of forming or repairing body tissues.

Iron

Iron has long been known to be an essential component of blood hemoglobin. Blood is not a static tissue but is constantly being re-formed as old red blood cells are trapped and destroyed by the spleen and other organs. Iron can be stored in the body, most notably in the bone marrow, but a dietary deficiency or a malabsorption problem in the intestinal tract soon manifests itself as an iron-deficiency anemia.

Iron-enriched infant formulas, such as Similac with Iron and Enfamil with Iron, have been designed to prevent this problem in very young children. Cow's milk is a very poor source of iron, and iron-deficiency anemia is a very frequent finding in infants from ages 6 months to 3 years. The problem is compounded if the infant is allowed to stay on the bottle after 1 year of age and to satisfy most of his or her appetite with a bottle of milk between meals, thus coming to mealtime with a poor appetite for the more nutritious meats and vegetables.

The teenage years are another time in life when iron-deficiency anemias are common. This is primarily due to the teenager's common pattern of fad diets and generally poor eating habits.

Menstruating women lose iron in the menstrual flow each month and are much more susceptible to deficiencies than males of the same age. Pregnancy is likewise a common time for anemia, because the developing fetus takes what it needs for development and can cause alarmingly low hemoglobin values in women whose diets are nutritionally inadequate.

Sources: meat, green vegetables, legumes, fortified cereals.

Commercial preparations:

Ferrous Sulfate, USP, BP (Feosol). This preparation is the most inexpensive and most commonly used form of iron supplement. It is available in tablet and liquid forms. Occasional abdominal cramping or discomfort is noted if it is taken on an empty stomach. The patient should be advised that all iron supplements will turn the stool black.

Dose: (Oral) 325 mg 3 times daily.

Ferrous Gluconate, USP, BP (Fergon). Very little therapeutic difference is noted between the gluconate and sulfate salts of iron. This preparation has the advantage of being slightly less irritating to the gastric mucosa but the disadvantage of being relatively more expensive.

Dose: (Oral) 435 mg once daily.

Iron Dextran Injection, USP, BP (Imferon). Designed for deep intramuscular injection, this preparation is reserved for cases of severe iron deficiency anemia and malabsorption problems. It should be administered with the Z-tract technique in the upper outer quadrant of the buttock to minimize skin discoloration and irritation at the site of injection. The primary disadvantage of this, as of any parenteral iron preparation, is the ever-present danger of iron overdosage. Hemosiderosis, fever, urticaria, and headache are among the symptoms of iron overload.

Dose: Calculated individually, based on the patient's hemoglobin level and weight. The range of dosage is generally 0.5 to 2 cc/day given IM or IV.

Calcium and Phosphorus

Unlike iron deficiencies, conditions arising from calcium and phosphorus deficiencies are usually due to metabolic problems rather than nutritional deficits. These elements perform a very dynamic and complex function in the body under the control of the parathyroid glands. They are in a constant equilibrium between the blood and calcified tissues of the body, primarily bone. Serum calcium levels should vary only slightly in healthy individuals. If calcium levels are too low, tetany occurs; if they are too high, cardiac irregularities are noted.

The kidneys are primarily responsible for the excretion of calcium, and severe or prolonged kidney damage can produce calcium deficiencies unrelated to the endocrine system. This condition is termed "renal rickets."

Vitamin D–deficient rickets, in which insufficient amounts of vitamin D limit proper calcium absorption, is extremely uncommon in the United States but may still be noted in underdeveloped countries.

Osteoporosis is a condition in which there is thinning of the calcified portions of bones owing to deficient formation of bone matrix. It may be seen in postmenopausal women as well as individuals with a severe protein-deficient diet. Osteoporosis in women may be alleviated by oral calcium supplements.

Commercial preparations:

Calcium Lactate, USP, BP

Dose: (Oral) 5 gm 3 times daily.

Calcium Gluconate, USP, BP

Dose: (Oral) 4 to 15 gm daily. (IV) 10 cc of 10% solution.

Calcium Chloride, USP, BP

Dose: (IV) 5 to 20 mL of a 5% solution.

Calcium Galactogluconate (Neo-Calglucon)

Dose: (Oral) 15 cc 2 or 3 times daily.

Calcium Carbonate, USP, BP (Os-Cal, Biocal)

Dose: (Oral) 2 to 4 500-mg tablets daily.

Potassium

Potassium, like sodium and chloride, has a dynamic function in the maintenance of water and electrolyte concentrations within the body tissues and cells. In addition, potassium has a unique function in the transmission of nerve impulses and the control of cardiac rhythm.

Potassium depletion results from the metabolic changes occurring in diabetic acidosis, in prolonged vomiting or diarrhea, and in the debilitation caused by surgery. It is often accidentally induced by prolonged administration of certain diuretics. Familial periodic paralysis is a hereditary disease characterized by bouts of muscular weakness and hypokalemia.

Commercial preparations:

Potassium Chloride, USP, BP

Dose: (Oral) 1 to 3 gm daily in divided doses. (IV) Based on potassium depletion. Maximum rate of administration would be 20 mEq/hr, usually 40 to 80 mEq in a 24-hour period.

Kaon Elixir

Dose: (Oral) 15 cc (20 mEq) in water 2 to 4 times daily after meals.

Kaon Tablets. Each one contains 1.17 gm (5 mEq) of potassium gluconate.

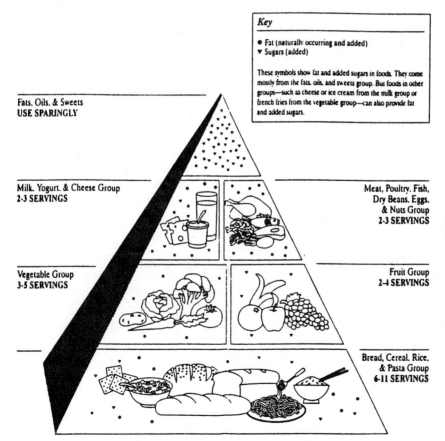

Key

● Fat (naturally occurring and added)
▼ Sugars (added)

These symbols show fat and added sugars in foods. They come mostly from the fats. oils. and sweets group. But foods in other groups—such as cheese or ice cream from the milk group or french fries from the vegetable group—can also provide fat and added sugars.

Fats. Oils. & Sweets
USE SPARINGLY

Milk. Yogurt. & Cheese Group
2-3 SERVINGS

Meat, Poultry. Fish, Dry Beans. Eggs. & Nuts Group
2-3 SERVINGS

Vegetable Group
3-5 SERVINGS

Fruit Group
2-4 SERVINGS

Bread, Cereal. Rice. & Pasta Group
6-11 SERVINGS

Figure 15–1. The food guide pyramid.

Dose: (Oral) 2 tablets 4 times daily after meals.

Potassium Triplex

Dose: (Oral) 5 cc (15 mEq) 3 times daily after meals.

Slow-K. This coated tablet has 600 mg (8 mEq) of potassium chloride in a wax matrix to minimize gastrointestinal irritation.

Dose: (Oral) 1 tablet 3 or 4 times daily.

CHANGES IN NUTRITION INFORMATION

For many years it was believed that proper nutrition could be attained by the eating administration of the basic food groups: proteins—meat, fish, and eggs; breads and grains; fruits; vegetables; and dairy products.

Increased information became available with regard to overnutrition, particularly in the red meat and fat groups, with resulting elevation of cholesterol and increased incidence of vascular diseases, cerebrovascular accidents (CVAs), and heart attacks. It has become important to control and reduce the amount of these food items in the diet.

The Food Guide Pyramid (Figure 15–1) shows the U.S. Department of Health and Human Services' current diet recommendations. The pyramid emphasizes that the most nutritious and healthy diet should stress food groups in different proportions in the diet, with complex carbohydrates as the base of the pyramid and then other foods in decreasing amounts.

Some nutritionists now recommend that fish or poultry be consumed only two or three times a week, with consumption of red meat being reduced to two or three times a month. It has been recommended that no more than 30% of the calories a person consumes come from fat.

Caloric requirements vary with age and activity. Children and active teenagers and adult males may need up to 2800 calories a day. Sedentary adults may require only 1600 calories.

Food labels can often be misleading. For instance,

- Cholesterol free does *not* mean fat free. Cholesterol only comes from animal sources. The food may still be fatty.
- Made with vegetable oil may or may not be a good sign. Good oil choices are canola, olive, corn, sunflower, and soybean oils. Saturated fats are in coconut oil, palm kernel oil, or any hydrogenated oil.

Look on the back of the package for the grams of fat or saturated fat per serving.

Implications for the Student

1. Discuss the patient's diet, and review the natural sources of vitamins. Be familiar with the basic food groups and the vitamins and minerals they supply.

2. In some cases a vitamin deficiency may be caused by a self-administered medication, such as mineral oil, which prevents absorption of the oil-soluble vitamins. Patients should be questioned about self-administered medications.

3. Self-administered medications such as vitamins can produce toxic effects, most notably the fat-soluble vitamins A, D, E, and K.

4. Patients and their families should be instructed to store all vitamins in a cool place and away from direct light and heat.

5. Individuals on a vegetarian diet should be advised of their special need for vitamin and mineral supplements.

6. Water-soluble vitamins can be destroyed by overcooking foods.

7. Certain vitamins, such as vitamin C, appear to have activities outside their "vitamin" status and may be useful in higher doses in the prevention of viral illnesses, such as the common cold.

8. Iron supplements may be used in the prevention of anemia, particularly in premeno-pausal women and children or adults with limited dietary preferences.

9. Calcium supplements are useful in the prevention of osteoporosis in postmeno-pausal women.

10. Certain minerals, such as calcium and potassium, may have cardiotoxic effects when their levels in the body are too high or too low.

11. Recognize the components of a healthy diet and the healthy effects of reduced fats in the diet.

CASE STUDIES

1. Mrs. J.D., age 72, has had difficulty eating since her dental extractions 1 year ago. She presented in the physician's office with a deep fissure on each side of her mouth and red irritated eyes. What vitamin deficiency is apparent?

2. Miss S.J., age 24, has many food allergies and intolerances. Her dentist referred her to her family physician because he could find no oral disease that would account for her loose teeth and gingival inflammation. What deficiency could account for her problem?

3. Susan L., age 6 years, was brought to the pediatrician's office by her mother because she was failing in school, pale, listless, and seemed to be tired all the time, even though she reportedly had 10 hours of sleep each night. Blood studies revealed a hemoglobin of 9.1, and other studies were within normal limits. How should her problem be handled?

4. Mrs. R.D. complained to the public health nurse that she has been having abdominal cramps and her stools are black. She had been taking an iron supplement for anemia. How would you identify the problem, and what instruction could you give her?

5. Mr. J.C., an unmarried construction worker, was noted to have a high cholesterol of 375 mg percent. He states he frequently eats out at fast-food restaurants. How could his diet be examined, and what advice could be given?

Review Questions

1. Discuss the importance of potassium in the diet.

2. Consult a textbook of medical-surgical nursing and discuss symptoms of potassium deficiency.

3. Discuss the problems related to vitamin deficiency in the older adult.

4. What measures do you recommend to improve the health status of older adults?

DRUG CLASSIFICATIONS

Antibiotics and Antifungal, Antiviral, and Antiparasitic Agents

Objectives for the Student

B E	
A B L E	
T O	■ 1. Identify the antibiotics and give their general uses.
	■ 2. Identify serious side effects of antibiotics.
	■ 3. Distinguish between a broad-spectrum antibiotic and a narrow-spectrum antibiotic.
	■ 4. Give examples of drugs of choice to treat specific conditions.
	■ 5. Identify common antiparasitic agents.
	■ 6. Identify antiviral agents and their general uses.

Antibiotics are substances produced by living cells that kill or inhibit the growth of microorganisms. The first knowledge of antibiotics was given to us by Sir Alexander Fleming in 1928, when he discovered that a product of the *Penicillium* mold had the power to destroy many disease-producing microorganisms.

Currently, we obtain many antibiotics from molds, bacteria, and yeasts, but an increasing number are now manufactured synthetically. Often only a small change in the structure of a naturally produced antibiotic can produce significant changes in the action and effect of a drug.

Each antibiotic has its own characteristic "spectrum" of activity against various microorganisms. A "broad-spectrum" antibiotic is effective against many microorganisms; a "narrow-spectrum" antibiotic is effective against only a few.

Much has been discovered in recent years about the growing resistance of many microorganisms to the action of antibiotics. It is believed that the use of antibiotics in many trivial infections has allowed microorganisms to develop mutant forms that are resistant to the drug. This is particularly true if an antibiotic is taken only for a few days instead of the generally prescribed 10-day minimum for antibiotic use. The organisms that are more naturally resistant to the drug are allowed to increase and multiply, whereas only the weaker ones are killed.

Allergic reactions to various antibiotics are also common. With repeated exposure to a drug, various defense mechanisms of the body begin to be sensitized, and allergic reactions result. Often these reactions are mild and may just produce a rash, which is easily treated. Subsequent exposures to the drug may produce severe and even fatal reactions, however.

THE PENICILLINS

Since its discovery as the first antibiotic, there have been many alterations in the structure of penicillin to increase its usefulness.

Penicillin G, USP, Benzylpenicillin, BP. Utilized as either the sodium or potassium salt to increase its water solubility, this early form of penicillin remains in common use for the treatment of streptococcal and pneumococcal infections as well as gonorrhea, syphilis, meningitis, and other infections caused by penicillin-sensitive organisms. Its main disadvantage is that in its crystalline form it has a short duration of action and must be injected, as it is destroyed when taken orally. Before any form of penicillin is given, the patient must be carefully questioned concerning allergic reactions to the drug.

Dose: Adults: (IV) 10 million to 100 million units daily in divided doses.
Children: (IM) 6000 to 12,500 units/kg four times daily. (IV) Up to 400,000 units/kg daily.
Neonates: (IM, IV) 30,000 units/kg twice daily.

Long-Acting Forms of Penicillin G

Because of the short duration of the crystalline form of penicillin G, several long-acting forms have been developed. These have the advantage of being given intramuscularly, whereby a repository of the drug remains in the muscle tissue and can be absorbed slowly by the body.

Penicillin G Procaine, USP, BP (Mycillin, Crysticillin, Duracillin). The addition of procaine to the penicillin molecule gives a product that provides good blood levels of penicillin for about 6 hours.

Dose: Adults: (IM) 600,000 to 4 million units in divided doses every 6 hours.
Children: (IM) 300,000 to 1.2 million units in divided doses every 6 hours.
Neonates: This form is not recommended.

Penicillin G Benzathine, USP, BP (Bicillin). By the addition of benzathine to the penicillin molecule, a very insoluble form of penicillin is formed. The drug is slowly leached from the repository in the muscle and may give prolonged but low doses of penicillin for as long as 1 month. This form is used in monthly injections for prophylaxis in patients who have had rheumatic fever and in the treatment of syphilis as well as in other cases when prolonged action is desired.

Bicillin L-A. Pure benzathine penicillin.

Dose: Adults: (IM) 1.2 million to 4.8 million units.
Children: (IM) 600,000 to 1.2 million units.

Bicillin C-R. A combination of equal parts of benzathine penicillin and procaine penicillin, so that a therapeutic blood level is reached sooner. Dosage range is similar to that of Bicillin L-A.

Bicillin A-P. This combination of benzathine, procaine, and crystalline penicillins gives yet more flexible blood levels. Dosage range is generally the same as that of other long-acting forms.

Penicillin V, USP, BP (V-Cillin, Pen Vee). By changing the structure of penicillin G, this form of penicillin is able to be absorbed orally. It is primarily used to treat respiratory infections.

Dose: Adults: (Oral) 250 mg every 4 hours.
Children: (Oral) 15 to 50 mg/kg daily in 4 divided doses.

Semisynthetic Penicillins

Considerable research and alteration of the penicillin molecule have resulted in new forms of penicillin that have a broader spectrum of activity than the parent molecule and greater effectiveness with oral administration. Table 16–1 gives an overview of this class of antibiotics.

General Toxicity and Side Effects

Hypersensitivity to the penicillins should always be considered. In some instances, however, individuals who are sensitive to penicillin G may be able to tolerate the altered forms of penicillin. When prescribed orally, abdominal cramping or diarrhea may result. Overgrowth of nonsusceptible organisms such as *Monilia* may occur, with resultant vaginal or perineal infections.

THE CEPHALOSPORINS

Also derived originally from a mold, the cephalosporins are structurally related to the penicillins. Like penicillin, these agents exert their activity against young, dividing cells by interfering with the formation of bacterial cell walls.

Because of their similarity to the penicillin molecule, there is a considerable cross-sensitivity with penicillin. Although it is thought that the cross-allergic reaction occurs only about 25 percent of the time, all patients with a history of allergy to penicillin should be given these agents with caution.

General toxic effects of these agents include gastrointestinal distress when they are administered orally as well as allergic skin rashes.

The cephalosporins are divided into three general groups, called the first, second, and third generations, on the basis of their spectrum of activity.

Table 16–1. SEMISYNTHETIC PENICILLINS

Generic Name	Trade Name	General Uses	Dose
Amoxicillin, USP, BP	Amoxil, Polymox, Wymox	Same as ampicillin	Adults: (Oral) 250–500 mg q8h Children: (Oral) 20–40 mg/kg/day divided to q8h
Amoxicillin and clavulanic acid	Augmentin	Same as ampicillin, but includes some ampicillin-resistant organisms	Adults: (Oral) 250–500 mg q8h Children: (Oral) 20 mg/kg/day in divided doses q8h
Ampicillin, USP, BP	Omnipen, Polycillin	Otitis media, respiratory infections, urinary tract infections, meningitis (in IV form)	Adults: (Oral, IM, IV) 500 mg–2 gm Children: (Oral) 50–400 mg/kg/day
Azlocillin sodium, USP	Azlin	Proteus infections of bone or soft tissue	Adults: (IV) 200–300 mg/kg/day in 4–6 divided doses Children: (IV) 300–600 mg/kg/day
Bacampicillin hydrochloride, USP	Spectrobid	Same as ampicillin	Adults: (Oral) 400 mg q12h Children: (Oral) 12.5 mg/kg q12h
Carbenicillin disodium, USP, BP	Geopen, Pyopen	Urinary tract infections	Adults: (IM, IV) 1–2 gm q6h, up to 30 gm/day Children: (IM, IV) 10–35 mg/kg q6h

Table continued on following page

Table 16-1. SEMISYNTHETIC PENICILLINS *Continued*

Generic Name	Trade Name	General Uses	Dose
Cloxacillin sodium, USP, BP	Tegopen	Respiratory tract and soft tissue infections	Adults: (Oral) 0.25–1 gm q4–6h Children: (Oral) 12.5–25 mg/kg/day in divided doses
Cyclacillin	Cyclacillin	Same as ampicillin	Adults: (Oral) 400 mg q12h Children: (Oral) 12.5 mg/kg q12h
Dicloxacillin sodium, USP, BP	Dynapen, Pathocil	Staphylococcal infections	Adults: (Oral, IM, IV) 250–500 mg q6h Children: (Oral, IM, IV) 12.5–50 mg/kg/day in divided doses
Methicillin sodium, USP, BP	Staphcillin	Staphylococcal infections	Adults: (IM, IV) 4–12 gm/day in divided doses Children: (IM, IV) 25 mg/kg 4 times daily
Mezlocillin sodium, USP, BP	Mezlin	Serious postsurgical abdominal, GI, and soft tissue infections	Adults: (IM, IV) 3–4 gm q4–6h Children: (IM, IV) 300 mg/kg/day in divided doses
Nafcillin sodium, USP, BP	Unipen	Staphylococcal infections	Adults: (Oral, IM, IV) 250 mg–1 gm 4–6 times daily Children: (Oral, IM, IV) 25–50 mg/kg/day in divided doses
Oxacillin sodium, USP, BP	Prostaphlin, Bactocil	Staphylococcal infections	Adults: (Oral, IM, IV) 250–500 mg q4–6h Children: (Oral, IM, IV), 50 mg/kg/day in 4 divided doses
Piperacillin sodium, USP	Pipracil	Serious postsurgical infections, some urinary tract infections	Adults: (IV) 3–4 gm q4–6h (IM) 2 gm q4–6h Children: Not recommended in those younger than 12 years
Ticarcillin disodium, USP, BP	Ticar	Urinary tract infections	Adults: (IM) 1 gm q6h (IV) 300 mg/kg/day Children: (IM) 50–100 mg/kg/day (IV) 150–200 mg/kg/day in 4–6 divided doses

IV = intravenous; IM = intramuscular; GI = gastrointestinal.

First-Generation Cephalosporins

These agents are effective against organisms such as streptococci and some strains of staphylococci. In addition, they are effective against some organisms that invade the urinary tract. They are listed in Table 16–2.

Second-Generation Cephalosporins

In addition to activity against the organisms of the first generation, these agents are also effective against *Haemophilus influenzae,* a common invader of the middle ear and respiratory tract. They are listed in Table 16–3.

Third-Generation Cephalosporins

This group is less effective against the streptococci and pneumococci than the early cephalosporins but more effective against the gram-negative invaders of the gastrointestinal and urinary tracts. They are generally reserved for serious infections that do not respond to other

Table 16-2. FIRST-GENERATION CEPHALOSPORINS

Generic Name	Trade Name	Dose
Cefazolin sodium, USP, BP	Ancef, Kefzol	Adults: (Oral, IM, IV) 250 mg–1.5 gm q6h Children: (Oral, IM, IV) 25–50 mg/kg/day in 3–4 divided doses
Cepfradroxil, USP, BP	Duracef	Adults: (Oral) 1–2 gm/day in 1–2 divided doses Children: (Oral) 10–15 mg/kg twice daily
Cephalexin, USP, BP	Keflex	Adults: (Oral) 250–500 mg q6h Children: (Oral) 25–50 mg/kg/day in divided doses
Cephalothin sodium, USP, BP	Keflin	Adults: (IM) 500 mg–100 gm (IV) q4–6h Children: (IM) 80–160 mg/kg/day in divided doses
Cephapirin sodium, USP, BP	Cefadyl	Adults: (IM, IV) 500 mg–1 gm q6h Children: (IM, IV) 40–80 mg/kg/day in 4 divided doses
Cephradine, USP, BP	Anspor, Velosef	Adults: (Oral) 250 mg q6h (IM, IV) 500 mg q12h Children: (Oral, IM, IV) 50–100 mg/kg/day in 4 divided doses

IM = intramuscular; IV = intravenous.

Table 16-3. SECOND-GENERATION CEPHALOSPORINS

Generic Name	Trade Name	Dose
Cefaclor, USP, BP	Ceclor	Adults: (Oral) 250 mg q8h Children: (Oral) 20 mg/kg/day in divided doses q8h
Cefamandole nafate, USP, BP	Mandol	Adults: (IM, IV) 500 mg–1 gm q4–8h Children: (IM, IV) 50–100 mg/kg/day in divided doses q4–8h
Cefmetazole sodium	Zefazone	Adults: 2 gm IV q6–12h Children: No dose established
Cefonicid sodium, USP, BP	Monocid	Adults: (IM, IV) 500 mg–1 gm diluted 1–2 times daily Children: No dose established
Ceforanide, USP, BP	Precef	Adults: (IM, IV) 0.5–4 gm q12h Children: (IM, IV) 20–40 mg/kg/day in 2 divided doses
Cefotetan disodium, USP, BP	Cefotan	Adults: (IM, IV) 1–2 gm q12h Children: (IM, IV) 40–60 mg/kg/day in 2 divided doses
Cefoxitin sodium, USP, BP	Mefoxin	Adults: (IM, IV) 1–2 gm q6–8h Children: (IM, IV) 80–160 mg/kg/day in 4–6 divided doses
Cefuroxime axetil, USP	Ceftin	Adults: 250–500 mg orally twice daily Children: 125–250 mg orally twice daily
Cefuroxime sodium, USP	Zinacef	Adults: 750 mg–1.5 gm IM or IV q8h Children: 50–100 mg/kg/day IM or IV in divided doses

IM = intramuscular; IV = intravenous.

agents. The third-generation cephalosporins are listed in Table 16–4.

THE TETRACYCLINES

The tetracyclines are broad-spectrum antibiotics that are effective against many organisms, particularly those infecting the respiratory system and soft tissues. Although many can be given parenterally, they are well absorbed orally and are generally given by mouth.

Tetracyclines are used principally in the treatment of infections caused by susceptible *Rickettsia, Chlamydia,* and *Mycoplasma* organisms and a variety of gram-negative and gram-positive bacteria. It is the drug of choice for Rocky Mountain spotted fever and Lyme disease.

General adverse effects include gastrointestinal irritation; the overgrowth of nonsusceptible organisms, such as yeasts, which may produce diarrhea; a perineal monilial rash; and vaginal infection. The tetracyclines should not be given during pregnancy or to any child younger than 8 years, because the drug concentrates in developing tooth enamel and produces a brown or yellow stain on the teeth. The tetracyclines are described in Table 16–5. All doses given are for adults and children older than 8 years.

THE ERYTHROMYCINS

Erythromycin is a relatively narrow-spectrum antibiotic, effective generally against the same organisms as penicillin. It is often used in penicillin-sensitive patients. Although effective parenterally, it is generally used orally, primarily for upper and lower respiratory tract infections.

General untoward effects include pain and cramping after oral administration as well as skin reactions. The erythromycins are given in Table 16–6.

QUINOLONE ANTIMICROBIAL AGENTS

The quinolones are a new class of orally effective antimicrobial agents that acts by inhibiting the bacterial enzyme DNA gyrase. They are effective against pathogens of the urinary and gastrointestinal tracts and against some organisms that cause sexually transmitted diseases. The quinolones are listed in Table 16–7.

Table 16-4. THIRD-GENERATION CEPHALOSPORINS

Generic Name	Trade Name	Dose
Cefixime, USP	Suprax	Adults: 400 mg daily orally in 1 or 2 daily doses Children: 8 mg/kg/day orally in 1 or 2 daily doses
Cefoperazone sodium, USP	Cefobid	Adults: 2–4 gm IV daily in divided doses q12h Children: no dose established
Cefotaxime sodium, USP, BP	Claforan	Adults: (IM, IV) 1–2 gm q6–8h Children: (IM, IV) 25–180 mg/kg/day in 4–6 divided doses
Cefpodoxime proxetil	Vantin	Adults: 100–400 mg orally q12h Children: 10 mg/kg/day orally in 2 divided doses
Cefprozil	Cefzil	Adults: 500 mg orally q12h Children older than 2 years: 7.5 mg/kg orally q12h
Ceftazidime sodium, USP, BP	Tazidime, Fortaz, Cepta z	Adults: (IM, IV) 1 gm q8–12h Children: (IV) 30–50 mg/kg q8h
Ceftizoxime sodium, USP, BP	Cefizox	Adults: (IM, IV) 1–2 gm q8–12h Children: (IM, IV) 50 mg/kg q6–8h
Ceftriaxone sodium, USP, BP	Rocephin	Adults: (IM, IV) 1–2 gm/day in 1 or 2 divided doses Children: (IM, IV) 50–75 mg/kg/day in 2 divided doses
Moxalactam disodium, USP, BP		Adults: (IV) 2–6 gm/day in 3 divided doses Children: (IV) 50 mg/kg q6–12h

IM = intramuscular; IV = intravenous.

Table 16-5. TETRACYCLINES

Generic Name	Trade Name	Dose
Demeclocycline hydrochloride, USP, BP	Declomycin	Oral: 150 mg q6h
Doxycycline hyclate, USP, BP	Vibramycin	Oral: 100–200 mg initially, then 100 mg 2–3 times daily
Methacycline hydrochloride, USP, BP	Rondomycin	Oral: 600 mg/day in 2–4 divided doses
Minocycline hydrochloride, USP, BP	Minocin	Oral, IV: 200 mg initially, then 100 mg q12h
Oxytetracycline hydrochloride, USP, BP	Terramycin	Same as tetracycline
Tetracycline hydrochloride, USP, BP	Achromycin, Panmycin, Steclin, Tetracyn	Oral: 250–500 mg q6h IM: 100 mg 2–3 times daily IV: 500 mg q12h

Note: All doses are for adults and children older than 8 years.

Table 16-6. ERYTHROMYCINS AND DERIVATIVES

Generic Name	Trade Name	Dose
Erythromycins		

Erythromycin, USP, BP	Ilotycin, Erythrocin	Adults: (Oral) 250–500 mg q6h
		    (IM, IV) 0.5–1 gm q6h
		Children: (Oral) 7–25 mg/kg/day in 4 divided doses
		    (IM, IV) 5–10 mg/kg twice daily

Erythromycin estolate, USP, BP	Ilosone	Adults: (Oral) 250–500 mg q6h Children: (Oral) 30–50 mg/kg/day in 4 divided doses
Erythromycin ethylsuccinate, USP, BP	EES, Ery-Ped	Adults: (Oral) 400 mg twice daily Children: (Oral) 30–50 mg/kg/day in 2–4 divided doses
Erythromycin gluceptate, USP, BP	Ilotycin	Adults: (IV) 250–500 mg q6h Children: (IV) 5–10 mg/kg q12h
Erythromycin lactobionate, USP, BP	Erythrocin lactobionate	Adults: (IV) 15–20 mg/kg/day in 4 divided doses Children: Same as adults
Derivatives		
Azithromycin	Zithromax	Adults (only): 250–500 mg orally once daily
Clarithromycin	Biaxin	Adults (only): 250–500 mg orally once daily

IM = intramuscular; IV = intravenous.

Table 16-7. QUINOLONE ANTIMICROBIALS

Generic Name	Trade Name	General Uses	Dose (Adult Only)
Ciprofloxacin hydrochloride, USP	Cipro	Respiratory, urinary tract, bone, soft tissue infections	250–500 mg orally q12h
Enoxacin	Penetrex	Sexually transmitted diseases and urinary tract infections	200–400 mg orally q12h
Lomefloxacin hydrochloride	Maxaquin	Infections of respiratory and urinary tracts	400 mg orally once daily
Norfloxacin, USP	Noroxin	Urinary tract and sexually transmitted infections	400 mg orally q12h
Ofloxacin	Floxin	Respiratory, prostate, urinary tract and sexually transmitted infections	200–400 mg orally q12h

These agents are analogues of nalidixic acid, USP (covered in the chapter on urinary tract drugs). These agents are entirely synthetic, and they act specifically on the DNA structure of the microorganism, causing abnormalities that result in death of the microbe.

Side effects are mild with these agents and usually do not cause them to be discontinued. The most common are gastrointestinal (i.e., nausea and vomiting). Rashes, insomnia, irritability, and arthralgia occur less commonly.

ANTIFUNGAL AGENTS

Fungi are members of the plant family that are obligatory parasites because they contain no chlorophyll for self-sustenance.

Fungal infections of humans can be as simple as tinea pedis (athlete's foot), tinea corporis (fungal rashes on the skin), or thrush (a superficial infection of the mouth often seen in infants).

When the immune system is impaired, fungal infections can become overwhelming and life threatening. AIDS and AIDS-related complex (ARC) are both caused by the human immunodeficiency virus (HIV), but owing to their severely compromised immune system, patients with these conditions are often subject to severe and life-threatening fungal infections. Cryptococcal meningitis, severe oropharyngeal candidiasis, and esophageal candidiasis can occur in these patients. Intravenous forms of the antifungal agents are generally used to treat these conditions (Table 16–8).

Other antibiotics are listed in Table 16–9.

ANTIVIRAL AGENTS

The discovery of antibiotics began a revolution in humans' ability to treat bacterial infections. It was anticipated that similarly effective antiviral agents would soon be identified as well.

A major problem in this drug development has been the more intimate relationship between viral and host metabolic activities. The search for selective inhibitors of viral activity

Table 16-8. ANTIFUNGAL AGENTS

Generic Name	Trade Name	Uses	Dose
Amphotericin B, USP, BP	Fungizone	Serious systemic fungal infections	Adults: (IV) 0.25 mg/kg in diluted infusion q2–4 days Children: (IV) 0.1 mg/kg in diluted infusion every 2–4 days
Fluconazole	Diflucan	Serious systemic infections	Adults: (Oral, IV) 50–100 mg/day Children: No dose established
Flucytosine, USP, BP	Ancobon	Serious systemic infections	Adults: (Oral) 50–150 mg/kg/day in 4 divided doses Children: Same as adults
Griseofulvin, USP, BP	Fulvicin, Grifulvin, Grisactin	Superficial fungal infections	Adults: (Oral) 250–500 mg/day Children: (Oral) 3.3 mg/kg 3 times daily
Ketoconazole, USP, BP	Nizoral	Serious systemic infections	Adults: (Oral) 200–400 mg/day as a single dose Children: (Oral) 50–100 mg/day
Miconazole, USP, BP	Monistat	Vaginally and topically for yeast infections Systemically for major infections	Adults: (IV) 1.2–3.6 gm/day (Topical) 2% cream Children: (IV) 20–40 mg/day
Nystatin, USP, BP	Mycostatin, Nilstat	Orally for moniliasis Topically and vaginally for skin monilia	Adults: (Oral) 500,000–1,000,000 U 3 times daily (Vaginal) 100,000 U suppository 3 times daily Children: (Oral) 100,000–200,000 U 4 times daily

IV = intravenous.

Table 16-9. OTHER ANTIBIOTICS

Generic Name	Trade Name	Uses	Toxic Effects	Dose
Amikacin sulfate, USP	Amikin	Serious infections of bone, soft tissues	Auditory and kidney damage	Adults: (IM, IV) 15 mg/kg/day in divided doses Children: Same as adults
Chloramphenicol, USP, BP	Chloromycetin	Meningitis, typhoid fever	Bone marrow depression	Adults: (Oral, IV) 12.5 mg/kg 4 times daily Children: (Oral, IV) 6 mg/kg 4 times daily
Clindamycin hydrochloride, USP, BP	Cleocin	Infections of respiratory tract, soft tissues	Leukopenia, vomiting, diarrhea, skin rash	Adults: (Oral) 150–300 mg q6h (IM, IV) 600 mg twice daily Children: (Oral, IM, IV) 10–40 mg/kg/day in divided doses
Colistimethate sodium, USP, BP Colistin sulfate, USP, BP	Coly-Mycin M Coly-Mycin S	Infections of urinary tract, soft tissues	Kidney damage	Adults: (Oral) 3–5 mg/kg/day in 3 divided doses (IM, IV) 1.5–5.0 mg/kg/day in 2–4 divided doses (Intrathecal) 5–15 mg every other day Children: Same as adults
Ethambutol hydrochloride, USP, BP	Myambutol	Tuberculosis	Optic neuritis, rash, mental changes	Adults: (Oral) 10–15 mg/kg/day Children: Same as adults
Gentamicin sulfate, USP, BP	Garamycin	Serious infections of soft tissue, GU tract, respiratory tract	Auditory and kidney damage	Adults: (IM, IV) 1–2 mg/kg/day in 2–3 divided doses Children: Same as adults
Imipenem and cilastatin sodium	Primaxin, ADD-Vantage	Serious infections of abdomen, respiratory tract, bone, kidneys	GI effects, seizures, bone-marrow suppression	Adults: (IV) Up to 50 mg/kg/day Children: (IV) 15–25 mg/kg q6h
Isoniazid, USP, BP	INH, Nydrazid	Tuberculosis	Neuritis, liver dysfunction	Adults: (Oral) 5–10 mg/kg/day Children: (Oral) 10–20 mg/kg/day
Kanamycin sulfate, USP, BP	Kantrex	Infections of bone, GU tract, respiratory tract, soft tissues	Auditory damage	Adults: (Oral) 1 gm 3–4 times daily (IM, IV) 7.5 mg/kg twice daily Children: (Oral) 12.5 mg/kg 4 times daily (IM, IV) 3–7.5 mg/kg twice daily
Lincomycin hydrochloride, USP, BP	Lincocin	Infections of soft tissue, bone, respiratory tract	Vomiting, diarrhea, skin rashes	Adults: (Oral) 500 mg 3 times daily (IM, IV) 600 mg q12h Children: (Oral) 30–60 mg/kg/day in 3–4 divided doses (IM, IV) 10–20 mg/kg/day in 2–3 divided doses
Metronidazole, USP, BP	Flagyl	Trichomoniasis, giardiasis, amebiasis	Metallic taste, diarrhea, intolerance to alcohol, rash	Adults: (Oral) Single dose of 2 gm or 250 mg 3 times daily for 7 days Children: (Oral) 15 mg/kg/day

Table continued on following page

Table 16-9. OTHER ANTIBIOTICS *Continued*

Generic Name	Trade Name	Uses	Toxic Effects	Dose
Polyxin B sulfate, USP, BP	Aerosporin	Serious infections of soft tissue or urinary tract	Neurologic and kidney damage	Adults: (IM) 6250–7500 U/kg 4 times daily (IV) 7500–12,500 U/kg twice daily (Intrathecal) 50,000 U once daily Children: Same as adults
Pyrazinamide, USP, BP	—	Tuberculosis	Liver toxicity, rash	Adults: (Oral) 20–35 mg/kg/day Children: (Oral) 15–30 mg/kg/day
Rifampin, USP, BP	Rifadin, Rifamate	Tuberculosis, carriers of meningitis organisms	Diarrhea, anemia, liver and kidney toxicity	Adults: (Oral) 600 mg/day Children: (Oral) 10–15 mg/kg/day
Spectinomycin hydrochloride, USP, BP	Trobicin	Gonorrhea	Chills, fever, nausea, dizziness, kidney damage	Adults only: (IM) 4 gm as a single injection
Streptomycin sulfate, USP, BP	Same	Tuberculosis	Auditory damage	Adults: (IM) 0.5–1.0 gm 4 times daily Children: (IM) 10 mg/kg 2–4 times daily
Tobramycin sulfate, USP, BP	Nebcin	Serious infections of bone, soft tissue, respiratory tract	Auditory and kidney damage	Adults: (IM, IV) 1 mg/kg q8h Children: Same as adults
Troleandomycin, USP, BP	Tao	Respiratory, GI, GU infections	Liver damage	Adults: (Oral) 250 mg q4–6h (IM) 200 mg q6h (IV) 1–2 gm/day in divided doses Children: (Oral IM, IV) 30–50 mg/kg/day in 2–4 divided doses
Vancomycin hydrochloride, vancocin, USP, BP	Vancocin	Severe septicemia, meningitis	Nausea, thrombophlebitis at IV site, skin rashes	Adults: (IV) 1 gm q12h Children: (IV) 5–10 mg/kg 4 times daily

GN = genitourinary; GI = gastrointestinal; IM = intramuscular; IV = intravenous.

that are not too toxic to the human host has been much more difficult than first appreciated.

All viruses and virus-infected cells have some characteristics that are different from uninfected cells. These differences offer ways to block viral division without affecting normal cells. The virus generally first fuses with the cell surface, then uncoats itself, gains entrance to the cell, and begins to synthesize its own viral nucleic acids within the cell. It then manufactures its own messenger viral RNA, and soon a new and free virion is released to attack yet another cell.

In the case of the HIV virus, latency poses an important problem. The virus may remain in the cell, but in a latent, undetectable form, so that the disease may occur years after the infection is transmitted. Now early changes are being detected in the T lymphocytes, and identification of ARC is detecting patients before total immunity is lost, when drug therapy may still be beneficial. Table 16–10 describes the currently available antiviral agents.

ANTIPARASITIC AGENTS

A number of parasites are able to invade the human body. The tropical parasites are not covered in this text.

Table 16-10. ANTIVIRAL AGENTS

Generic Name	Trade Name	Uses	Dose
Acyclovir sodium	Zovirax	Herpes simplex infections, oral or genital varicella zoster (shingles), varicella (chickenpox) in immunocompromised patients	Adults: (Oral) 200–800 mg q4h 5 times daily (IV) 5 mg/kg Children: (IV) 5–15 mg/kg q8h
Amantadine hydrochloride, USP, BP	Symmetrel, Symadine	Prevention and treatment of influenza A infections	Adults: (Oral) 100–200 mg/day Children: (Oral) 4.4–8.8 mg/kg/day in 1–2 doses
Didanosine (dd1)	Videx	Advanced HIV	Adults: 125–200 mg bid orally
Foscarnet sodium	—	Cytomegalovirus retinitis Herpes simplex and varicella zoster	Adults: 60 mg/kg IV q8h for 14–21 days Adults: 40 mg/kg IV q8h
Ganciclovir sodium	Cytovene	Cytomegalovirus, retinitis in immunocompromised patients	Adults: (IV) 5 mg/kg q12h Children: Some as adults
Idoxuridine, USP, BP	Herplex	Topically for herpes simplex ulcers of eye	Adults: (Topical) 0.1% solution of 0.5% ointment to eyes Children: Same as adults
Ribavirin	Virazole	Respiratory syncytial virus infections, adenovirus pneumonia	Adults: (Nasal) Aerosol mist containing 190 µg/L for 12–18h/day for 3–7 days Children: Same as adults
Rimantadine hydrochloride	—	Influenza A prophylaxis	Adults: 100 mg orally twice daily for up to 6 weeks Children: 5 mg/kg/day up to 150 mg/day maximum for under age 10 years
Trifluridine	Viroptic	Herpes simplex conjunctivitis, keratitis of eye	Adults: (Topical) 1% solution applied to eye for 7–14 days Children: Same as adults
Vidarabine, USP, BP	Vira-A	IV: herpes simplex encephalitis, neonatal herpes infections, varicella in immunocompromised patients, herpes zoster Topically to eyes for herpes simplex keratitis	Adults: (IV) 15 mg/kg/day for 5–10 days Children: Same as adults Adults: (Topical) 3% ointment applied 5 times a day Children: Same as adults
Zalcitabine (ddC)	Hivid	HIV	Adults: 0.75 mg tid orally
Zidovudine (AZT)	Retrovir	Treatment of AIDS and ARC	Adults: (Oral, IV) 200–300 mg q4h Children: (IV) 100–180 mg/M^2 q6h

IV = intravenous; AIDS = acquired immunodeficiency syndrome; ARC = AIDS-related complex; HIV = human immunodeficiency syndrome.

Anthelminthic Drugs

Worm infestations appear throughout the world but are particularly prominent in the warmer climates. Cultural hygienic practices are important in the prevention of worm infestations, because in every case they are spread by a feces-to-mouth route. Day care centers, where the diaper changer is also the food handler, have been important sources for the spread of worms and other parasites.

Mebendazole, USP, BP (Vermox). This agent is used in the treatment of roundworm, hookworm, threadworm, pinworm, and many tropical parasites.

Dose: Adults: (Oral) 1 100-mg tablet twice daily for 3 days.
Children: Same as adults.

Niclosamide, USP (Niclocide). This agent is used for the treatment of all tapeworm infestations.

Dose: Adults: (Oral) 2 gm/day for 7 days.
Children: (Oral) 1–1.5 gm/day for 7 days.

Piperazine Citrate, USP (Vermizine). This agent is used to treat roundworm (*Ascaris*) and pinworm infestations.

Dose: Adults: (Oral) 65 mg/kg for 7 days.
Children: Same as adults.

Pyrantel Pamoate, USP, BP (Antiminth). This agent is used for roundworm, hookworm, and pinworm infestations.

Dose: Adults: (Oral) 11 mg/kg.
Children: Same as adults.

Thiabendazole, USP, BP (Mintezol). This agent is used for cutaneous larva migrans (creeping eruption) and threadworm infestations.

Dose: Adults: (Oral) 25 mg/kg twice daily for 2 days. A 10% suspension of the drug may be applied topically to cutaneous larva migrans as well.
Children: Same as adults.

Medication for Lice and Scabies

Lice and scabies occur indiscriminately among all socioeconomic groups. Outbreaks of head lice in school systems create a public health challenge, particularly in the fall. It is often not possible to see the lice themselves, but the infestation is characterized by pruritus and the presence of nits, or the small, silver eggs attached to the hair shaft.

Scabies is caused by a mite that burrows under the skin and causes intense body pruritus. It is often spread by shaking hands, because the thin skin between the fingers is a typical spot for infestation.

Lindane, USP, BP (Kwell). This agent may be used as a shampoo for head lice or as an application to the entire body for scabies.

Dose: Adults: (Topical) 1% solution applied to the body or scalp once. Treatment may be repeated 1 more time in a week if necessary.
Children: Same as adults.

Permethrin Creme Rinse (Nix). This product is recommended as a single-dose treatment for head lice.

Dose: Adults: (Topical) After the hair has been washed, rinsed, and towel dried, the creme rinse is applied and left on the hair for 10 minutes.
Children: Same as adults.

Implications for the Student

1. All injectable antibiotics should be carefully checked for the expiration date before administration.

2. The patient should be carefully questioned concerning previous allergic reactions to antibiotics.

3. After administration, the patient should be checked for possible untoward effects, such as a skin rash, respiratory distress, or other allergic responses.

4. Become familiar with the special tags placed on patients' charts noting drug allergies.

5. Remember to check for Medic-Alert tags that an unresponsive patient may be wearing.

6. The nurse should be aware of cross-sensitivity reactions of the antibiotics, such as those between penicillin and the cephalosporins.

7. Patients should be carefully instructed to take their entire supply of antibiotics to prevent the development of resistant strains of bacteria.

8. Old antibiotic prescriptions should be discarded if they are not finished, because antibiotics quickly outdate.

9. Aseptic technique is still the most effective way to prevent infection. Antibiotics cannot be relied on to correct infections caused by disregard for asepsis.

10. Many antibiotics are irritating when given by injection. Intramuscular injections should be given deeply in large muscles.

11. Resolution of fever is a sign used to check the early effectiveness of an antibiotic against an infection.

12. The student should be aware of possible side effects of the anti-infective agents.

13. Superinfection by organisms not susceptible to antibiotics is a common sequela to antibiotic therapy. Superinfections may occur as a rash, commonly monilia in the oral or genital region, or as diarrhea.

14. Good nutrition, adequate rest, and general cleanliness are important to the overall well-being of a patient recovering from an infection.

15. Instruct patients in the importance of hygiene in preventing the spread of parasites. Short fingernails that are kept very clean, good hand-washing techniques, and the avoidance of "mouthing" of objects, such as pencils, and nailbiting should be stressed.

16. Become familiar with steps used to prevent head lice cross-infection. Combs, brushes, and other toilet articles should not be shared. Outer garments hung in cloakrooms can spread the infestation from garment to garment.

17. Stools should be inspected for the presence of worms. Transmission of infestations by toilet seats and bedpans should be considered and avoided.

18. Superinfections with fungal and bacterial agents are common in immunocompro-

mised patients. These patients should be observed carefully and instructed to report changes in skin, mucous membranes, or bowel habits.

19. Infections such as chickenpox and common colds can have life-threatening implications for the immunocompromised patient. The patient and the family should be instructed to avoid infected persons.

CASE STUDIES

1. Mr. S.L., 48, was referred by his family doctor to a local ear, nose, and throat specialist for his hearing deficit. The physician took the following case history: The patient had been well until age 35 when he had suffered a severe case of lobar pneumonia that did not resolve on appropriate penicillin therapy. Further studies showed that he had tuberculosis and was treated effectively in a sanitarium. In the past few years he has had gouty arthritis and a spastic colon but no other notable illnesses. What further inquiries might be made as to the cause of his deafness?

2. Mrs. S.A., 32, was treated for recurrent and persistent sinusitis with tetracycline and the decongestant Ornade. On the eighth day of medication her condition improved, but she presented with complaints of diarrhea and abdominal griping discomfort. What recommendations should be made?

3. Mrs. Jones brought her 2-month-old infant in for a routine well-baby exam. Her height and weight had increased normally. She appeared healthy except for a yellowish-white plaque that covered most of her tongue, and a few spots were noted on the buccal mucous membranes. What is this? How is it treated? Is it serious?

4. David N., age 3, was placed on ampicillin 3 days ago for otitis media. Today his mother called to report that she noted a very pale-pink flat rash on his chest when she bathed him. The rash did not appear to itch. She also reported that his fever was gone now, and he did not complain of his earache any more. Should the medication be discontinued? What precautions should be taken?

Review Questions

1. Why should the use of antibiotics be restricted to serious infections?

2. What is meant by the term "broad spectrum"?

3. Discuss the disadvantages of prolonged oral administration of the tetracyclines.

4. What side effects may result after prolonged use of Chloromycetin?

5. What is the drug of choice in treating fungal infections?

6. Why are drugs used in combination to treat tuberculosis?

7. Give an example of prophylactic use of penicillin.

8. Name two drugs that are effective in treating infections caused by staphylococci.

9. What is the primary advantage of giving amoxicillin instead of ampicillin?

10. List antibiotics that should not be used for young children.

11. Name two drugs that may be given to children for pinworm infestation.

12. What antiviral drug is most effective thus far against AIDS?

13. Name two antiviral drugs used for varicella zoster (shingles).

14. What drug is used for Lyme disease?

Sulfonamides

Objectives for the Student

B E

A B L E

T O

■ 1. Explain the reason for the limited use of sulfonamides.
■ 2. List symptoms of toxic effects of sulfa drugs.
■ 3. Identify intermediate and long-acting sulfa drugs.
■ 4. Discuss nursing responsibilities related to the care of patients on sulfonamides.

Sulfonamide drugs, more commonly called the "sulfa drugs," combat infection in the body by checking the growth of bacteria and other microorganisms, thus enabling the body's own defenses to cope with the infection.

These are synthetic drugs and are made to resemble para-aminobenzoic acid (PABA), a substance that the microorganisms need for the synthesis of folic acid, an essential enzyme. The microorganism cannot assimilate the sulfa drug; thus, it is prevented from growing and multiplying.

The sulfa drugs are less effective in the presence of a large amount of PABA because the microorganisms prefer PABA to the drug. For this reason the patient must not be taking medications containing PABA (e.g., Pabalate, an agent used for rheumatic conditions) when taking sulfa drugs.

These drugs are usually administered by mouth, the method of choice from the standpoint of convenience and because they are well absorbed from the intestinal tract.

Although sulfa drugs obviously aid in controlling infections, they now have been largely replaced by the antibiotics, which have faster action and fewer side effects.

The Department of Health, Education, and Welfare has stated concern over the increasing frequency of bacterial resistance to the sulfonamides. In addition, the development of newer and more effective agents has sharply limited the usefulness of sulfonamides in many instances. They recommend the use of sulfonamides for the following conditions only:

1. Chancroid
2. Trachoma
3. Inclusion conjunctivitis
4. Nocardiosis
5. Uncomplicated urinary tract infections caused by susceptible organisms
6. Toxoplasmosis
7. Malaria, as adjunctive therapy in some cases
8. Meningococcal meningitis due to susceptible organisms

9. *Haemophilus influenzae* infections of the middle ear

It is important that a patient taking sulfa drugs maintain an adequate fluid intake. Sulfonamides have a tendency to crystallize in the urine and deposit in the kidneys, resulting in a painful and dangerous condition. The chances of crystallization in the urine are minimized if the urine is kept dilute by a high fluid intake.

Sulfa drugs used today produce fewer symptoms of toxicity than the older compounds. However, toxic reactions may result from the use of any drugs that are absorbed and exert systemic effects. In this case toxic reactions include nausea, vomiting, cyanosis, drug fever (often confused with a recurrent fever from the infection), rash, acidosis, jaundice, blood complications, and kidney damage. In a few cases fatal Stevens-Johnson syndrome has occurred.

The general treatment of the toxic symptoms includes discontinuing the drug and forcing fluids. The severity of the symptoms determines whether the drug is permanently discontinued. The high incidence of toxicity associated with the sulfonamides explains why they have been largely supplanted by the antibiotics.

Sulfisoxazole, USP, BP (Gantrisin). Sulfisoxazole is one of the more commonly used sulfonamides at present. It has a relatively high solubility, and the incidence of crystalluria is low if fluid intake is reasonably adequate. It is indicated primarily in the treatment of acute or recurrent urinary tract infections caused by susceptible organisms.

In its injectable form it may be used in the treatment of meningitis along with antibiotic therapy. It is of little use in the treatment of streptococcal infections and other invaders of the upper respiratory tract. It may be used safely in infants older than 2 months. The dose is calibrated by weight for use in children.

Dose: Adults: (Oral) 2 to 4 gm initially, then 1 to 2 gm four times daily.
(IV) In diluted solution by slow IV drip, a total daily dose of 4 to 8 gm is given in four divided doses.
(IM) No dilution of the ampule is necessary for IM administration. The total

daily dose of 4 to 8 gm is divided into two or three injections per 24 hours.
Children: (Oral) 75 to 150 mg/kg/day in four divided doses.

Azo Gantrisin. Each tablet of this combination drug contains 500 mg of sulfisoxazole and 50 mg of phenazopyridine (Pyridium). The combination provides a urinary antiseptic property as well as the local anesthetic property of phenazopyridine, which relieves the symptoms of dysuria and urgency that often accompany urinary tract infections. The patient should be informed that the urine will be bright red-brown in color when the combination is administered.

Dose: Adults: (Oral) 4 to 6 tablets initially, then 2 tablets four times daily.
Children: This combination is not available in pediatric dosage forms.

Sulfamethizole, USP, BP (Thiosulfil). When given orally, sulfamethizole is rapidly absorbed and excreted via the kidneys. It is very useful in the treatment of kidney infections.

Dose: Adults: (Oral) 75 to 100 mg/kg/day in four divided doses.
Children: (Oral) 30 to 45 mg/kg/day in four divided doses.

LONG-ACTING SULFONAMIDES

Because most of the sulfonamides are excreted fairly rapidly, until recently it has been necessary to give relatively high doses at short intervals to maintain an effective blood level of the drug. The use of the newer long-acting sulfonamides, however, permits lower doses to be given, because the drug remains in effective concentrations for a longer time in the blood. Often only one dose is needed daily to maintain effective blood levels. Because a lower dose may be used, side effects occur less frequently than with other sulfa drugs.

Sulfamethoxazole, USP, BP (Gantanol). Chemically this drug is closely related to sulfisoxazole, but its rate of excretion from the body is much slower. It has the same uses as sulfisoxazole.

Dose: Adults: (Oral) 2 gm initially, then 1 gm twice daily.

Children: (Oral) 50 to 60 mg/kg/day in four divided doses.

Sulfacytine (Renoquid). This agent is used for uncomplicated infections of the urinary tract caused by susceptible organisms. It is administered only by the oral route.

Dose: Adults: (Oral) 250 mg four times daily.

Children: No children's dose has been established.

Sulfasalazine, USP, BP (Azulfidine). Sulfasalazine is used orally in the treatment of ulcerative colitis and Crohn's disease. It is often used in conjunction with corticosteroid therapy.

Dose: Adults: (Oral) 3 to 4 gm daily in divided doses.

Children: (Oral) 40 to 60 mg/kg/day in three to six divided doses.

Trimethoprim and Sulfamethoxazole, USP, BP (Bactrim, Septra, Bactrim DS, Septra DS). This combination of agents blocks two successive steps in bacterial growth and has become one of the more successful antibacterial agents in the sulfonamide groups.

The regular strength of the two brands of this combination contains 80 mg of trimethoprim and 400 mg of sulfamethoxazole. The DS noted for both of these signifies the double strength of the tablet. The suspension contains 40 mg of trimethoprim and 200 mg of sulfamethoxazole per teaspoonful.

In addition to considerable effectiveness in the treatment of urinary tract infections, this combination is now used successfully in the treatment of acute otitis media, particularly when routine antibiotic therapy has been ineffective. It should not be used in the treatment of streptococcal pharyngitis, because it has been shown to have little effectiveness.

Dose: Adults: (Oral) Regular strength, 2 tablets every 12 hours. Double strength, 1 tablet every 12 hours.

Children: (Oral) 8 mg/kg of trimethoprim and 40 mg/kg of sulfamethoxazole per 24 hours in two divided doses.

Implications for the Student

1. During administration of the sulfonamides, observe the patient for signs of improvement of the urinary tract infection. The improvement may be manifested by reduction of the fever, increased urine output, or clearing of the appearance of the urine.

2. The urine should remain acid for the optimum effectiveness of the sulfonamides. Prunes and cranberries in any form promote an acid urine, as does vitamin C in high doses. Carbonated beverages and citrus fruits should be avoided because they produce an alkaline urine.

3. Sulfonamides have as their primary side effect the production of allergic skin rashes. The patient should be observed carefully for signs of untoward skin eruptions.

4. To treat an infection of the urinary tract effectively, medication should be given for a 2-week period. Patients should be carefully instructed to take all the medication prescribed to prevent the development of subsequent, more resistant, urinary tract infections.

5. Abdominal distress may be a side effect of the orally administered sulfonamides.

6. The patient should be encouraged to maintain an adequate fluid intake during the administration of sulfonamides to prevent the crystalluria that is a side effect of these drugs in concentrated urine.

CASE STUDIES

1. Judy D., 21, has had recurrent urinary tract infections for many years. She was treated this time with Gantrisin tablets. Although her dysuria has subsided after 5 days of treatment, she awoke this morning unable to go to work because she has a headache and a temperature of 103° F. She didn't want to bother her doctor, so she mentioned this problem to you, her neighbor. What would your advice be?

2. Mrs. H., 22, received Azo Gantrisin from her physician yesterday afternoon. This morning she calls the office in total panic, saying that she urinated "pure blood." The doctor is not in yet. Should you tell her to come into the office immediately for an emergency appointment?

3. Jason F., age 5, is in the hospital for evaluation of his urinary tract infections. He had been taking Bactrim and was doing well. Yesterday morning, however, while being bathed, he complained that his back was "itching." A pink rash was apparent on his back, but it seemed to bother him less after a backrub. You obtained an order for Calamine lotion. This morning Jason presented with a bright red, very pruritic rash over his whole body and a temperature of 102° F. What are the possible reasons for this problem? Was it handled properly from the start?

Review Questions

1. What toxic reactions may occur from drugs that are absorbed and exert systemic effects?

2. What accounts for the decrease in use of sulfa drugs?

3. Discuss the instructions you would give to an individual who is taking one of the sulfonamides.

4. What information would you give to a patient who will be taking Azo Gantrisin?

5. What nursing action is indicated when toxic symptoms occur?

6. What is the advantage of the use of long-acting sulfonamides?

7. Name three drugs from this group that are effective in treating urinary tract infections.

CHAPTER 18

Antihistamines

Objectives for the Student

BE ABLE TO

- 1. Identify the symptoms of an allergic reaction.
- 2. Discuss information the nurse should give to a patient taking antihistamines.
- 3. Describe the symptoms of anaphylaxis.
- 4. Distinguish between "over-the-counter" and prescribed drugs for nasal congestion.
- 5. List precautions to be observed by the physician when prescribing an antihistamine.

Early in the twentieth century it was discovered that the release of histamine from body tissues was in large part responsible for symptoms that occurred after certain viral infections or the introduction of sensitizing foreign substances into the body.

Histamine is an amino acid that is found in many plant and animal tissues. Under normal circumstances it is probably bound to an intracellular protein.

When an antigen (the general term for a sensitizing foreign substance) is introduced into the body, it evokes a tissue response in the form of an antibody, which is synthesized specifically to combat the particular antigen. It is believed that the complex reactions and interactions that follow cause the release of histamine. It is the histamine, then, that evokes the symptoms, more commonly known as the "allergic reaction," which may be manifested by red watery eyes, urticaria, sneezing, coryza, rash, bronchiolar constriction of asthma, and so forth.

Anaphylaxis is the term used to signify the presence of a severe allergic reaction, which is marked by an extreme drop in blood pressure and body temperature, a decrease in the circulating blood volume, and cardiac abnormalities. If emergency measures are not taken immediately (i.e., administration of epinephrine or corticosteroids and the rapid administration of intravenous fluids), death may occur.

The emotional component of allergic reactions is less well understood. It is a well-established fact that certain persons can experience urticaria, or hives, after severe emotional stress. It has likewise been observed that asthmatic children and, occasionally, adults develop severe and even life-threatening attacks of asthma in times of emotional upheaval and stress, when no precipitating antigen can be demonstrated.

DETERMINING THE CAUSE OF THE ALLERGY

In some cases the source of the allergy can be determined by a little investigation or attention to circumstances prevailing when allergic symptoms appear. For instance, persons allergic to certain animal dander often determine this fact for themselves, noting that symptoms arise shortly after contacting dogs, cats, or other animals. Likewise, an individual who sneezes uncontrollably after contact with a certain flower is likely to remember the circumstances and avoid the allergen in the future.

Food allergies are somewhat more difficult to determine in some instances, but if suspected they can often be discovered if the individual keeps a careful record of all food eaten. Allergic reactions to a food may occur within a 3-day period after the offending food is eaten; thus the meals of this time span should be investigated. Seafood, chocolate, wheat, and nuts are common offenders, but any food may be involved.

Skin tests may be used to determine the offending allergen, but these are often disappointing. Obviously, it is impossible to prepare testing solutions of every existing antigen. It is also rare to have one or even two allergens defined as the offending substance even under optimum conditions. Many persons react to multiple allergens with wheals of varying size. At best, a diagnostic impression can be obtained, and some improvement in severe allergic reactions can be achieved following regular injection of desensitizing vaccine.

Antihistamines, then, by virtue of their effect in counteracting the symptoms of allergic reactions, remain a very useful, though not curative, form of drug therapy. Mild or seasonal allergies may often be controlled satisfactorily by the use of antihistamines alone. The ability of these agents to modify the symptoms of viral upper respiratory infections or the "common cold" is also well established.

The most troublesome, if not dangerous, side effect of the antihistamines in general is drowsiness. For this reason they should not be taken when working around machinery, when driving, or at any other time when drowsiness could be hazardous. The sedative effect of these agents is greatly increased when they are combined with alcohol, tranquilizers, hypnotics, narcotics, and many antihypertensive medications; thus the combination of these agents is to be avoided.

Diphenhydramine Hydrochloride, USP, BP (Benadryl). This agent is useful both orally and intramuscularly to control moderately severe allergic reactions, such as those occurring in serum sickness, urticaria, and drug reactions.

In addition, it is used occasionally as a mild sedative, particularly in the elderly, in whom more potent agents are not advisable.

Dose: Adults: (Oral) 50 mg three to four times daily. (IM) 10 to 50 mg three times daily.
Children weighing more than 20 lb: (Oral) 12.5 to 25 mg three to four times daily.

Chlorpheniramine Maleate, USP, BP (Chlor-Trimeton, Teldrin). This agent is available in both tablet form and delayed-action preparations, which allow effective release of the antihistamine for up to 8 hours. As a general rule, drowsiness is more troublesome in the delayed-release forms.

Dose: Adults: (Oral) 4-mg tablets every 3 to 4 hours. Delayed-release forms: 8 to 12 mg every 8 hours.
Children: (Oral) ¼ to ½ the adult dose of tablets.

Dimenhydrinate, USP, BP (Dramamine). This agent is used primarily for the relief of motion sickness and is quite successful in this respect if taken ½ hour before air or ground travel. No doubt the sedative effect of this agent is in part responsible for its success. It may be administered parenterally as well for nonspecific nausea and vomiting.

Dose: Adults: (Oral) 50 mg two to four times
daily. (IM) 50 mg as necessary.
Children: (Oral) ¼ to ½ the adult dose.
(IM) 1.25 mg/kg four times daily.

Tripelennamine Hydrochloride, USP, BP (Pyribenzamine). In addition to its use as an oral antihistamine for mild allergic symptoms, tripelennamine is also available in some topical ointments. Its use as a topical antihistamine is quite disappointing, however, and it is now largely replaced by corticosteroid creams if symptoms warrant local therapy.

Dose: Adults: (Oral) 50 mg four times daily.
Children: (Oral) 5 mg/kg/day in four
divided doses.

Meclizine Hydrochloride, USP, BP (Bonine). Although long used to control nausea and vomiting of pregnancy, federal regulations now restrict this drug and most other antinausea preparations from use in pregnant women. It is quite effective in the prevention of motion sickness. This drug is not recommended for children.

Dose: Adults: (Oral) 25 to 50 mg one to three
times daily.
Children: Not recommended.

Promethazine Hydrochloride, USP, BP (Phenergan). The drowsiness and antisecretory effects caused by promethazine make it particularly useful in preoperative patients. If this drug is administered parenterally with a narcotic agent, the sedative effect is increased. Oral forms and rectal suppositories are available as well.

Dose: Adults: (Oral) 25 mg three to four
times daily. (IM) 25 to 50 mg as necessary.
Children: (Oral) 6.25 to 12.5 mg three
to four times daily. (IM) 0.5 mg/lb as
necessary.

Brompheniramine Maleate, USP, BP (Dimetane). Very similar in action and uses to

chlorpheniramine, this agent is available in tablets as well as delayed-action dosage forms.

Dose: Adults: (Oral) 1 4-mg tablet every 4 to
6 hours. Delayed-action form: 8 to 12
mg every 8 hours.
Children: (Oral) 0.5 mg/kg/day in three
or four divided doses.

Trimethobenzamide Hydrochloride, USP, BP (Tigan). This agent is used in the form of capsules, rectal suppositories, and intramuscular injections to control nausea and vomiting in children and adults. It is not recommended for use in pregnant women. Side effects have been infrequent, but occasional hypersensitivity reactions have occurred. Hypotension, coma, disorientation, dizziness, headaches, blurred vision, and opisthotonos have been reported. Because the suppositories contain benzocaine, they should not be administered to individuals known to be sensitive to local anesthetics.

Dose: Adults: (Oral) 250 mg three to four
times daily. (Rectal suppository) 200
mg three to four times daily. (IM)
200 mg three to four times daily.
(This form not recommended for use
in children.)
Children weighing more than 30 lb:
(Oral) 100 mg three to four times
daily.
Children: (Rectal suppository) 50 to
1200 mg three to four times daily.

Cyclizine Hydrochloride, USP, BP (Marezine). Cyclizine is available in oral form for the prevention of motion sickness and in rectal suppository and intramuscular forms for the treatment of nausea and vomiting from nonspecific causes as well as in the postsurgical patient. It is not recommended for pregnant women. Drowsiness is the only significant side effect noted. This agent is not recommended for children.

Dose: Adults: (Oral) 50 mg every 4 to 6 hours.
(IM) 50 mg every 4 to 6 hours as
necessary. (Rectal suppository) 100
mg every 4 to 6 hours.

Terfenadine (Seldane). The main advantage of terfenadine is that it does not cause the usual side effect of antihistamines (i.e., drowsiness). It is used for the relief of seasonal allergic symptoms. New reports of severe cardiovascular adverse effects have been received regarding this drug. Seizures and syncope have been reported with overdoses.

Terfenadine is contraindicated in patients taking ketoconazole, erythromycin, clarithromycin, or troleandomycin because these enable accumulation of high terfenadine levels, which leads to cardiac irregularities.

Dose: Adults: (Oral) 60 mg every 12 hours.
   Children older than 12 years: Same as adults.

Astemizole (Hismanal). This long-acting selective antihistamine is used for the relief of symptoms of seasonal rhinitis and chronic idiopathic urticaria. Its main advantage is that it does not cause the sedation usually associated with antihistamines. It can be given conveniently as a once-daily oral dose.

Like terfenadine, this drug will have serum accumulation of toxic levels of the drug if it is given with ketoconazole, erythromycin, clarithromycin, or troleandomycin. Cardiac irregularities occur with high serum levels.

Dose: Adults and children older than 12 years: 10 mg orally once daily.

Antihistamine Combinations. Antihistamine combinations vary greatly in composition. The proprietary "cold capsules" generally contain a small dose of antihistamine in combination with a decongestant and often aspirin or other salicylate compound. Examples are Allerest, Contac, Coricidin D, Dristan, Novahistine, Sinutab, and Vicks Tri-Span.

Other combinations are available on prescription only and generally have higher doses of the respective drugs, for example, Ornade and Tuss-Ornade.

Implications for the Student

1. Allergic conditions can best be treated by avoidance of the suspected allergen. Animals should be removed from the home, as should items that collect dust, such as curtains, carpets, and collectibles, particularly in the bedroom.

2. Feather pillows should be avoided and foam pillows used instead. All pillows and mattresses should be covered in vinyl material.

3. Become familiar with the Medic-Alert tags and remember to check them for potential allergies.

4. The symptoms of a mild allergic reaction include rhinitis, coryza, conjunctival injection, and skin rashes.

5. Anaphylaxis is an acute emergency and has as its onset respiratory distress with wheezing and bronchospasm, leading to edema of the face and extremities, hypotension, and even death.

6. The primary side effect of the antihistamines is drowsiness. The patient should be instructed not to work around machinery or to drive long distances after taking antihistamines.

7. The sleepiness produced by the antihistamines is an individual variation; certain people become rapidly resistant to the drowsiness induced by these agents and can take them routinely without drowsiness.

8. Bed rails and assistance with ambulation may be indicated when an individual, particularly an elderly person, has been administered an antihistamine.

9. The antihistamines potentiate the central depression of many other agents, such as alcohol, tranquilizers, sedatives, and hypnotics.

10. Antihistamines are useful in the prevention of motion sickness and should be given 30 minutes before entering the vehicle for optimum effect.

CASE STUDIES

1. Mr. H., a machinist, has been miserable since his daughter bought a cat. He has coryza, excessive sneezing, and rhinitis. Because his daughter insists on keeping the cat, Mr. H. wants to control his allergies with antihistamines. What health teaching is indicated here?

2. You have a part-time job in a drug store as a drug clerk. A pregnant woman comes in and asks your advice as to which over-the-counter antihistamine she can safely take for her spring allergies. How would you respond to this situation?

3. Mr. Z., a construction worker, stepped in a nest of fire ants and has a severe local reaction over both lower legs. It is 10 o'clock in the morning, and you detect a strong odor of alcohol on his breath. The physician decides to prescribe Benadryl 50 mg four times a day, and the man reports that he has to go back to work. What suggestions might be made?

Review Questions

1. What are the symptoms of an allergic reaction?

2. What are the symptoms of anaphylaxis?

3. Name some sources of allergies.

4. What information should be given to an individual who will be taking an antihistamine?

5. Define allergen.

6. What is the most dangerous side effect of antihistamines?

7. List other side effects of antihistamines.

8. List five examples of antihistamines.

9. Give examples of antihistamine combinations that do not require a prescription.

10. Give examples of antihistamine combinations that require a prescription.

11. Which two antihistamines do not cause drowsiness?

Drugs that Affect the Skin and Mucous Membranes

Objectives for the Student

BE

ABLE

TO
- 1. List functions of the skin.
- 2. Distinguish between emollient and demulcent and give an example of each.
- 3. State the purpose for which irritants are used and give an example of each type.
- 4. Describe the action of astringents.
- 5. Give examples of local anesthetics and the purpose for which each one is used.
- 6. Identify agents used to treat *Candida* infections.
- 7. Identify agents used to treat fungal infections.
- 8. Distinguish between a bacteriostatic and a bactericidal substance.
- 9. Identify local anti-infectives.

The skin is a complex structure that serves many functions. Chief among these are regulation of body temperature, maintenance of electrolyte and water balance, protection, excretion of waste substances, and some metabolic activity, such as formation of vitamin D, the "sunshine vitamin."

Drugs applied to the skin may likewise serve many functions and may be intended for either a local effect or a systemic effect following absorption through the skin. The drugs may be conveniently divided into the following classes:

Soothing Substances

These agents are applied to irritated and abraded areas to protect them and alleviate itching.

Emollients. These fatty or oily substances are applied to soothe the skin or mucous membranes. Irritants, air, and air-borne bacteria are excluded by an oily layer, and the skin is rendered softer and more pliable by penetration of the emollient into the surface layers. Emollient substances are used chiefly as vehicles for oil-soluble drugs and as protective agents. Some commonly used emollients are as follows:

Petrolatum
Rose water ointment (cold cream)
Hydrous wool fat (lanolin)

Demulcents. These protective agents are employed primarily to alleviate irritation, particularly of mucous membranes and abraded tissue. They are generally applied to the surface in viscid preparations that cover the area rapidly. Demulcents may be incorporated in lozenges to soothe oral and throat mucosa and are swallowed in liquid form as an antidote for corrosive poisons.

A variety of substances possess demulcent properties; some common demulcents are as follows:

Gums and mucilages (e.g., acacia and tragacanth)
Starch
Cream, milk
Egg white

Astringents

These agents precipitate protein but ordinarily do not penetrate beyond cell surfaces; thus, the cell remains viable. This action is accompanied by contraction and blanching of skin, and mucus and other secretions may be reduced so that the affected area becomes drier.

These agents are used to arrest minor hemorrhage, check perspiration, reduce inflammation, promote healing, and toughen skin. The principal astringents are as follows:

Salts of aluminum, zinc, and other heavy metals
Tannins (e.g., tannic acid in alcohol, witch hazel)
Alcohols, phenols

Irritants

These agents produce irritation; the degree of irritation is determined by the concentration and the duration of action.

Counterirritants. Agents used to irritate unbroken skin to relieve deep pain in muscles, joints, bursae, and other areas.

Rubefacients. These produce local vasodilation, redness, and a feeling of warmth.

Vesicants. Cause a strong irritation; blisters may be produced.

The following agents may be either counterirritants, rubefacients, or vesicants, depending upon the concentration used and the length of application:

Camphor, menthol, chloroform
Mustard
Oil of wintergreen

Keratolytics

These agents cause sloughing of hardened epithelium. They are used to cauterize ulcers and to destroy excess tissue such as calluses and warts. Common keratolytics are as follows:

Benzoic and salicylic acids
Resorcinol
Lactic acid

Local Anesthetics

These agents may be applied directly to the skin or injected. Many ointments contain local anesthetics and are applied topically for minor conditions, such as sunburn and insect bites, as well as for more serious dermatoses, burns, hemorrhoids, and other conditions. A few of the local anesthetics are as follows:

Cocaine, USP, BP. Used especially in ointments and nasal preparations. It is quite habit forming and comes under the restrictions of the Dangerous Drug laws.
Procaine, USP, BP (Novocain). Used in dentistry and before minor surgery. Because it is not effective topically, it must be injected.
Dibucaine, USP, BP (Nupercaine). Applied topically in ointments.

Benzocaine, USP, BP. Used in throat lozenges and topical preparations.

Medicone rectal ointment

Unguentine ointment

Surfacaine ointment

Antifungal Agents

Fungal infections of the skin are a common problem in both warm and temperate climates. They particularly affect areas of the skin that tend to remain warm and moist, such as the feet, underarms, breasts, and perineal area (*intertrigo*). Topical therapy is often sufficient in uncomplicated infections, but systemic therapy, such as oral griseofulvin, may be necessary to treat long-standing infections.

Haloprogin, USP, BP (Halotex). This synthetic antifungal agent is applied topically for the treatment of fungal infections of the skin. It is also used for tinea versicolor. Adverse effects may include burning and local irritation at the site of application.

Dose: 1% cream or solution.

Ketoconazole, USP, BP (Nizoral). This agent is used topically for the treatment of fungal and yeast infections. It is also effective for seborrheic dermatitis. Local application is generally well tolerated, but there may be some local irritation at the site of application.

Dose: 2% topical cream.

Ciclopirox, Olamine, USP, BP (Loprox). This agent may be applied topically for the treatment of various fungal and yeast infections. It has a low toxicity but may show some burning at the site of application.

Dose: 1% cream or lotion.

Tolnaftate, USP, BP (Tinactin). When applied twice daily to topical fungal infections, tolnaftate is quite effective against ringworm, athlete's foot, and similar conditions. To prevent recurrences, care must be taken to continue the use of this preparation for 2 weeks after all visible signs of the infection have cleared. Sensitivity reactions are rare.

Dose: 1% cream, solution, powder, or aerosol.

Triacetin, USP, BP (Enzactin). Particularly useful in the treatment of athlete's foot, this preparation has also been used for topical therapy of other superficial fungal infections. Occasional sensitivity reactions have been reported following prolonged use.

Dose: 25 to 33% in ointment, powder, solution, or aerosol.

Zinc Undecylenate Ointment, USP, BP (Desenex, Undesol, Undex). Zinc undecylenate was one of the first topical antifungal agents and continues to be a popular over-the-counter preparation for the treatment and prevention of athlete's foot. It has been surpassed in effectiveness by tolnaftate and other preparations, however.

Dose: 20% (often in combination with varying amounts of undecylenic acid).

Clotrimazole, USP, BP (Lotrimin). Clotrimazole has a broad spectrum of activity against fungi as well as yeasts. It is available in the form of a solution or cream for topical application.

Erythema, blistering, peeling, pruritus, and general skin irritation have been observed in sensitive persons; thus, the application should be discontinued if these symptoms occur.

Dose: 1% in solution or cream.

Clioquinol, USP, BP (Iodochlorhydroxyquin, Vioform). The antibacterial as well as antifungal properties of this agent make it extremely useful in nonspecific or mixed infections. It is also available in combination with hydrocortisone to suppress local inflammatory reactions.

Topical application is helpful in some cases of eczema, athlete's foot, or intertriginous rashes.

Dose: 3% iodochlorhydroxyquin. The combination forms contain 0.5 or 1% hydrocortisone.

Econazole Nitrate (Spectazole). A once-daily application of this topical antifungal agent will cure many topical tinea infections. Candida (monilial) infections will need twice-daily application.

Dose: 1% in ointment once or twice daily.

ACNE PREPARATIONS

Acne occurs in most adolescents and many adults and can cause both physical and emotional scars when severe. There are many new preparations to treat this troublesome disorder.

A variety of factors can aggravate acne. Young women should be counseled to avoid oily cosmetics and creams and opt for makeup that is hypoallergenic and water based. The hair should be clean and worn in a style off the face. The use of styling gels, creams, or sprays may clog pores.

Dietary theories regarding food's relationship to acne come and go. Seafood contributes iodine, an irritant, to the perspiration and may enhance folliculitis, according to some theories. There may also be an individual intolerance to chocolate or acid fruits when eaten in excessive amounts.

Cleansing Agents. It is recommended that the patient cleanse the face twice daily with a mild, nonirritating soap, such as Dove or Neutrogena, or a product containing triethanolamine. Astringent drying lotions (Stri-Dex Pads, Clearasil Medicated Astringent) help to accelerate the resolution of lesions.

Tretinoin (Retinoic Acid, Retin-A). This drug appears to act as a follicular irritant, preventing cells from sticking together. A mild inflammatory reaction is produced with peeling and extrusion of the comedo.

Topical tretinoin has been shown to enhance the repair of skin that has been damaged by ultraviolet radiation. It is used cosmetically for this effect to reduce the wrinkling of aging, sun-damaged skin.

Dose: (Topical) Applied once daily at bedtime in the form of a cream, gel, or solution. Strengths of 0.025 to 0.1% are prescribed.

Isotretinoin, USP, BP (Accutane). The principal effect of this drug appears to be the regulation of cell proliferation in addition to exhibiting anti-inflammatory and antineoplastic activities. It is used in nodular acne to reduce the size of sebaceous glands and inhibit sebum production. It inhibits the adhesion of epithelial cells and permits them to be sloughed more easily. Its side effects include conjunctivitis, thinning of the hair, photosensitivity, and hyperlipidemia.

Dose: Adults: (Oral) 0.5 to 1 mg/kg/day in two divided doses.
Children over 12: Same as adults.

Benzoyl Peroxide, USP, BP (Benzac, Benzagel, Desquam-X). Also a peeling agent, benzoyl peroxide is usually applied to the face in the morning after washing. Some irritation or inflammation is common; severe forms force discontinuing the product. It will take 6 to 8 weeks to determine whether treatment is effective.

Dose: Applied locally in strengths of 2.5, 5, and 10% in a variety of vehicles.

Erythromycin Topical Solution, USP, BP (T-Stat). This antibiotic solution should be applied twice daily for the local treatment of acne. Peeling will occur. Severe dryness and irritation will necessitate discontinuing the product.

Dose: 2% topical solution in applicator bottle.

Clindamycin Phosphate Solution, USP, BP (Cleocin-T). A topical antibiotic applied directly to acneiform lesions, clindamycin has been shown to be effective against *Propionibacterium acnes,* one of the agents contributing to acne. Some systemic absorption does occur, however, and the side effects of diarrhea and colitis will cause the product to be discontinued.

Dose: Solution form equivalent to 10 mg clindamycin per milliliter to be applied once daily.

Antimonilial Preparations

Like fungal infections, topical monilial or yeast infections due to *Candida albicans* tend to occur in warm, macerated areas. Monilial diaper rash is common in infants, particularly after antibiotic therapy, when the normal intestinal flora is disturbed. Monilial vaginitis and perineal and intertriginous infections tend to occur with increased frequency in diabetics and obese individuals.

Mycolog Cream and Ointment. This commercial preparation consists of a combination of nystatin, neomycin, gramicidin, and triamcinolone acetate. The topical antibiotics and corticosteroid included in this product have been demonstrated to be highly effective in all forms of topical *Candida* infections and aid in clearing secondary infections caused by local irritation and scratching of the areas. When applied two to three times daily, noticeable improvement is seen within 1 week in most cases. Topical sensitivity reactions have been noted but are rare.

Dose: 100,000 U nystatin ⎫
2.5 mg neomycin ⎪ per gram of
0.25 mg gramicidin ⎬ cream or
1 mg triamcinolone ⎪ ointment
acetate ⎭

Nystatin Vaginal Tablets, USP, BP (Mycostatin). Vulvovaginal *Candida* infections may be treated topically with the use of vaginal tablets. Very rarely irritation or sensitization to this agent may occur.

Dose: (Vaginal) 1 tablet containing 100,000 U daily for 2 weeks.

Miconazole Nitrate Vaginal Cream (Monistat). This water-miscible cream is indicated for vaginal use in the treatment of vulvovaginal *Candida* infections.

Very rarely, vaginal burning, pelvic cramps, hives, skin rash, and headache are observed.

Dose: (Vaginal) One applicator of the 2% cream once daily for 7 days.

Terconazole (Terazole). This agent is used for the treatment of vulvovaginal monilial infections.

Dose: (Vaginal) Cream 0.4% daily for 7 days.
(Vaginal) Suppository daily for 3 days.

Clotrimazole, USP, BP (Lotrimin, Gyne-Lotrimin). This is used intravaginally for monilial infections.

Dose: (Vaginal) 1% cream inserted daily for 7 days.
(Vaginal) 2 100-mg tablets daily for 3 days.

LOCAL ANTI-INFECTIVES

The development of the germ theory of disease directly heralded a dramatic revolution in medicine and was responsible for the development of entirely new aseptic procedures and antiseptic drugs.

Several classifications may be distinguished among the anti-infectives, however, and a single agent may fit into more than one category, depending on the strength used and the duration of application to the area.

Antiseptic: a substance that inhibits the growth of microorganisms.

Bacteriostatic or *antibacterial:* a substance that inhibits the growth of bacteria.

Bacteriocidal: a substance that kills bacteria.

Disinfectant or *germicide:* a substance that destroys microorganisms on objects. (Often these are too destructive to living tissue to use on the body.)

TOPICAL ANTIBIOTIC OINTMENTS

Mupirocin (Bactroban). This topical antibiotic ointment is used for the treatment of local infections, such as impetigo. Few adverse effects occur; burning or local irritation are indications for discontinuing the drug.

Dose: 2% ointment applied three times daily.

Over-the-Counter Antibiotic Ointments

These products are too numerous to list, but include polymyxin B sulfate, neomycin, lidocaine

(Neosporin); bacitracin; triple-antibiotic ointments; and many brand names of combinations. They all effectively kill or inhibit the organisms causing skin infections.

Examples of Other Anti-Infectives

Ethyl Alcohol, USP, BP (Alcohol). The alcohol most frequently used is ethyl alcohol; the optimum antiseptic activity is obtained from a 70% solution. Higher concentrations have a decreased antiseptic action. In addition to its antiseptic activity, alcohol has an astringent effect when applied topically and is frequently used in the treatment of decubitus ulcers; it is commonly utilized to cleanse the skin before giving hypodermic injections and while dressing wounds.

Isopropyl alcohol is approximately twice as germicidal as ethyl alcohol and is much less corrosive to instruments. Isopropyl alcohol is more toxic, however. It is used in full strength.

Benzalkonium Chloride, USP, BP (Zephiran Chloride). A rapid-acting, nonirritating antibacterial agent, this compound may be used safely on skin and mucous membranes in concentrations from 1:10,000 to 1:2000. One precaution to be observed with this agent, however, is that all soap or detergent must be completely removed before application of Zephiran, because it is inactivated by anionic agents.

Hexachlorophene, USP, BP (Incorporated in Gamophen and Dial Soaps, Septisol, and pHisoHex). Preparations containing this agent in 3% concentrations are used widely as antiseptic scrubs. When it is used regularly, a residual layer of the antiseptic forms on the skin and reduces the normal bacterial flora. Its activity is lessened by the presence of serum and organic materials.

Because hexachlorophene has been found to be systemically absorbed from skin surfaces, it is no longer recommended for the routine bathing of infants. It should be used in its more concentrated forms (e.g., pHisoHex) only on the advice of a physician.

Saponated Cresol Solution, USP, BP (Lysol, Creolin). Used in strengths of approximately 2%, this solution is used for disinfection of contaminated utensils such as bedpans, basins, and linens. The presence of organic material does not interfere with its action. In very weak dilutions it may be used for vaginal douches.

Gentian Violet, USP, BP. This antiseptic dye may be applied to surface areas for many infectious conditions. In strengths of 1:1000 to 1:100, it is used to combat impetigo, thrush, fungus infections, cystitis, urethritis, and similar conditions.

Iodine Tincture, USP, BP. One of the oldest and most effective of the germicides and fungicides, this tincture is used in 2% solution for application to wounds and abrasions. It is not safe for application to large wounds. The agent of choice for application to mucous membranes is a 2% solution of iodine in glycerin.

Povidone-Iodine Solution, USP, BP (Betadine). The iodine compound content of this preparation furnishes the germicidal activity of iodine without the locally irritating effect of the tincture. The iodine is released more slowly than from the tincture, but the prolongation of action compensates for this in large part. It is used in 1 to 1.5% solutions and has a variety of applications in aerosol, douche, vaginal gel, shampoo, and topical forms.

Mercury Bichloride. Although extremely poisonous if taken internally, the germicidal activity of this agent still renders it useful in some instances as a disinfectant of inanimate objects and unbroken skin. It is commonly prepared in the form of dispensing tablets that are angular in shape and marked with a skull and crossbones and the word "Poison." These are dissolved in water to prepare 1:1000 solutions.

Merbromin Solution (Mercurochrome). A mildly active antiseptic, this agent has a variety of uses as a skin antiseptic and as a treatment for urethritis and cystitis. It is used in 2% concentrations. The tincture shows more antiseptic activity than the solution, owing to the added presence of alcohol in the tincture.

Hydrogen Peroxide Solution, USP, BP. The antiseptic activity of this agent depends on the liberation of oxygen, which destroys many anaerobic bacteria and produces an effervescent action, which cleans wounds of dead tissue and pus. It deteriorates upon standing, however, and should be stored in a cool, dark place. The 3% solution is most frequently used.

Amphyl. An effective, nontoxic disinfectant, this preparation may be used in specific dilutions for various purposes, such as body cavity irrigations, cleansing of wounds, antiseptic rinsing of hands, and general disinfection of inanimate objects. It is used in concentrations of 0.25 to 2%.

Staphene. This general-purpose disinfectant has a wide range of activity against many types of microorganisms. Although it is relatively noninjurious to the skin, prolonged skin contact should be avoided. As a general disinfectant it is used in strengths of 0.5 to 2.5%. It may be used in the foot bath in a 2.5% solution as an aid in controlling athlete's foot.

Potassium Permanganate, USP, BP. The anti-infective activity of this agent depends on its strong oxidizing property. As an antiseptic agent it is utilized in 1% solutions, but in 1:5000 solutions it may be used for vaginal and urethral irrigations as well as for topical application in a variety of conditions. After ingestion of barbiturates, chloral hydrate, or alkaloids, a gastric lavage with potassium permanganate helps to destroy the poison. The crystals may be applied locally to a widely opened snake bite to aid in the destruction of the venom.

SUN DAMAGE TO SKIN

In the past two decades or so, knowledge of sun-induced skin disorders has expanded tremendously. The radiant energy from the sun produces a thermal burn, giving light-skinned persons a coveted tan for the temporary reaction; but over the years sun damage produces premature aging and leathery skin and greatly increased chances of skin cancer.

It is now believed that one significant sunburn in early life will measurably increase the risk of skin cancer later. Sun exposure effects are cumulative; thus, even belated awareness to sun protection will help.

Many commercial sunscreen products are available, labeled with a sun protection factor (SPF) number. The higher the number, the more sun protection there is. To have significant protection, the SPF number should be 15 or higher.

Unfortunately, many individuals became sensitized or allergic to many components of sunscreen. There are para-aminobenzoic acid (PABA)–sensitive individuals and those who are allergic to the replacements for PABA.

Many drugs, chemicals, and foods also act as photosensitizers; it is not possible to give a complete list, but they include the following:

Cosmetics (lipsticks, many perfumes)
Pigments and dyes in clothes and tattoos
Plants (buttercup, carrots, celery, dill, fennel, figs, limes, mustard, parsley, parsnip)
Some soap deodorants containing hexachlorophene, bithionol
Drugs:

Acetazolamide	Ibuprofen
Acetohexamide	Imipramine
Amantadine	Indomethacin
Amiloride	Ketoconazole
Amitriptyline	Methyldopa
Astemazole	Nalidixic acid
Azathioprine	Naproxen
Barbiturates	Nifedipine
Captopril	Nitrofurantoin
Carbamazepine	Nonsteroidal anti-
Chlordiazepoxide	inflammatory
Chloroquine	drugs
Chlorothiazide	Nortriptyline
Chlorpromazine	Ofloxacin
Chlorthalidone	PABA
Cephalosporin	Phenothiazine
Contraceptives, oral	Phenylbutazone
Coumarin	Promazine
Desipramine	Promethazine
Diflunisal	Quinidine
Diltiazem	Retinoic acid
Diphenhydramine	Sulfa drugs
Doxycycline	Tetracycline
Fluorescein	Tolazamide
Fluorouracil	Tolbutamide
Furosemide	Trazodone
Glyburide	Triamterene
Griseofulvin	Trimethoprim
Haloperidol	Vinblastine
Hydrochlorothiazide	Warfarin

Implications for the Student

1. For the desired effect when topical application of medications is ordered, the skin should be cleansed before application.

2. The site of application should be observed for edema and inflammation. The physician should be informed if the patient complains of discomfort during or after the application of topical medications.

3. Signs of healing in skin lesions are the development of a healthy, pink color and granulation tissue.

4. Orders should be followed carefully as to the application of dressings after administration of topical medications. In some cases untoward effects can be obtained by bandaging the area after application.

5. To prevent cross-contamination, no topical medications should be used on more than one patient.

6. Aerosol containers should be stored in a cool, dry place. The aerosol container should be at least 6 inches from the skin at the time of application. Care should be taken that the aerosol does not spray into the eyes.

7. If improper hygiene contributed to the formation of skin lesions, the patient should be carefully instructed in proper hygiene.

8. It is often advisable to put on gloves before application of topical medications to infected areas.

9. The nurse should be aware of the psychological effects of severe and disfiguring skin disorders. Counseling may be advisable in some patients.

10. Many skin disorders are worsened by self-treatment by the patient. If improper application of proprietary medications has occurred, the patient should be counseled against self-treatment.

11. This student should become familiar with means to improve acne by proper use of cosmetics and hygienic aids.

12. Topical acne agents have severe side effects in some cases. The student should take time to read the product literature on all preparations.

CASE STUDIES

1. J.S. came home from college with a severe case of athlete's foot. She has not seen a doctor because of her heavy class schedule. She stated that she did not have time to go to the health nurse. What advice would you give her?

2. An 80-year-old woman complains of dry, itchy skin. She states that she is a very clean person because she takes a bath daily and always uses plenty of soap. What health teaching is indicated?

3. Your roommate returned from the dentist after a tooth extraction. She stated that the dentist gave her a "lot of Novocain." Later

in the day her face was markedly swollen. She had difficulty talking and appeared very nervous.

On the basis of your knowledge of pharmacology, what do you think might have been the cause of the problem?

Review Questions

1. Define bacteriostatic.

2. Define bactericidal.

3. Distinguish between an antiseptic and a disinfectant.

4. Special assignment: Prepare a list of the agents discussed in this chapter that are used in the hospital where you are assigned for clinical experience.
   A. Observe the labels for instructions for use and precautions.
   B. Be prepared to discuss the agent used to:
      1. disinfect thermometers, when individual thermometers are not supplied.
      2. clean the floors.

5. Define and give an example of each of the following:
   emollient   antifungal agent
   demulcent   antimonilial preparation
   vesicant   astringent
   local anesthetic agent

6. What drug is used systemically to treat a long-standing fungal infection?

7. What is a common factor in the development of monilial infections?

8. What determines the degree of irritation produced by irritants?

9. How do astringents achieve their effects?

10. Discuss the purposes of astringents.

11. What is acne? What are its causes?

12. What proprietary or over-the-counter products are available for the treatment of acne?

Drugs that Affect the Respiratory System

Objectives for the Student

B E

A B L E

T O

- 1. Discuss the action of respiratory stimulants and give three examples.
- 2. Identify important drug groups that produce respiratory depression.
- 3. Define expectorant and give three examples.
- 4. Discuss the action of bronchodilators and give three examples.
- 5. Identify side effects produced by bronchodilators.
- 6. Discuss nursing measures related to assisting patients with respiratory tract disorders.

The respiratory system in humans includes the nasal cavity, larynx, pharynx, trachea, bronchi, lungs, muscles of the larynx, intercostal muscles and diaphragm, and the respiratory center in the medulla.

The chief functions of respiration are to supply oxygen to the tissues and remove carbon dioxide as well as to aid in the evaporation of water from the respiratory passages, a function that helps to regulate body temperature.

Figure 20–1 shows a cross-section of the upper respiratory organs. Figure 20–2 illustrates a cross-section of the lungs, showing the bronchial tree. Figure 20–3 shows a cross-section of the terminal respiratory unit.

Drugs that act on the respiratory system may be classified as those that

a. Act on the respiratory center in the brain.

b. Affect the mucous membrane lining of the respiratory tract.

c. Affect the size of the bronchioles.

DRUGS THAT ACT ON THE RESPIRATORY CENTER IN THE BRAIN

Respiratory Stimulants

Carbon Dioxide, USP, BP. This gas is used as a respiratory stimulant in the treatment of

121

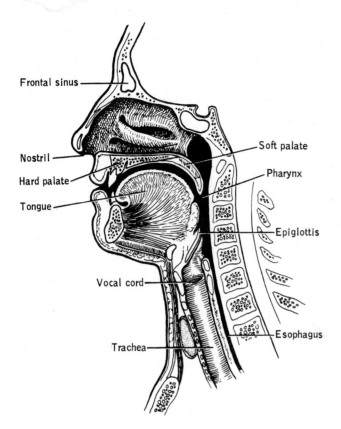

Figure 20–1. The upper respiratory organs.

asphyxia of all types. It is the natural respiratory stimulant because it is actually the increase in carbon dioxide in the blood that influences the respiratory center in the brain to cause the individual to take a breath. The lack of oxygen in the tissues does *not* stimulate respiration. During strenuous exercise more carbon dioxide is produced, the respiratory center is stimulated, and breathing becomes deeper and more frequent.

Caffeine, USP, BP. An alkaloid found in coffee and tea, caffeine is the cause of the so-called "coffee nerves" produced by excessive central nervous system stimulation. Coffee nerves are characterized by irritability, restlessness, and insomnia; however, the response of individuals to this stimulation varies greatly. In large doses caffeine increases respiration by stimulating the respiratory center. Caffeine is contraindi-

cated for patients with peptic ulcers because it stimulates the flow of pepsin and hydrochloric acid in the stomach.

Commercial preparation: Caffeine and sodium benzoate ampules.

Dose: Adults only: (IM, IV) 0.5 gm as necessary. This product has some usefulness in the treatment of respiratory depression induced by alcohol or depressant drugs.

Doxapram Hydrochloride, USP, BP (Dopram). This central nervous system stimulant is used to treat the respiratory depression of chronic obstructive pulmonary disease and, less frequently, neonatal hypoxia. There is a very narrow margin of safety with this drug, and even small overdoses can lead to convulsions. It may also be used to hasten arousal after overdoses of depressant drugs.

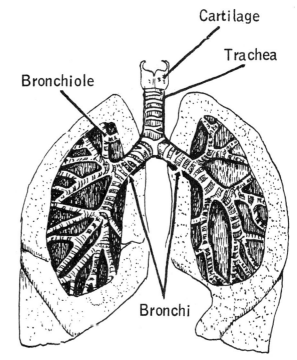

Figure 20–2. The lungs.

SECTION OF LUNGS

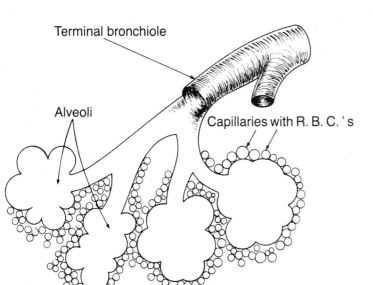

Figure 20–3. The terminal respiratory unit.

Dose: Adults: (IV) 1 to 2 mg/kg in two initial doses at 5-minute intervals. The dose may be repeated after 1 to 2 hours according to patient response.
Children: Same as that for adults.

Respiratory Depressants

The most important of these agents are the central depressants of the opium group (e.g., morphine, codeine) and the barbiturate group (e.g., phenobarbital, secobarbital). Respiratory depression, however, is an undesirable side effect of these drugs. They are not given therapeutically to produce respiratory depression.

DRUGS THAT AFFECT THE MUCOUS MEMBRANE LINING OF THE RESPIRATORY TRACT

Agents in this group are used chiefly to relieve coughing. A cough is a reflex action produced by irritation in the upper portion of the respiratory tract. This can be a foreign body (e.g., a particle of food accidentally inhaled), excessive mucus, a malignant growth, and so forth. Treatment of the cough is, of course, only secondary to the treatment of the underlying cause of the cough.

Expectorants are drugs that liquefy the mucus in the bronchi and facilitate the expulsion of sputum. They are used for coughs resulting from the common cold, bronchitis, and pneumonia.

Many of the remedies used to treat colds contain codeine or codeine and morphine derivatives to depress the cough reflex. These agents are not given to patients with tuberculosis, however, because coughing is desired to expel the sputum.

Benylin Expectorant
Robitussin Cough Syrup
Cheracol Cough Syrup
Conar Expectorant
Vicks Formula 44

Potassium Iodide Solution, USP (SSKI).
Small amounts of this solution are given orally to irritate the stomach to aid in the expulsion of mucus.

Dose: (Oral) 20 drops in water three or four times daily.

ASTHMA

Asthma, for reasons not perfectly understood, appears to be a disease on the rise. The prevalence of asthma increased 29% from 1980 to 1987. The death rate from asthma increased 31% and health care costs for the disease increased as well. Treatment is best aimed at prevention of the attacks as well as care of the episode. To this end, then,

■ Educate the patients and family members.
■ Control the patient's environment to control triggers.
■ Institute drug therapy to prevent and treat episodes.

Allergies have a significant role in the development of asthma. It has been shown that 75 to 85% of asthmatics have positive immediate skin test reactions to common inhalant allergens. Continuous exposure to these allergens will worsen the asthma, causing more symptoms, increasing the medication requirement, and diminishing the quality of life.

Environmental Control

■ Smoke from personal smoking and second-hand smoke should be eliminated. In addition, smoke from wood-burning stoves is a trigger.
■ Pet dander is a common allergen. Animals should not be in the home of an asthma patient.
■ Dust: The dust harbors the dust mite, which is the culprit.
■ Cockroaches should be controlled as much as possible.
■ Air filtration and air conditioning should be used.
■ Seasonal factors should be evaluated, including grass, ragweed, and other plants.
■ Occupational concerns: Farmers are around

molds and mites in hay and fungal agents in silage. Asbestos, dust, chemical allergens are implicated. Latex allergies are developing in health care workers and in patients.

DRUGS THAT AFFECT THE SIZE OF THE BRONCHIOLES

Epinephrine Injection, USP, BP (Adrenalin). The rapid action of this drug makes it best for an acute attack. It has a short duration of action, however, so it is not suitable for long-term therapy. It must be given by injection.

A rapid heart rate and an acute rise in blood pressure may be observed after administration; thus, caution must be used when administering this agent.

Dose: Adults: (SC, IV) 0.3 mg, often repeated three times at 20-minute intervals.
Children: (SC) 0.01 mg/kg as above.

Sus-Phrine. This aqueous suspension of epinephrine is administered subcutaneously for prolonged release of epinephrine. After an acute attack of asthma has been brought under control with aqueous epinephrine, it is often administered to prevent rebound of the bronchiolar constriction.

Dose: Adults: (SC) 0.1 to 0.3 mL
Children: (SC) 0.005 mL/kg

Ephedrine Sulfate, USP, BP. Although not as potent as epinephrine, this agent has the added advantages of being active when taken orally and having a longer duration of action. Nervousness and central stimulation may occur.

Dose: Adults: (Oral) 25 mg three to four times daily.
Children: (Oral) 15 mg three to four times daily.

Isoproterenol Hydrochloride, USP, BP (Isuprel). This agent is similar in its effects to epinephrine and can be administered orally, by injection, or as an aerosol for inhalation. It is used for asthma and also as a cardiac stimulant.

Side effects are similar to those of epinephrine, with some patients experiencing anginal pain, nervousness, heart palpitations, and excitability.

Dose: Adults: (Oral) 5 mg in elixir form three to four times daily. (Sublingual) 10 mg as glosset four times daily. This drug is used primarily as a cardiac stimulant at a dose of 0.01 to 0.02 mg of a diluted solution. (Inhalation) 5 to 15 inhalations of the 1:200 solution at 3- to 4-hour intervals.
Children: (Oral) 1 to 2.5 mg in elixir form three to four times daily. (Sublingual) 5 to 10 mg as glosset three times daily. (Inhalation) Up to 0.25 ml of the 1:200 solution for treatment three to four times daily.

Terbutaline Sulfate, USP, BP (Brethine). Terbutaline has a dilating effect on the smooth muscles of the bronchioles and may be administered for the treatment of acute asthma attacks or chronic obstructive pulmonary disease.

Side effects are similar to those of epinephrine and isoproterenol.

Dose: Adults: (SC) 0.25 mg with a second dose in 15 to 30 minutes. Other agents should be used if two doses are not effective.
Children: (SC) 0.01 to 0.04 mg/kg in two doses over 15 to 30 minutes.

Theophylline Ethylenediamine, USP, BP (Aminophylline). A very effective bronchodilator, theophylline may be used to treat asthma attacks and aid in the prevention of further attacks by daily oral administration.

The primary side effect is central nervous system stimulation, which may be shown by nervousness, excitation, or tachycardia. Some gastric distress may be produced by oral administration.

Dose: Adults: (Oral) 300 to 600 mg two to three times daily. (IV) 500 mg over a

20-minute period. (Rectal) 0.25 to 0.5 gm two to three times daily.

Children: (Oral, IV) Initial dose: 5 to 7.5 mg/kg. Subsequent administration: 20 to 24 mg/kg/day in divided doses.

Because of alterations in absorption and elimination of this agent, the dose is often periodically adjusted according to the blood level of theophylline. A therapeutic level is 10 to 20 μg/mL.

Various forms of pure theophylline are available commercially. In all cases the dose is as outlined previously. Most of these preparations are designed to provide prolonged theophylline levels in the blood.

Theo-Dur
Theo-Dur Sprinkle
Slo-Phyllin
Slo-Bid
Theo-24
Theovent
Uniphyl
Elixophyllin

See Table 20–1 for combination forms of theophylline.

Albuterol Sulfate, USP, BP (Proventil). Albuterol is indicated for the relief of bronchospasm in adults and children older than 2 years with reversible airway obstructive disease. It should be used with caution in patients with coronary disease, because it may have a cardiovascular stimulatory effect.

Dose: Adults: (Oral) 2 to 4 mg four times daily.
Children: (Oral) 0.1 mg/kg, increased to 0.2 mg/kg three times daily.

Metaproterenol Sulfate, USP, BP (Alupent). This agent is a potent beta-adrenergic stimulator and rapidly acts to reverse bronchospasm. It is contraindicated in patients with cardiac arrhythmias.

Dose: Adults: (Oral) 20 mg three to four times daily.
Children: (Oral) 10 mg three times daily.

Terbutaline Sulfate, USP, BP (Brethine). Terbutaline stimulates the beta-adrenergic receptors of the sympathetic nervous system and thus relaxes the bronchioles and the peripheral vasculature. Adverse effects include an increased heart rate, dizziness, and tremor.

Dose: Adults: (Oral) 2.5 to 5 mg three times daily.
Children older than 12 years: (Oral) 2.5 mg three times daily.

ADMINISTRATION OF DRUGS BY INHALATION

Various drugs may be administered by inhalation directly to the respiratory tract to exert local bronchodilator effects. These agents may be used in the treatment of asthma or chronic obstructive pulmonary diseases such as emphysema.

A hand nebulizer may be used for self-administration of these agents, or, if greater depth within the respiratory tract is desired, the drugs may be administered under pressure by means of an intermittent positive-pressure breathing machine. Respiratory therapists generally monitor the use of these machines. The settings may be varied to obtain the desired pressure (usually 15 to 20 cm of water). The patient should breathe slowly and must be observed for side effects of the drugs, such as nausea, vomiting, dizziness, and tachycardia.

Agents administered by inhalation include the following:

Metaproterenol Sulfate Inhaler, USP, BP (Alupent). When inhaled, this agent produces a direct bronchodilator effect. It is used in the treatment of asthma and emphysema.

Dose: Adults only: (Inhalation) Two to three inhalations every 3 to 4 hours. Total daily dose should not exceed 12 inhalations.

Table 20-1. COMBINATION FORMS OF THEOPHYLLINE

Trade Name		Ingredients		Dose
Bronkolixir	Each 5 cc contains:	Ephedrine sulfate Guaifenesin Theophylline Phenobarbital	12 mg 50 mg 15 mg 4 mg	Adults: (oral) 2 teaspoonfuls 4 times daily Children over 6 years: (oral) 1 teaspoonful 4 times daily
Bronkotabs	Each tablet contains:	Ephedrine sulfate Guaifenesin Theophylline Phenobarbital	24 mg 100 mg 100 mg 8 mg	Adults: (Oral) 1 tablet 3–4 times daily Children over 6 years: (Oral) ½ tablet 3–4 times daily

Marax syrup	Each 5 cc contains:	Ephedrine sulfate
		Theophylline
		Hydroxyzine HCl
			6.25 mg
			32.5 mg
			2.5 mg
				Children over 5 years: (Oral)
				  1 teaspoonful 4 times daily
				Under 5 years: (Oral) ½ teaspoonful
				  4 times daily

Marax tablets	Each tablet contains:	Ephedrine sulfate Theophylline Hydroxyzine HCl	25 mg 130 mg 10 mg	Adults: (Oral) 1 tablet 2–4 times daily

Tedral
  suspension
	Each 5 cc contains:	Theophylline
		Ephedrine HCl
		Phenobarbital
			65 mg
			12 mg
			4 mg
				Adults: (Oral) 2–4 teaspoonfuls q4h
				Children: (Oral) 1 teaspoonful per 60 lb
				  body weight q4–6h

Tedral elixir	Each 5 cc contains:	Theophylline Ephedrine Phenobarbital	32.5 mg 6 mg 2 mg	Children: (Oral) 1 teaspoonful per 30 lb body weight q4–6h
Tedral tablets	Each tablet contains:	Theophylline Ephedrine HCl Phenobarbital	130 mg 24 mg 8 mg	Adults: (Oral) 1 tablet 4 times daily

Albuterol, USP, BP (Proventil, Ventolin). Each activation of the inhaler releases 90 μg albuterol. The onset of action occurs within 15 minutes by aerosol compared with 30 minutes by the oral route. Duration of action is 3 to 4 hours.

Dose: Adults: (Inhalation) Two inhalations every 4 to 6 hours.
    Children older than 12 years: Same as that for adults.

Terbutaline Sulfate (Brethaire). Each activation of the inhaler releases 0.2 mg terbutaline sulfate. The onset of action is within 5 to 30 minutes and has a duration of 3 to 6 hours.

Dose: Adults: (Inhalation) Two inhalations 60 seconds apart every 4 to 6 hours.
    Children older than 12 years: Same as that for adults.

Bitolterol Mesylate (Tornalate). Each activation releases 0.37 mg bitolterol. The onset of action is within 3 to 4 minutes and will last 5 to 6 hours.

Dose: Adults: (Inhalation) Two inhalations 1 to 3 minutes apart every 8 hours.
    Children older than 12 years: Same as that for adults.

Beclomethasone Dipropionate, USP, BP (Beclovent Oral Inhaler). This corticosteroid preparation does not directly relax the bronchioles but acts as an anti-inflammatory steroid to aid in the treatment of asthma. It is not used in the primary treatment of asthma because, like all the steroids, it exerts its effect slowly and is generally more useful for its sustained effect.

Dose: Adults: (Inhalation) Two inhalations three to four times daily. Maximum daily intake should not exceed 20 inhalations.
    Children older than 6 years: (Inhalation) One to two inhalations three to four times daily.

Flunisolide Nasal Solution, USP, BP (Nasalide). Intended for use as a spray to the nasal mucosa, this anti-inflammatory corticosteroid reduces the symptoms of rhinitis and swollen nasal mucous membranes resulting from allergic rhinitis. Although relief is generally apparent after a few days of therapy, it may take as long as 2 weeks before a full therapeutic effect is obtained.

Dose: Adults: (Nasal) Two sprays in each nostril two times daily.
Children older than 6 years: (Nasal) One spray in each nostril three times daily.

Acetylcysteine, USP, BP (Mucomyst). A derivative of the amino acid cysteine, this agent is effective by inhalation when the liquefaction of mucous and purulent material is desired. It loosens pulmonary secretions and aids in their removal by postural drainage.

Dose: Adults: (Inhalation) 3 to 5 mL of a 10 to 20% solution three to four times daily.
Children: Same as that for adults.

Tergemist. This combination product contains 0.125% 2-ethylhexyl sulfate sodium (a detergent-like substance) and 0.1% potassium iodide. It decreases the viscosity of pulmonary secretions and can be used in many acute and chronic pulmonary conditions.

Dose: Adults: (Inhalation) 3 to 5 mL four times daily for periods of up to 30 minutes per treatment.
Children: Same as that for adults.

Alevaire. Alevaire is a commercial preparation containing 0.125% tyloxapol (a detergent) and 2% sodium bicarbonate with 5% glycerin in a preparation for administration by inhalation.

Dose: Adults: (Inhalation) This may be used for continuous aerosol therapy in amounts not to exceed 500 mL every 12 to 24 hours.
Children: Same as that for adults.

Cromolyn Sodium, USP, BP (Aarane, Intal). Although ineffective in the treatment of acute asthma, this drug is useful in the prevention of asthma attacks. It is believed to stabilize the membranes of the mast cells, which are responsible for liberating histamine and initiating the allergic reaction.

Dose: Adults: (Inhalation) 20 mg four times daily.
Children: Same as that for adults.

CORTICOSTEROIDS

Although covered more completely in the chapter on endocrine drugs, the corticosteroids are often used for their effect on the respiratory tract, particularly in severe asthma attacks.

In an acute asthma attack, often aminophylline is given after epinephrine and similar drugs are used. Corticosteroids are administered intravenously to aid in the management of the acute attack, but it must be realized that their effect is not exerted immediately. The anti-inflammatory effect to aid in bronchodilation generally takes 6 hours. For initial therapy an intravenous form of hydrocortisone is usually used (e.g., Solu-Cortef). For prolonged effect against recurrence of wheezing, an oral synthetic form of the corticosteroids is used (e.g., prednisone). Systemic effects are not noted after the administration of corticosteroids for asthma unless the drug is given for longer than 2 weeks. Prolonged administration of therapeutic corticosteroids will have an inhibitory effect on the body's own natural hydrocortisone and must be adjusted for if necessary.

Implications for the Student

1. An adequate fluid intake is necessary during the treatment of respiratory infections or wheezing to liquefy mucus and aid in its expulsion.

2. Coughing is beneficial in some cases to clear secretions from the respiratory tract. Antitussives are often prescribed if the coughing is excessive or nonproductive.

3. Because coughing is often increased when the patient is lying flat, greater comfort is attained if the patient is placed in a sitting position.

4. Cough preparations, particularly those with codeine or similar drugs, cause drowsiness. The patient should be cautioned against combining cough preparations with self-prescribed antihistamines, because increased central nervous system sedation may result.

5. In patients with severe, chronic respiratory conditions, such as emphysema or late forms of cystic fibrosis, respiration is stimulated by low blood oxygen levels. High levels of oxygen administered suddenly to these patients may result in respiratory arrest and death.

6. Arterial blood gases are useful in monitoring the severity of an acute asthma attack and are often used as a guideline in adjusting the oxygen and the drug dose necessary for the treatment of asthma.

7. Cyanosis, particularly on the lips and perioral area, is a sign of decreased blood oxygen level. A decrease in cyanosis and less respiratory distress can be used to quickly assess improvement in the patient's condition.

8. Theophylline has as its major side effect central nervous system stimulation and tachycardia. The patient should be monitored for these effects during administration of these medications.

9. Blood levels of theophylline are generally used to monitor dosage levels because individual absorption of this agent will vary.

10. Nursing measures should be directed toward relief of anxiety in patients with respiratory conditions.

CASE STUDIES

1. Jimmy P., 6 years old, is brought to the physician's office after his mother noticed he had some wheezing after a strenuous soccer game in the backyard. He has had wheezing a few times before after playing outside but has never been brought to his doctor for this. What drugs do you think may be prescribed?

2. Jennifer L., 21, had one of her infrequent asthmatic spells last night, but in the office today she has only scattered and mild wheezing. She reports that she cannot take theophylline because it always gives her palpitations. What other medications could be used for her asthma? Would any other procedures be of benefit here?

Review Questions

1. What structure is common to both the respiratory and digestive systems?
2. Why would morphine or codeine not be given to a person with a head injury?
3. Discuss the disadvantages of over-the-counter preparations for colds and coughs.
4. What special precaution must be taken when administering Adrenalin?
5. Name drugs used to treat an acute asthmatic attack.
6. What drugs are given intravenously to treat status asthmaticus?
7. What teaching is indicated for patients with respiratory tract obstruction?
8. Discuss nursing observations important to effective care of the patient with a respiratory tract problem.
9. What nursing measures are indicated in caring for these patients?

Drugs that Affect the Circulatory System

Objectives for the Student

B E

A B L E

T O

1. Discuss the ways drugs may affect the heart.
2. Identify digitalis preparations.
3. State the action of digitalis.
4. List side effects of digitalis toxicity.
5. Explain the action of antiarrhythmic agents.
6. Explain the action of vasoconstrictors.
7. Explain the action of vasodilators.
8. Identify drugs used to hasten the process of coagulation.
9. Discuss the uses of anticoagulants.
10. Identify the specific antidote for an overdose of sodium heparin.
11. Identify the specific antidote for an overdose of sodium warfarin.
12. Discuss nursing responsibilities related to care of patients taking cardiovascular drugs.
13. Identify the classes of antihypertensive drugs and the general mechanism of action.
14. Become familiar with side effects of antihypertensive drugs.
15. Understand the role of platelets in cardiovascular complications.
16. Identify drugs used in antiplatelet therapy.
17. Identify drugs used as thrombolytic agents.
18. Identify drugs used in antilipemic therapy.

The circulatory system includes the heart and all the blood vessels. Figure 21–1 is a diagrammatic sketch of the system.

The heart is a hollow, muscular organ that is roughly cone shaped; it is situated near the center of the thoracic cavity in close relation to the lungs. It is divided by partitions (septa) into four chambers: the right and left atria and the right and left ventricles. The left ventricular wall has a thickness that is about twice that of the right ventricle because the work it must perform is much greater than that performed by the right ventricle.

In normal circulation of blood throughout the body, the oxygenated blood comes into the left atrium from the lungs and passes into the left ventricle upon contraction of the atrium. The ventricle contracts shortly after the atrium and the blood is forced into the aorta, which branches into other major arteries. The blood is

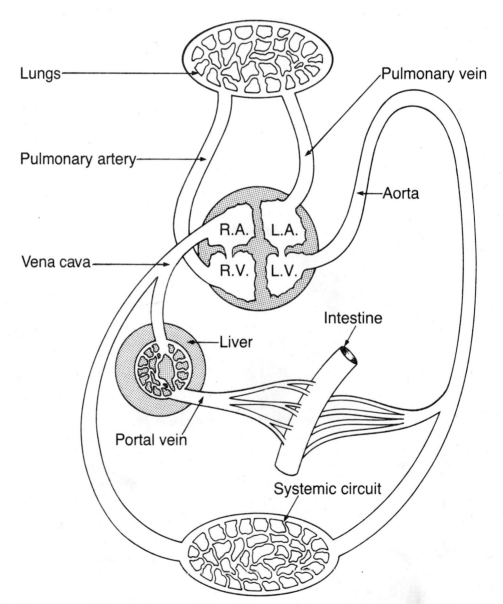

Figure 21–1. The circulatory system. (R.A. = right atrium; L.A. = left atrium; R.V. = right ventricle; L.V. = left ventricle.)

then carried to the gastrointestinal tract, liver, and the capillary beds in the systemic circuit. In this capillary region the objectives of circulation are fulfilled: Oxygen and nutritive materials are carried to the tissues, and carbon dioxide and waste products are carried away.

The venous capillaries merge to form larger veins; the blood returns to the heart via the vena cava and enters the right atrium. Contraction of the atrium forces blood into the right ventricle; the ventricle's subsequent contraction forces the blood to the lungs, where it is oxygenated and then returned again to the left atrium to begin the cycle anew.

Cardiac drugs may affect (1) the rate of the heart; (2) the rhythm of the heartbeat; (3) the amount of output of blood; or (4) the strength of contraction. In general, there are two main conditions for which the cardiac drugs are used: heart failure and arrhythmias.

HEART FAILURE

Heart "failure" means that the heart, for one reason or another, is not circulating blood at a satisfactory rate. When a person is in good health, the heart accomplishes the circulation of blood without faltering. Thus, it does not allow an abnormal amount of blood to accumulate in the veins of the body, in the chambers of the heart, or in the lungs. The rate of flow is sufficient to provide a normal pressure in the systemic arteries and the veins in the vascular bed of the lungs.

A diseased heart may have such a handicap that it is unable to move the blood satisfactorily. If this defect is moderate, it may occur only during physical exertion (e.g., running or climbing stairs). Under these circumstances the muscles of the legs need a faster moving bloodstream because of their greater workload.

If, by reason of a mechanical handicap (such as leaking or constricted valves), the heart cannot increase its output to meet the demands of the muscles, the body will suffer from the inadequacy. The same is true when the heart is weak because of a diseased condition of its fibers.

The following changes may take place during the period of heart failure:

The capillaries and all veins contain more than the normal amount of blood.

The hydrostatic pressure is greater than normal in these areas, forcing fluid into the lungs and body tissues.

The blood in these areas has a greater amount of carbon dioxide and waste products of the muscles.

The blood has less oxygen combined with hemoglobin.

Respiration in the lungs may be so reduced that the blood pumped into the aorta may contain carbon dioxide and less oxygen than it should.

Cyanosis.

Edema.

Drugs used in the treatment of heart failure are known as ionotropic drugs. They increase the contractility of the myocardium.

Digitoxin, USP, BP (Purodigin, Crystodigin)

Dose: Adults: (Oral) 0.1 to 0.3 mg daily (maintenance dose).
Children: Not generally used.

Digoxin, USP, BP (Lanoxin). The most important action of digitalis on the heart is the strengthening of the heart musculature. The digitalized fibers contract more vigorously and enable the heart to empty more completely. The result is an increase in the amount of blood propelled with any contraction of the ventricles.

Another manner in which heart action is improved by digitalization is the slowing of the rate of contraction. The dosage should be adjusted to bring the pulse rate down to the normal range of 60 to 80 beats per minute. Excessive doses of digitalis depress the heart rate still further; therefore, the pulse must always be taken before administering a dose. If the pulse is below 60 the medication should not be given.

Side effects that warn of early overdosage are nausea, vomiting, and visual disturbances (objects appear brighter than they actually are; green objects may appear almost white). At this point the digitalis dose is usually decreased or even discontinued for a few days. A lethal dose of digitalis causes death by stopping the heart.

Dose: Adults: (Oral, IM, or IV) Digitalizing dose: 8 to 15 µg/kg/day. Maintenance, 0.25 to 0.5 mg/day.

Children: (Oral, IM, or IV) Digitalizing dose: 10 to 15 µg/kg/day. Maintenance, 20 to 30% of the digitalizing dose.

Dopamine Hydrochloride, USP, BP (Dopastat). Dopamine exerts an ionotropic effect on the myocardium of the heart. This is accompanied by an increased renal blood flow and sodium excretion. Adverse effects include anginal pain, ectopic heartbeats, headache, and hypotension.

Dose: Adults only: (IV) A 200-mg ampule is diluted in 250 to 500 cc of IV diluent. The flowmeter is individually titrated to obtain the desired effect.

Dobutamine Hydrochloride, USP, BP (Dobutrex). Dobutamine is a direct-acting ionotropic agent that stimulates the beta receptors of the heart. It also produces a mild antiarrhythmic and vasodilative effect. It is indicated in the short-term treatment of cardiac decompensation.

Dose: Adults only: (IV) 250 mg of dobutamine is diluted in IV solution for drug delivery at rates of 2.5 to 15 mg/kg/min.

Isoproterenol Hydrochloride, USP, BP (Isuprel). Isoproterenol increases the strength of cardiac contraction and, to a limited extent, the rate of contraction. Systolic blood pressure may increase, and diastolic pressure may decrease. Isoproterenol is also useful to treat mild or transient episodes of heart block.

Dose: Adults: (IV) Infusion at a rate of 5 µg/min.

Children: (IV) Infusion at a rate of 0.1 µg/kg/min.

ARRHYTHMIAS

The rate of heartbeat and rhythm of the heart are controlled by the "pacemaker," known as the sinoatrial (SA) node, in the right atrium. This node generates tiny electrical impulses to the adjacent muscle of the atrium, causing the atria to contract and pump blood into the ventricles.

The impulses sent out by the SA node are received by the atrioventricular (AV) node, travel down the bundle of His, and are transported to the ventricular muscles by a network of nerves. The ventricles contract shortly after the atria.

The SA node as well as the AV node receives autonomic innervation that controls the rate of the heart to a certain extent.

Any deviation from the normal orderly sequence is a disturbance of the rhythm and is called an "arrhythmia." Sometimes an area of muscle in one of the atria becomes more excitable than the SA node and fires more rapid impulses. The rest of the heart then responds to this new pacemaker, and the resulting arrhythmia is known as atrial tachycardia.

Such a new focus may discharge impulses at extremely rapid rates of 180 to 250 impulses per minute. The atria, instead of beating in unison, are swept by wave upon wave of contraction and relaxation known as atrial fibrillation. When fibrillation occurs, the AV node is literally bombarded with impulses and is unable to let them all through. The result is that the ventricles, which are the more important chambers, are irregularly stimulated and, consequently, beat less efficiently.

Three drugs are used most often to treat arrhythmias.

Quinidine Sulfate, USP, BP. This drug is used to decrease the number of times the atrial muscle can contract in a given period of time; hence, it is used to treat atrial fibrillation. It is administered orally or intravenously.

Dose: Adults: (Oral, IV) 200 to 400 mg three to five times daily for 1 to 3 days.

Children: No standard dose is established.

Procainamide Hydrochloride, USP, BP (Pronestyl). Although also effective in atrial fibrillation, this drug is used more commonly in ventricular arrhythmias in which premature contractions occur. Generally, it is administered orally or intravenously.

> Dose: Adults: (Oral) 250 mg three or four times daily. (IM) 500 mg to 1 gm every 6 hours. (IV) 2 to 6 mg/min in diluted solution. Total daily dose ranges from 200 mg to 1 gm.
> Children: (IV) 20 to 80 μg/kg/min in diluted solution.

Lidocaine Hydrochloride, USP, BP (Xylocaine). When administered intravenously, lidocaine has been shown to be extremely effective in controlling and preventing ventricular fibrillation. The drug must be administered by a physician and must be monitored carefully with electrocardiograph tracings. It is often used in cardiac intensive care units, particularly in patients who have recently had a severe myocardial infarction, to prevent arrhythmias.

Side effects of lidocaine primarily affect the central nervous system and include drowsiness, disorientation, confusion, visual disturbances, and, very rarely, convulsions or coma.

> Dose: Adults: (IV) 50 to 100 mg at a rate of 25 to 50 mg/min. Maximum dose per hour is 300 mg. Prophylactic intravenous infusions are administered to deliver a dose of 1 to 4 mg/min.
> Children: (IV) Bolus of 1 mg/kg. After 2 minutes a second dose of 0.5 mg/kg may be given. Maintenance infusions: 0.3 mg/kg/min.

Propranolol Hydrochloride, USP, BP (Inderal). Propranolol is an antiarrhythmic agent that exerts its influence by blocking the effect of circulating norepinephrine on the myocardium of the heart. By blocking the receptor sites, this agent reduces cardiac irritability. It is used to treat and prevent atrial flutter and fibrillation and to control extrasystoles, both originating from the atria and the ventricles.

Side effects include nausea, vomiting, diarrhea, skin rash, hallucinations, and blood disorders.

> Dose: Adults: (Oral) 10 to 30 mg three times daily. (IV) 1 to 3 mg administered slowly at a rate not over 1 mg/min.

> Children: No pediatric dose has been established.

Bretylium Tosylate (Bretylol). Bretylium is used in the treatment of ventricular arrhythmias that are unresponsive to the first-line drugs lidocaine and procainamide.

Side effects include diarrhea, hiccups, sweating, tongue and parotid gland swelling, and hypotension.

> Dose: Adults: (IM) 5 to 10 mg/kg, first repeated in 1 to 2 hours, then at 6- to 8-hour intervals. (IV) 5 mg/kg over 1 minute; may be repeated at 15- to 30-minute intervals.
> Children: (IM) 2 to 5 mg/kg as a single dose.

Disopyramide Phosphate, USP, BP (Norpace). The antiarrhythmic activity of this agent is similar to that of quinidine and procainamide in the treatment of arrhythmias.

> Dose: Adults only: (Oral) 150 mg every 6 hours.

Nadolol, USP, BP (Corgard). This beta-blocking agent has a mechanism of action similar to that of propranolol. It is used to prevent arrhythmias and treat hypertension.

> Dose: Adults only: (Oral) 40 mg daily, increased as necessary to 320 mg daily.

DRUGS THAT AFFECT THE BLOOD VESSELS

Abnormal conditions affecting the arteries, arterioles, capillaries, and veins are many in number and variety. Drugs may be used to increase or decrease the lumina of the blood vessels and thus affect the flow of blood through them.

Vasoconstrictors

These agents bring about constriction of the muscle fibers in the walls of the blood vessels either by direct action on the vessels or by stimulation of the vasomotor center in the medulla. They may be used to (1) stop superficial hemorrhage; (2) relieve nasal congestion; (3) raise the blood pressure; or (4) increase the force of heart action. Some of the drugs that act as vasoconstrictors follow.

Epinephrine Injection, USP, BP, Epinephrine Solution, USP (Adrenalin). The chief use of epinephrine is to constrict peripheral blood vessels by local application. It is commonly used in the eye for this purpose. Although used to control bleeding from capillaries or small arteries, it does not stop bleeding from a larger vessel.

Given hypodermically, epinephrine produces powerful vasoconstriction, which, in turn, causes a marked rise in blood pressure. The heart is stimulated as well, which also contributes to the rise in blood pressure. The peak of this elevation is rarely sustained for more than a few minutes, and the blood pressure returns to normal limits usually ½ hour after the dose has been given. Because of this transitory action, epinephrine is not the agent of choice when a gradual, sustained elevation of blood pressure is desired. It is quite effective in emergency situations, however. When used with local anesthetics, the vasoconstricting properties prolong the action of the anesthetic.

Dose: Adults: (SC) 0.3 mg.
Children: (SC) 0.01 mg/kg.

Levarterenol Bitartrate Injection, USP, BP (Levophed). A potent pressor substance, this drug is used to raise and sustain the blood pressure in acute states of hypotension. One ampule is usually added to the intravenous fluid, and the rate of flow is carefully regulated to maintain the desired effect. The blood pressure should be checked regularly to avoid overdosage. The drug should be administered in the lowest effective dosage for the shortest possible time to control hypotension.

Dose: Adults: (IV) 5 μg/min.
Children: (IV) 2 μg/min.

Metaraminol Bitartrate, USP, BP (Ara-mine). Also a potent vasopressor with a prolonged duration of action, this compound has an advantage over levarterenol in that it may be given intramuscularly or subcutaneously in addition to the intravenous route. Levarterenol is too irritating to the tissues to be used this way.

Dose: Adults: (IM, IV, SC) 5 mg.
Children: (IV, IM, SC) 10 μg/kg.

Ephedrine Sulfate, USP, BP. Small doses of ephedrine stimulate the heart, increase the rate and strength of the contraction, and raise the blood pressure. Ephedrine is used to sustain the blood pressure in some types of hypotension, but it is of no benefit in shock, circulatory collapse, and hemorrhage. It is used more often for local application to cause vasoconstriction in mucous membranes. It is frequently incorporated in nose sprays for this purpose but may also be administered orally.

Dose: Adults: (Oral) 25 mg six to eight times daily.
Children: (Oral) 0.75 mg/kg four times daily.

Vasodilators

Vasodilators bring about an increase in the size of the blood vessels and as such play a part in the treatment of peripheral vascular diseases, heart conditions, and hypertension. Many vasodilators are used currently.

The Nitrites. These agents cause relaxation of the muscle fibers in the walls of the blood vessels. The relaxation increases the width of the vessels and lowers the pressure of the bloodstream through the mucous membranes of the mouth, stomach, or lungs. Many times the tablets are prescribed to be dissolved under the tongue rather than swallowed.

One of the chief uses of the nitrites is in the treatment of angina pectoris (a painful condition caused by spasm of the coronary vessels). The nitrites are also used to relax the smooth-muscle spasm in bronchial asthma, to relieve cramps, and to treat hypertension.

Amyl Nitrite, USP. This agent is conveniently prepared in the form of perles or cloth-covered ampules that the patient may crush into a handkerchief to inhale the fumes when he or she feels an attack coming on. Prompt relief is obtained in this manner.

> Dose: Adults: (Inhalation) 0.3 mL as necessary.
> Children: No standard dose established.

Glyceryl Trinitrate, USP (Nitroglycerin). This drug is used in the form of small soluble tablets that are dissolved under the tongue to prevent or relieve attacks.

> Dose: Adults: (Sublingual) 0.4 mg as necessary.
> Children: No standard dose established.

Papaverine Hydrochloride, USP, BP (Cerespan). Although this drug is one of the alkaloids of the opium poppy, it is not subject to the restrictions placed on narcotics because it is singularly free from narcotic action; neither tolerance nor habituation has been reported with this drug. The main action of papaverine is to relax smooth muscles, especially those of the blood vessels. It may be administered orally or parenterally.

> Dose: Adults: (Oral, SC, IM, IV) 100 mg four to six times daily.
> Children: (Oral, SC, IM, IV) 6 mg/kg/day in four divided doses.

Ethyl Alcohol, USP, BP (Alcohol). Vasodilation is produced by a direct depression of the vasomotor center in the medulla. The skin becomes warm and flushed as a result of this vasodilation. Some authorities consider moderate amounts of alcohol taken orally to be beneficial in the relief or prevention of angina pectoris because of its action on the coronary vessels.

> Dose: Adults: (Oral) 30 cc (approximately).

Rauwolfia Serpentina, USP, BP. Extracts of this large climbing shrub grown in India, Malaysia, and Java have been used for some time to treat insanity, insomnia, and, more recently, hypertension. The alkaloids of this plant are recommended for the oral treatment of mild to moderate forms of hypertension. Their maximal effects are achieved rather slowly (over a period of weeks), and when administration is stopped, the hypotensive action continues for some time.

Reserpine is one of the most active alkaloids of this plant and is sold under various trade names, including Serpasil, Rau-Sed, and Reserpoid.

> Dose: Adults: (Oral) 0.25 mg three or four times daily for treatment of hypertension. 5 to 10 mg/day for treatment of mental illness.
> Children: Not generally administered.

ANTIHYPERTENSIVE AGENTS

Although there will be some repetition and overlap with drugs discussed in the chapter on the autonomic nervous system, the antihypertensive agents primarily affect the cardiovascular system and are covered here also.

In the United States about 58 million people suffer from hypertension. Nearly one third do not take their medication properly, and many stop the medication altogether because of unpleasant side effects. Hypertensive patients, particularly in the early stages of the disease, feel well; thus, they have the tendency to take their medication irregularly or not at all. From the patient's point of view the treatment often seems worse than the illness.

Diuretic Therapy. The individual diuretics used in the treatment of hypertension are discussed in the chapter on diuretics and urinary antiseptics. Although diuretics were long believed to be the first line of treatment for newly diagnosed hypertensives, today physicians are realizing that other agents are often more effective as a first line of approach. Diuretics are still commonly used in the treatment of hypertension, however, owing to their ability to remove excess sodium from the body and reduce the vascular volume.

Drugs that Act Via the Autonomic Nervous System

The treatment of hypertension has significantly changed over the past decade with the development of more specific agents that treat hypertension by activating or suppressing certain portions of the autonomic nervous system.

It is beyond the scope of this text to treat each activity in detail, but to know generally what these agents do and their purpose in the treatment of hypertension is important.

Central Alpha Agonists

These agents generally stimulate central alpha-adrenergic receptors, resulting in a decreased sympathetic outflow from the brain to the peripheral circulatory system.

Guanabenz Acetate, USP, BP (Wytensin). This agent may be used alone or in combination for the treatment of hypertension. Side effects are generally dry mouth, sedation, and occasionally dizziness or weakness.

Dose: Adults: 4 to 8 mg orally twice daily.
    Children older than 12 years: 0.08 to 0.2 mg/kg/day in divided doses, orally.

Clonidine Hydrochloride, USP, BP (Catapres). This agent has a rapid onset of activity, with lowering of blood pressure within 30 to 60 minutes after an oral dose. Dry mouth and drowsiness are the most common side effects.

In addition to its use as an antihypertensive agent, this drug has been found to be helpful in controlling impulsivity in the hyperactive child or child with attention deficit hyperactivity disorder. It has been used when methylphenidate (Ritalin) has not been helpful with these children. Clonidine, unlike methylphenidate, does not seem to improve school performance and may need to be combined with methylphenidate in some cases. This indication is still under study.

Dose: Adult: (Oral) 0.1 to 0.3 mg every 12 hours.
    Children: No dose established; lower doses are being tried experimentally.

Catapres TTS. This transdermal delivery system consists of patches of clonidine that may be applied and are effective for 1 week of therapy. The patches are noted as Catapres-TTS–1, –2, or –3 to deliver 0.1, 0.2, or 0.3 mg daily transdermally. These are used experimentally in children as well.

Guanfacine Hydrochloride (Tenex). This agent is similar in effect to the other agents in this class and may be given orally for the treatment of hypertension. Side effects are mild and include dry mouth and sedation.

Dose: Adults (only): 1 to 2 mg daily at bedtime.

Alpha Blockers

The agents in this group are believed to work through blockade of the postsynaptic alpha adrenoreceptors. This causes a vasodilator effect and a lowering of peripheral resistance. It is usually not accompanied by an increased heart rate. All are given to adults only; no children's doses are established.

Prazosin Hydrochloride (Minipress). Prazocin is generally well tolerated and effective orally with few systemic side effects after treatment is established. Its most notable problem is known as the "first dose effect" in a few patients. This occurs as a sudden, severe postural hypotension and a sudden syncopal episode or drop attack. This occurs in a *very* small percentage of patients and is generally avoided by stressing that the first dose be taken after the patient is in bed for the night.

Dose: 1 to 5 mg three times daily orally to a maximum of 20 mg/day.

Terazosin Hydrochloride (Hytrin). Action and effects are similar to those of prazosin, including the first dose effect.

Dose: 5 mg once daily orally. Maximum daily dose is 20 mg.

Doxazosin Mesylate (Cardura). Action and effects are similar to those of prazosin, including the first dose effect.

Dose: 1 to 16 mg orally daily in one dose.

Angiotensin-Converting Enzyme Inhibitors

The angiotensin-converting enzyme (ACE) inhibitors are drugs that inhibit ACE. This enzyme is important in hypertension because it enables angiotensin I (a precursor) to be converted to angiotensin II, a vasoconstrictor substance produced by the body.

These agents are specific antihypertensive agents and generally work well with good patient tolerance. They do not cause sedation, a common side effect with antihypertensives.

The most distressing side effect that occurs is a chronic, irritating, and nonproductive cough. When this cough occurs, treatment must be changed to another class of drugs because all will produce the cough. The cough may persist for up to 2 weeks after the drug is withdrawn. Angioedema, although rare, is another side effect that necessitates withdrawal of the drug. No children's doses are established.

Enalapril Maleate (Vasotec)

Dose: 5 to 40 mg orally daily in one or two divided doses.

Quinapril Hydrochloride (Accupril)

Dose: 10 to 80 mg orally daily in one or two divided doses.

Captopril (Capoten)

Dose: 25 to 50 mg orally three times daily.

Lisinopril (Prinivil)

Dose: 10 to 40 mg orally daily in one dose.

Ramipril (Altace)

Dose: 2.5 to 20 mg orally daily in one or two divided doses.

Fosinopril Sodium (Monopril)

Dose: 10 to 80 mg orally once daily.

Benazepril Hydrochloride (Lotensin)

Dose: 10 to 40 mg orally daily in one to two divided doses.

Beta Blockers with Intrinsic Sympathomimetic Activity

These agents block the beta-adrenergic receptor sites. They also possess the intrinsic sympathomimetic activity (ISA), which has a partial agonist activity aimed at the adrenergic sites. This technicality is academic as far as the scope of this text. Suffice it to say, there are two groups of beta blockers, one with ISA and one without ISA, the effects of which are noted particularly in the side effects of these agents.

Heart failure may be precipitated by these agents as well as by precipitation of an acute asthma attack. They should not be withdrawn abruptly because doing so can result in the onset of angina or myocardial infarction.

All of these agents may be used in the treatment of hypertension alone or in combination with other drugs. They are used only for adults.

Pindolol, USP, BP (Visken)

Dose: 5 mg twice a day orally. Total daily dose may be increased to 60 mg/day.

Acebutolol (Sectral)

Dose: 200 to 1200 mg daily in one or two divided doses, orally.

Crateolol Hydrochloride (Cartrol)

Dose: 2.5 to 5 mg orally once daily.

Penbutolol Sulfate (Levatol)

Dose: 20 to 40 mg orally once daily.

Beta Blockers Without Intrinsic Sympathomimetic Activity

These agents are nonspecific beta-adrenergic blocking agents that are used in the treatment of hypertension and other disorders.

Decreased cardiac output and cardiac failure may occur during administration of these agents. They may precipitate asthma attacks, and their sudden withdrawal may precipitate angina pectoris or myocardial infarction.

They may be used alone or with other antihypertensive agents.

Propranolol Hydrochloride, USP, BP (Inderal). Propranolol may be used alone or in combination with other agents in the treatment of hypertension. It is often used in the treatment of cardiac arrhythmias and prophylactically to prevent the onset of migraine headaches.

Dose: Adult: doses are highly individualized and range from 40 to 640 mg/day. The L-A (long-acting) tablets facilitate the higher doses. For life-threatening arrhythmias, IV doses of 1 to 3 mg.

Children: IV doses are not recommended. Orally: 1 to 2 mg/kg/dose given twice daily.

Metoprolol Tartrate, USP, BP (Lopressor, Toprol XL). Metoprolol is used for the treatment of hypertension and in the long-term management of patients with angina pectoris.

Dose: Adults only: 100 to 450 mg orally daily in two divided doses.

Atenolol, USP, BP (Tenormin). Atenolol is used in the treatment of hypertension and in the long-term management of angina pectoris. It may be given acutely intravenously to treat acute myocardial infarction.

Dose: Adults only: 50 to 200 mg orally as one daily dose. IV 5 mg over 5 minutes, followed by another 5-mg injection 5 minutes later.

Nadolol, USP, BP (Corgard). This agent is used for hypertension, to slow the cardiac rate, and for the treatment of angina pectoris.

Dose: Adults only: 40 to 240 mg orally once daily.

Timolol Maleate, USP, BP (Blocadren). Timolol is used in the treatment of hypertension and in patients who are over the acute phase of myocardial infarction to reduce the risk of reinfarction.

Dose: Adults only: 10 mg one to two times daily to a total daily dose of 30 mg orally.

The Calcium Channel Blockers

This class of antihypertensive agents acts by blocking the entry of extracellular calcium ions into the myocardial and vascular smooth-muscle cells. This leads to reduced cardiac output and reduced total peripheral resistance, with the subsequent reduction in blood pressure. They are also effective for angina pectoris, supraventricular arrhythmias, and cardiomyopathy.

Nifedipine, USP, BP (Procardia, Adalat). This agent is particularly effective in managing hypertension in patients with coexisting angina or peripheral vascular disease. Hypotension, dizziness, and nausea are included in its side effects.

Dose: Adults: (Oral) 10 mg three times daily. As extended-release capsules, 30 to 60 mg once daily.

Children: Pediatric dose not established.

Verapamil Hydrochloride, USP, BP (Calan). This agent is used for hypertension, angina, and tachyarrhythmias. Bradycardia, heart block, and constipation are included in its side effects.

Dose: Adults: (Oral) 40 to 80 mg three times daily.

(IV) 0.075 to 0.2 mg/kg, repeated once in 30 minutes.

Children: (IV) 0.1 to 0.3 mg/kg, repeated in 30 minutes.

Diltiazem Hydrochloride, USP, BP (Cardizem). This agent is used in hypertension and angina pectoris. Nausea, dizziness, and bradycardia are among its side effects.

Dose: Adults only: (Oral) 60 to 180 mg twice daily.

Miscellaneous Agents

Methyldopa Hydrochloride, USP, BP (Aldomet). This agent's actions are primarily due to its effect on the central nervous system. The hypotensive effect is attributed to a decrease in peripheral resistance with little change in heart rate. Side effects include drowsiness, impotence, and gynecomastia.

Dose: Adults: (Oral) 250 to 500 mg four times daily.
(IV) 350 to 500 mg every 6 hours.
Children: (Oral, IV) 10 to 40 mg/kg/day in divided doses.

DRUGS THAT AFFECT THE BLOOD

Coagulants

These agents hasten the process of coagulation.

Calcium Salts. Needed for the reactions in blood coagulation, these salts may be given orally just before surgery to prevent excessive bleeding. Calcium salts may also be given intravenously to treat tetanic convulsions. The salts used are calcium gluconate, calcium chloride, and calcium lactate.

Dose: Adults: (Oral, IV) 1 gm as necessary.

Vitamin K. This is a fat-soluble vitamin that is needed for normal blood coagulation. Bile salts must be present in the gastrointestinal tract for absorption of natural vitamin K; hence, in the event of a bile obstruction, oral preparation of natural vitamin K would be of no avail. Among the commercial preparations of vitamin K are:

Phytonadione, USP, BP (Vitamin K_1 Oxide) (Mephyton). This emulsion of the vitamin may be given intravenously to control hemorrhage. It is also available in tablet form.

Dose: Mephyton: Adults: (IV) 50 mg two to three times daily.
(Oral) 5 mg four times daily.

Phytonadione Injection, USP, BP (Aquamephyton). This colloidal solution of the vitamin has smaller particles that permit this preparation to be given intramuscularly or subcutaneously as well as by the intravenous route.

Dose: Aquamephyton: Adults: (SC, IM) 10 mg two or three times daily.
Children: (SC, IM) 0.5 to 1.0 mg is administered to newborns to prevent hemorrhagic disease of the newborn.

Menadiol Sodium Diphosphate, USP, BP (Synkayvite), Menadione Sodium Bisulfite (Hykinone). These preparations, water-soluble analogues of vitamin K, are absorbed without the aid of bile salts; therefore, they may be given orally when the natural vitamin is of no use. Menadione is also prepared in injectable form.

Dose: Adults: (Oral, SC, IM, IV) 5 to 15 mg once or twice daily.
Children: (Oral, SC, IM, IV) 1 to 5 mg/day.

Anticoagulants

These agents increase the blood coagulation time. They are used to prevent coagulation of blood that will be used for transfusions; preserve blood; and prevent postoperative thrombi and emboli. Some of the common anticoagulants follow.

Sodium Heparin Injection, USP, BP (Liquaemin). Known as the "natural anticoagulant," it is obtained for commercial use from the liver and lungs of domesticated animals. It is the blood component that prevents coagulation within the vessels under ordinary conditions.

Heparin is not active orally and must be given parenterally. If given subcutaneously or intramuscularly, extra care must be taken to prevent hematoma formation. The preferred method of administration is by intravenous infusion. Although it has no effect on clots already formed, heparin prevents extension of the clot and the formation of new clots.

Dose: Adults: (IM, IV) 5000 U as needed.

Bishydroxycoumarin, USP, BP (Dicumarol). Like heparin, this agent does not affect an already formed clot, but it retards or prevents the extension of one already formed. The main advantage of this drug over heparin is that it may be given orally.

The dosage must be adjusted to the individual patient's needs, and the prothrombin time of the blood must be taken at frequent intervals to prevent overdosage. Symptoms of overdosage are nosebleed, small areas of bleeding into the skin, and massive hemorrhage on injury. Overdosage may be treated with vitamin K.

Dose: Adults: (Oral) 100 mg two to four times daily.

Sodium Warfarin, USP, BP (Coumadin). Very similar in action to Dicumarol, this agent may be absorbed orally and is used to prevent clot formation and extension. The onset of action is a little faster than that of Dicumarol; Coumadin takes 12 to 18 hours compared with the 24 to 72 hours needed for Dicumarol to take effect. When immediate action is desired, heparin is given intravenously, followed by one of the oral forms for prolonged anticoagulant therapy. Overdosage may be treated with vitamin K.

Dose: Adults: (Oral) 10 to 30 mg initially; then 2.5 to 5 mg two or three times daily.

THROMBOLYTIC THERAPY FOR MYOCARDIAL INFARCTION

Myocardial infarction, in which a blood clot has formed in a coronary artery, is a life-threatening condition. Advances have been made in aggressively pursuing therapy to dissolve the blood clot before extensive anoxia and tissue damage to the myocardium of the heart occur. Thrombolytic therapy has been shown to salvage myocardium, reduce mortality in patients with acute myocardial infarction, and improve left ventricular function.

Streptokinase, USP, BP (Kabikinase). Streptokinase is a protein produced by group C beta-hemolytic streptococci. It promotes thrombolysis, or dissolution of blood clots. It is used by intravenous infusion to lyse coronary artery thrombi. Benefit has been greatest when ther-

apy has been instituted within 6 hours after onset of symptoms. The most frequent side effects are hemorrhage, fever, and allergic reactions.

Dose: Adults: (IV) 10,000 to 30,000 U given in a bolus with a small volume of diluent, followed by a maintenance infusion of 2000 to 4000 U/min. The infusion is maintained until lysis occurs or the predetermined maximum dose has been given (around 500,000 U).

Urokinase, USP, BP (Abbokinase). This agent is most effective in lysing recently formed thrombi and should be instituted as soon as possible but no longer than 5 days after clot formation. When used for coronary thrombi, treatment should be given within 6 hours. For pulmonary emboli there is a longer span of effectiveness. Hemorrhage, hypersensitivity, and fever are reported as untoward reactions.

Dose: Adults: (IV) For coronary perfusion 750,000 U in 500 mL diluent. For pulmonary emboli 4400 U/kg over 10 minutes, followed by a continuous infusion of 4400 U/kg/hr for 12 hours.

Alteplace (Activase, rt-PA, t-PA). This biosynthetic form of the human enzyme tissue-type plasminogen activator (t-PA) is a thrombolytic agent. Unlike streptokinase and urokinase, t-PA is a relatively fibrin-selective plasminogen activator. For maximum effectiveness, it should be administered within 3 to 5 hours after myocardial infarction. The most frequent complication is hemorrhage.

Dose: Adults: (IV) 100 mg in a small amount of diluent over a 3-hour period, and a subsequent maintenance infusion of 0.25 mg/kg/hour for the next 2 hours.

ANTIPLATELET THERAPY IN CARDIOVASCULAR DISEASE

Blood platelets are small granular bodies that number about 250,000 to 350,000 per milliliter of blood. They have three functions:

1. They stick to the inner surfaces of damaged blood vessels, plug up leaks, and cement over injured tissues.
2. When they rupture they release thromboplastin, a substance that begins a series of reactions that form a blood clot.
3. Once a clot is formed, platelets make it shrink or retract, during which the clot is changed from a soft mass to a firm one. This helps to stop bleeding from damaged vessels.

Obviously platelet activity and blood clot formation are important functions in the body. In certain circumstances, however, when a patient has atherosclerosis and the linings of many of the blood vessels are ragged with plaques of cholesterol, the formation of clots is unwanted. Antiplatelet therapy is designed to prevent clots in damaged blood vessels.

Antiplatelet Drugs

Aspirin, USP, BP. By inhibiting enzymes within the platelet, aspirin prevents platelet aggregation. When given daily to patients after a myocardial infarction, there is a reduction in the incidence of recurrent myocardial infarction and cardiovascular death.

> Dose for antiplatelet effect: (Oral) 65 to 325 mg daily. Higher doses were not more effective than lower doses.

Dipyridamole, USP, BP (Persantine). Dipyridamole inhibits platelet aggregation caused by platelet-released agents. It is often used in conjunction with aspirin therapy after myocardial infarction.

> Dose: Adults only: (Oral) 75 to 400 mg daily in divided doses.

ANTILIPEMIC DRUGS

The measuring of cholesterol and the definition of "good" and "bad" cholesterol have become a matter of public concern in recent years.

As recently as the 1960s, if the total cholesterol was under 300 mg percent, no one became excited. As the understanding of the relationship between blood cholesterol levels and atherosclerotic vessel diseases became known, the "optimum" cholesterol was moved down to 250 mg, then 225 mg, then 200 mg percent. Most recent studies have shown that we should be looking at 160 mg percent for optimum vessel health.

A blood cholesterol even less than 200 mg percent is an unattainable goal for many on diet restriction alone, because cholesterol can be manufactured by the body also, and this activity is genetically determined.

After dietary restrictions have been tried, drug therapy is used to attain acceptable cholesterol levels. Many agents have been used and continue to be developed.

Cholestyramine for Oral Suspension, USP, BP (Questran). Cholestyramine is used orally to bind with bile acids in the intestine, forming an insoluble complex that is excreted in the feces. Cholesterol is the precursor of bile acids; thus, when the bile acid loss is accelerated, this stimulates for cholesterol to form bile acids, resulting in a net loss of cholesterol from the blood stream. It is ineffective, and thus contraindicated, in patients with bile duct obstruction.

The most common adverse effect is constipation. Abdominal pain and flatulence may also be noted. This may be treated with conventional laxative therapy.

> Dose: 15 gm (one packet or one scoopful) two to four times daily.

Colestipol Granules (Colestid). Like cholestyramine, this agent acts to remove bile acids from the gastrointestinal tract, thus causing more cholesterol to be converted to bile acids and lowering the serum cholesterol. Constipation is the most common side effect.

> Dose: 5 to 30 gm daily in divided doses. It should always be mixed with fluids.

Pravastatin Sodium (Pravachol). Through a complex mechanism of action involving enzymes and membrane transport complexes, this agent acts to clear the serum of cholesterol and triglycerides.

The most significant side effect is alteration

of liver function; thus, liver enzymes should be tested before therapy and every 6 weeks.

Dose: 10 to 40 mg orally daily at bedtime for 3 to 6 months.

Gemfibrozil (Lopid). This lipid-lowering agent acts to reduce serum levels of triglycerides and very-low-density cholesterol. Renal and liver abnormalities have occurred with prolonged treatment; thus, the patient should be followed frequently.

Dose: 1200 mg orally daily in two divided doses.

Lovastatin (Mevacor). This agent was isolated from a strain of *Aspergillus terreus,* a fungus. Through complex enzyme activation, it in-

terferes with the biosynthesis of cholesterol. Liver dysfunction must be guarded against.

Dose: 20 to 80 mg daily in single or divided doses orally.

Simvastatin (Zocor). Also derived from *Aspergillus,* this agent lowers cholesterol by interfering with its biosynthesis. Hepatic, renal, and cardiac complications may occur with prolonged use.

Dose: 5 to 40 mg daily orally in the evening.

Probucol (Lorelco). Probucol lowers serum cholesterol but has very little effect on triglycerides. Ventricular arrhythmias are the most serious side effect noted.

Dose: 500 mg orally twice daily.

Implications for the Student

1. Care should be taken to monitor the pulse of a cardiac patient before each dose of medication. If the pulse is less than 60, digitalis should be withheld and the physician notified.

2. Blood levels of digoxin provide an accurate method of determining digoxin dose for an individual patient.

3. An increase in urine output is generally seen as an early sign of improvement in a patient being treated for congestive heart failure.

4. A decrease in visible edema from fluid retention is generally noted as a sign of improvement in patients with congestive heart failure.

5. Patients with congestive failure are generally more comfortable in a sitting position and should be placed in this position to minimize dyspnea.

6. Cardiac patients are generally prescribed a low-sodium diet to minimize fluid retention. The patient should be carefully instructed in the importance of the diet.

7. Alterations in the serum calcium and potassium will affect the performance of digitalis. Severe changes in the serum concentration of these electrolytes may be responsible for toxic effects from digitalis.

8. The patient should be monitored for any change in the cardiac rhythm during administration of cardiac drugs. An irregular pulse rate should be reported to the physician.

9. The patient should be instructed to take the cardiac medication exactly as prescribed when he or she returns home. He or she should be told to report any weight gain, shortness of breath, or edema to the physician.

10. The prothrombin time (pro time) is generally used as a measure of the effectiveness of anticoagulants. The ideal pro time is twice that of the control when a patient is on anticoagulants. With less than this time the desired anticoagulation is generally not affected. With more than doubled time there is a danger of bleeding. The dose of medication is generally based on the patient's current pro time.

11. Hypertensive agents may have severe side effects. All untoward symptoms should be reported to the physician.

CASE STUDIES

1. Mrs. L.M., 58, is admitted to the hospital emergency room with shortness of breath; cold, clammy skin; a heart rate of 100; and a cough producing pink, frothy sputum. A probable diagnosis of heart failure and pulmonary edema has been established. What nursing procedures might be taken immediately to make her more comfortable? What drugs are likely to be needed?

2. Mr. J.B., 32, comes into the emergency room in a state of extreme anxiety, expressing a fear that he is dying. His pulse is thready, rapid, and irregular but is continued at about 150. A probable diagnosis of atrial fibrillation is established. What drugs are likely to be needed? What other techniques are known to be useful in stopping an attack such as this?

3. Mr. K.A., 67, is chronically ill. He has recurrent chest pain and reports shortness of breath. The probable diagnosis is angina. What drugs are likely to be useful in managing his condition?

4. After a heart attack Mr. H.A., 62, was placed on Coumadin, 10 mg a day. He has returned to work and feels well. However, he is annoyed that he has to have periodic blood tests and checkups. Could you help him understand the need for these tests?

Review Questions

1. List the ways drugs may affect the heart.

2. What precaution is necessary in giving digitalis?

3. What is the most important action of digitalis?

4. What instructions would you give to a person taking nitroglycerin?

5. How would you classify vitamin K preparations?

6. What is the main advantage of Coumadin over heparin?

7. What is the antidote for an overdose of heparin?

8. Name three drugs frequently used to treat arrhythmias.

9. What is the antidote for an overdose of sodium warfarin?

10. Discuss the importance of observation in the care of patients with cardiovascular problems.

11. Discuss the importance of observation in the care of patients on antihypertensive drugs.

12. Why is compliance so important when taking antihypertensives? What side effects can occur if the patient is careless about taking the medicine?

13. What are the functions of blood platelets?

14. Why is platelet aggregation a disadvantage after a heart attack?

15. What is a myocardial infarction?

16. What is the difference between an anticoagulant and a thrombolytic drug?

17. What is the normal cholesterol level?

18. Why is cholesterol important?

19. Name two drugs used to treat elevated cholesterol levels.

Drugs that Affect the Central Nervous System

Objectives for the Student

BE

ABLE

TO

- 1. Classify and give an example of drugs that affect the central nervous system.
- 2. Differentiate between the narcotic and non-narcotic analgesics.
- 3. Identify three narcotic analgesics.
- 4. State the precautions to be observed when narcotic analgesics are administered.
- 5. List the symptoms of drug dependence.
- 6. Explain the action of general anesthetic agents.
- 7. Discuss the therapeutic uses of alcohol.
- 8. List eight drugs that are classified as anticonvulsants.
- 9. Discuss problems associated with abuse of stimulants.

The central nervous system, including the peripheral nerves, constitutes the body's equipment for rapid coordination of many of its activities. These activities must often be set into play and governed to needs in a fraction of a second. An example is the very rapid closing of the eyes when they are unexpectedly touched (e.g., by a grain of sand). We move ourselves at will by sending electrical signals from the central nervous system to our skeletal muscles.

The nervous system is composed of the brain and spinal cord; together they coordinate many functions such as blood pressure, heart rate, the flow of saliva and gastric juices, and skin temperature.

In addition, the brain serves to store knowledge and to cause conscious and unconscious reactions to stimuli and conditions on the basis of past experience. Our awareness of our environment, our satisfaction or dissatisfaction with it, happiness, love, and all emotions or moods are seated in the brain.

It has long been known that the brain can be depressed and stimulated. The use of alcoholic beverages and plants with depressant effects has its origin in antiquity. The discovery of anesthesia may be cited as one of the greatest boons to humankind, for it made possible life-saving surgical procedures that were hitherto impossible.

A noteworthy advance of the twentieth century has come in the past decade owing to the discovery of drugs that give truly effective treatment to the mentally ill. After centuries of study, the first big steps have been taken in unraveling the mysteries of mental illness. Although Chapter 23 is devoted exclusively to drugs used in the management and treatment of mental illness, many of the agents discussed in this chapter have also been used therapeutically in this area.

CENTRAL NERVOUS SYSTEM STIMULANTS

Central stimulants are drugs that increase the activity of the brain and spinal cord. They are used to counteract the depressant effects of such drugs as opium, morphine, and alcohol as well as to speed up vital processes in instances of shock and collapse.

Caffeine, USP. Obtained from tea leaves, coffee beans, and other plants, this drug is used to produce mild cerebral stimulation. Its use as a respiratory stimulation has been discussed previously. Some side effects are noted with this drug, chiefly tachycardia and irritability accompanied by insomnia.

Dose: Adults: (Oral) 200 mg three to four times daily. (IM or IV) Caffeine and sodium benzoate injection 0.5 gm as necessary.

Amphetamine Sulfate, USP, BP (Benzedrine). More powerful than caffeine in stimulating the cerebral cortex, this agent produces brighter spirits and may cause restlessness, talkativeness, and insomnia. Psychic stimulation may be followed by depression or fatigue. Although amphetamine may superimpose excit-

ability on fatigue, it does not obliterate the need for rest. In normal individuals it does not facilitate mental performance, and the nervousness produced may be quite uncomfortable. Repeated administration may cause hypertension, restlessness, irritability, and gastrointestinal distress. Collapse may result.

The main action of this agent is stimulation of the cerebral cortex, but it is a useful aid in the treatment of obesity. By depressing the senses of smell and taste, it helps to curb the appetite (a conditioned reflex originating in the higher cerebral centers). The brighter spirits strengthen determination to stay on a diet with few calories, and the stimulation also gives rise to increased physical activity, which is beneficial.

Dextroamphetamine sulfate (Dexedrine) is more often used than amphetamine because its greater activity permits the use of a lower dose.

This drug is controlled under the Dangerous Drug Act.

Dose: Adults: (Oral) Amphetamine 10 mg two to four times daily. Dextroamphetamine 5 mg two to four times daily.

Pentylenetetrazol Injection, USP, BP (Metrazol). This drug stimulates the higher centers of the cerebrum as well as the medullary centers and the reflex activity in the spinal cord. Because of the respiratory stimulation produced, it is sometimes used as an antidote for barbiturate poisoning. It is incorporated in various tonics for its stimulating effect, including Niatric and VitaMetrazol.

Dose: Adults: (Oral) 100 mg three times daily.

Doxapram Hydrochloride, USP, BP (Dopram). This central stimulant acts on all levels of the central nervous system but is used primarily as a respiratory stimulant to hasten arousal in individuals who have taken depressants.

There is a small margin of safety with this agent, and hypertension, tachycardia, and seizures have occurred with its use.

Dose: Adults: 1 to 2 mg/kg with the first two

Table 22-1. VOLATILE ANESTHETICS

Generic Name	Trade Name	Uses	Concentration
Ether, USP, BP	—	Major surgical procedures	10–15 vol %
Vinyl ether, USP, BP	Vinethene	Major procedures	2–4 vol %
Nitrous oxide, USP, BP	—	Short procedures	80 vol %
Halothane, USP, BP	Fluothane	Major procedures, particularly when vasoconstriction is desired	1–3 vol %
Enflurane, USP, BP	Ethrane	General use	1.5–4 vol %
Methoxyflurane, USP, BP	Penthrane	Obstetrics, short procedures	2–3 vol %

doses at 5-minute intervals and then repeated as necessary at 1- to 2-hour intervals.

Children: Same as that for adults.

Methylphenidate Hydrochloride, USP, BP (Ritalin). The primary use of methylphenidate is in the treatment of the minimal brain dysfunction (MBD) or hyperactivity syndrome. Although the drug is a central stimulant, it causes a slowing of the hyperactive individual and increases the ability to concentrate. It is occasionally used in the treatment of narcolepsy and mild depressive states.

The side effects, when they occur, are generally mild and include nervousness, headache, and insomnia. They can generally be controlled by alteration of the dose.

Dose: Adults: (Oral) 5 to 20 mg two to three times daily.
Children: Same as that for adults.

Pemoline (Cylert). Like methylphenidate, this agent is used in the treatment of MBD. It has a gradual onset of action, however, and therapeutic effects may not be evident for 2 to 3 weeks. It has the advantage of being taken once daily instead of in divided doses.

Dose: Adults: (Oral) 37.5 mg daily in the morning. The dose may be increased at weekly intervals to a maximum of 112.5 mg daily.
Children: Same as that for adults.

CENTRAL NERVOUS SYSTEM DEPRESSANTS

The action of central nervous system depressants may be general, depressing the central nervous system more or less as a whole, or they may act in a more specific way on one or more centers of the brain.

General Anesthetics

The general anesthetics produce a loss of sensation throughout the body by cutting off all sensory impulses to the brain, thus causing unconsciousness. General anesthetics are most commonly administered by inhalation, although a few, such as sodium penthothal, are administered intravenously (Tables 22–1 and 22–2).

Table 22-2. GENERAL ANESTHETICS ADMINISTERED INTRAVENOUSLY

Generic Name	Trade Name	Uses	Concentration
Thiopental sodium, USP, BP	Pentothal	Short procedures or to facilitate induction with volatile anesthetics	2.5% solution
Ketamine hydrochloride, USP, BP	Ketalar	Obstetrics, short procedures	2–3% solution
Diazepam, USP, BP	Valium	Anticonvulsant, induction aid, preoperative medication	0.2–1.5 mg/kg Not to exceed 10 mg/min

The stages of anesthesia provide guidelines as to the level or depth of anesthesia. The anesthetist controls the depth of anesthesia for various procedures by observing the stages. All stages of anesthesia are passed through during induction; the order is then reversed during the recovery period.

Stages of Anesthesia

I. Analgesia

This stage begins when the anesthetic is administered and lasts until loss of consciousness. It is characterized by analgesia, euphoria, perceptual distortions, and amnesia.

II. Delirium

This stage begins with loss of consciousness and extends to the beginning of surgical anesthesia. There may be excitement and involuntary muscular activity. Skeletal muscle tone increases, breathing is irregular, and hypertension and tachycardia may occur.

III. Surgical Anesthesia

This stage lasts until spontaneous respiration ceases. It is further divided into four planes based on respiration, the size of the pupils, reflex characteristics, and eyeball movements.

IV. Medullary Depression

This stage begins with cessation of respiration and ends with circulatory collapse. The pupils are fixed and dilated, and there are no lid or corneal reflexes.

Local Anesthetics

The local anesthetics are presented in this section for completeness and clarity, but they are not central depressants. Rather, local anesthetics interfere with nerve conduction from an area of the body to the central nervous system. In this way they interfere with pain perception by the central nervous system. Table 22–3 presents a summary of the local anesthetics.

Hypnotics and Sedatives

Hypnotic and sedative agents may generally be used in smaller doses for daytime sedation and in larger doses for the induction of sleep at bedtime.

Patients who are taking these agents must be cautioned not to take other central depressants, such as alcohol. The antihistamines, with their side effect of drowsiness, can also give untoward effects when administered concurrently with these agents. In some cases when these agents are used for their hypnotic effect, a morning

Table 22-3. LOCAL ANESTHETICS

Generic Name	Trade Name	Uses	Concentration
Cocaine hydrochloride, USP, BP	—	Mucous membranes of the nose and throat	1–20% topically
Procaine hydrochloride, USP, BP	Novocaine	Local nerve block	0.25–2% solution SC
Lidocaine hydrochloride, USP, BP	Xylocaine	Local nerve block	1–2% solution SC
Bupivacaine hydrochloride, USP, BP	Marcaine	Epidural or caudal block Local nerve block	0.25–0.5% solution SC
Chloroprocaine hydrochloride, USP, BP	Nesacaine	Epidural, caudal, local nerve block	1–2% solution SC
Mepivacaine hydrochloride, USP, BP	Carbocaine	Dental and local block	1% solution SC
Tetracaine hydrochloride, USP, BP	Pontocaine	Spinal anesthesia	1% solution subarachnoid

SC = subcutaneously.

"hangover" or sedative effect may be obtained. In many cases this can be minimized by using one of the shorter acting hypnotics or reducing the dose.

Barbiturates. These agents are prescribed more frequently than any other class to produce sedation of the central nervous system. The response to the barbiturates may be mild sedation, hypnosis, or general anesthesia, depending on the dose and the method of administration. All of these agents are controlled under the Dangerous Drug Act.

The barbiturates are not analgesics, however, and cannot be depended on to produce sleep when insomnia is caused by pain. These drugs are definitely habit forming, will produce tolerance, and may lead to addiction if large doses are taken over a long period of time. The symptoms of barbiturate poisoning are similar to those of chronic alcoholism. There is impairment of mental efficiency, confusion, belligerence, blurred speech, and tremors. The skin is clammy and cyanotic, the temperature drops, and respiratory depression continues, causing death.

Severe poisoning results from 5 to 10 times the hypnotic dose, and death results from 15 to 20 times the hypnotic dose. Treatment of poisoning in the past consisted of the administration of a respiratory stimulant such as Megimide, nikethamide, or caffeine sodium benzoate. A more recent treatment is preferred to the administration of stimulants, however. This is known as dialysis. The patient's blood is run through an artificial kidney in which the barbiturate is diffused out of the blood. Fewer dangerous aftereffects are reported from this treatment of poisoning.

There are many commonly used barbiturates. They differ in onset of action, duration of action, and method of administration, but for all practical purposes the pharmacologic effects on the body are the same.

Phenobarbital, USP, BP (Luminal)

Dose: Adults: (Oral, IM, IV) 30 mg four times daily.

Pentobarbital, USP, BP (Nembutal)

Dose: Adults: (Oral) 100 to 200 mg at bedtime.

Amobarbital, USP, BP (Amytal)

Dose: Adults: (Oral) 200 to 300 mg at bedtime.

Secobarbital, USP, BP (Seconal)

Dose: Adults: (Oral) 100 to 200 mg at bedtime.

Butabarbital, USP, BP (Butisol)

Dose: Adults: (Oral) 30 mg four times daily.

Chloral Hydrate, USP, BP. Sleep is produced in a relatively short time after administration of this drug and lasts from 5 to 8 hours. The sleep greatly resembles natural sleep, and the patient can be awakened without difficulty. There is no analgesic effect from this drug, so it is not used when the restlessness or insomnia is due to pain. It is controlled under the Dangerous Drug Act.

Dose: Adults: (Oral) 500 mg at bedtime.
Children: (Oral) 50 mg/kg at bedtime.

Glutethimide, USP, BP (Doriden). This is a fast-acting hypnotic with few side effects. The onset of action is usually within 15 to 20 minutes, and it gives 4 to 8 hours of sleep with no morning "hangover." It is used in smaller doses for daytime sedation and has been used safely in elderly patients and individuals with cardiovascular diseases in whom other types of sedatives may be tolerated poorly or contraindicated. It is controlled under the Dangerous Drug Act and is not recommended for children.

Dose: Adults: (Oral) 0.5 gm at bedtime. (Daytime dose is 0.25 gm three to four times daily.)

Ethchlorvynol, USP, BP (Placidyl). This agent may be used in smaller doses as a sedative and in larger doses as a hypnotic.

Dose: Adults only: (Oral) As a sedative, 100 to 200 mg two to three times daily. As a hypnotic, 500 mg at bedtime.

Ethinamate, USP, BP. Because of its short

4-hour activity in the body, this agent may give satisfactory hypnosis with little or no hangover.

Dose: Adults only: (Oral) 0.5 to 1 gm at bedtime.

Methyprylon, USP, BP (Noludar). With a duration of action of 6 to 7 hours, this agent is comparable to the barbiturates in its effect. It can be used as a sedative or hypnotic.

Dose: Adults: (Oral) As a sedative 50 to 100 mg three to four times daily. As a hypnotic 200 to 400 mg at bedtime.
Children: (Oral) As a hypnotic 50 mg at bedtime.

Flurazepam Hydrochloride, USP, BP (Dalmane). This agent is used to treat all types of insomnia and is a hypnotic of moderate activity.

Dose: Adults only: (Oral) 15 to 30 mg at bedtime.

Narcotic Analgesics

In ancient times, analgesia, or relief of pain, was attributed to the opium poppy. Opium is described in Chinese literature written long before the time of Christ. It is obtained from the hardened, dried juice of the unripened seeds of the species of poppy grown in Asia Minor. Three alkaloids derived from opium are in use today: morphine, codeine, and papaverine.

Although undoubtedly the most powerful and effective pain relievers known to humans, these agents are also the most addicting. After repeated doses, the dose must be continually increased to obtain relief of pain. In the case of the narcotic addict, the desired euphoria is also subject to dose tolerance, and the dosage levels must be continually increased to obtain the desired effect. For these reasons, all agents in this class are strictly controlled by the Bureau of Narcotics and Dangerous Drugs.

Morphine Sulfate, USP, BP. Morphine depresses the cerebral cortex; sensation and perception are dulled. Anxiety and apprehension disappear, and euphoria may occur. When ad-

ministered for painful situations, such as postsurgery, the drug is most effective if administered before the pain becomes severe. As long as time intervals are strictly observed and the drug dose is reduced as the pain becomes less severe, addiction is not seen as a frequent problem in short-term indications for this agent.

Some of the other effects of morphine include the following:

- The respiratory center is depressed, which is seen as the most dangerous effect of drug overdose.
- The pupils contract and become "pinpoint" in size.
- The emptying time of the stomach is delayed.
- Peristalsis is decreased (these last two effects explain why the patient may often experience abdominal pain, distention, and constipation when given morphine for pain).
- The cough center is depressed and coughing is lessened.
- The patient may experience interference with motor coordination. He or she may have difficulty handling a glass of water, may misjudge distances when attempting to pick up articles, and may stagger when walking.

Some of the uses of opium and its derivatives are as follows:

- The chief use, as before stated, is as a potent pain reliever.
- As a preliminary medication before general anesthesia, morphine is usually given with atropine. Atropine is used mainly to prevent excessive salivation and respiratory tract secretion, but it also antagonizes the depressant action of morphine upon the respiratory center and tends to speed the heart. This combination promotes a relaxed state, which favors a more satisfactory induction of anesthesia and decreases the amount of general anesthetic needed for the induction.
- Opium derivatives are frequently used in cough preparations. These syrups or expectorants usually contain codeine, dihydrocodeinone, or dihydromorphinone, but paregoric has been found useful as well.

■ To check diarrhea, paregoric (camphorated opium tincture) may be used alone or in combination with an absorbent. Laudanum (opium tincture) has also been used as well as synthetic derivatives of opium (Lomotil).

■ Because of the relaxant effect of morphine on the smooth muscles, opium derivatives may be used as antispasmodics.

Poisoning caused by opium or morphine results from overdoses that have been taken with a therapeutic or suicidal intent. Death usually results from asphyxia brought on by respiratory failure. The pupils are constricted at first and later become dilated as asphyxia deepens. As a rule, the patient perspires freely and increasingly as poisoning advances. The body temperature falls, and the skin feels cold and clammy and appears cyanotic or gray. Attention must be focused especially on respiration in the treatment of poisoning. Respiratory stimulants such as nikethamide, caffeine, sodium benzoate, or a mixture of carbon dioxide and oxygen are given. The specific antidote for morphine poisoning, however, is Narcan, because this agent counteracts the effects of morphine in the body.

The toxic dose of morphine is 60 mg in a normal individual, and the fatal dose is about 240 mg. Addicts become tolerant of the drug, however, and can take much higher doses without severe toxic effects.

Addiction to opiates is characterized by tolerance, physical dependence, and habituation. Repeated doses of these drugs lead not only to marked tolerance but also a very strong desire for the drug that the victim seems powerless to resist. The results vary in individuals, but long use leads to depression and weakness not only of the body but also of the mind and morals. The patient suffers a loss of appetite and various other digestive disturbances and, before long, becomes thin and anemic. The addict seems particularly incapable of telling the truth and will resort to almost any method to obtain the drug. Ill health, crime, and low standards of living are the result not of the effects of morphine itself but of the sacrifices of money, social position, food, and self-respect made to obtain the daily dose of the drug.

Dose: Adults: (SC, IM, IV) 10 mg, repeated up to six times daily.

Children: (SC, IM, IV) 0.1 mg/kg, up to six times daily.

Codeine Phosphate, USP, BP, and Codeine Sulfate, USP, BP. Codeine, like morphine, is a narcotic controlled under the Dangerous Drug Act. It is a mild analgesic, but the respiratory depression in overdose and the potential for drug abuse require that the usual precautions for narcotic analgesic therapy be taken.

Because the analgesic activity of this drug is potentiated when it is combined with other analgesics, it is probably most often prescribed in a combination form with aspirin, acetaminophen, or other analgesic agents.

Its antitussive activity is well known; thus, it is included in many cough preparations.

Dose: Adults: (Oral, SC) 30 mg four to six times daily.
Children: (Oral, SC) 0.5 mg/kg four to six times daily.

Meperidine Hydrochloride, USP, BP (Demerol). This is one of the synthetic substitutes for morphine. It does cause addiction, but tolerance develops at a slower rate and the withdrawal symptoms are not as severe as those of morphine. Unlike morphine it does not produce sleep but is an effective analgesic agent. Because the respiratory depression produced is less than that caused by morphine, it is preferred to morphine in obstetrics. Meperidine is a narcotic and is subject to the Dangerous Drug laws.

Dose: Adults: (Oral, SC, IM) 100 mg one to six times daily.
Children: (Oral, SC, IM) 1 mg/kg four to six times daily.

Fentanyl Transdermal System (Duragesic). This transdermal delivery system consists of patches that are applied to the skin and provide a continuous systemic delivery of fentanyl, a potent opiate narcotic. The patches have the same concentration of drug per area of patch. Increased doses are obtained by using the larger patches for greater surface area of delivery. They may be used for acute and chronic pain conditions such as cancer, Paget's disease of the bone, and postoperative pain from many types of surgery.

After removal of the patch, serum concentrations of fentanyl decline gradually and reach an approximate 50% reduction 17 hours after removal. The patch should be applied to a nonirritated area of skin on a flat surface or the upper torso. Each patch is to be worn for 72 hours.

Side effects are similar to those associated with opiates along with the potential for addiction.

Dose: Duragesic-25, -50, -75, -100. Patches will deliver 2.5, 5, 7.5, 10 mg of fentanyl, respectively.

Non-Narcotic Analgesics

The drugs of this category, although some remain habit forming, generally do not have the addicting properties of the narcotic analgesics. They also are not as effective as the narcotic agents.

Pentazocine Hydrochloride, USP, BP (Talwin). Pentazocine is a very effective nonnarcotic analgesic that may be used for moderate to severe pain. It is effective orally and parenterally. It should not be stopped suddenly after prolonged use, because some withdrawal effects may occur.

Dose: Adults: (Oral, SC, IM, IV) 30 mg every 3 to 4 hours.

Nalbuphine Hydrochloride (Nubain). Although it is believed to be equivalent to morphine on a milligram-to-milligram basis for analgesia, this agent does not produce euphoria.

Dose: Adults only: (SC < IM, IV) 10 mg every 3 to 6 hours.

Florital. This commercial preparation for oral use contains in each tablet or capsule: butalbital 50 mg, caffeine 40 mg, aspirin 200 mg, phenacetin 130 mg. It is used orally for the relief of mild to moderate pain.

Dose: Adults only: (Oral) One to two tablets every 4 to 6 hours.

Acetaminophen, USP, BP (Tylenol, Tempra). Acetaminophen has been shown to be an effective and safe analgesic and antipyretic. Unlike aspirin, however, it has no antirheumatic or anti-inflammatory activity; thus, it is of limited benefit in the treatment of pain arising from joint disorders. It is not as irritating to the gastric mucosa as aspirin, so it is useful in patients who do not tolerate aspirin well.

Acetaminophen has been found to be of great benefit in the treatment of fevers in infants and young children. Even a slight overdose of aspirin in children, when repeated doses are necessary to control fevers, has produced mild to severe symptoms of salicylate toxicity.

Sensitivity reactions are rare, and acetaminophen is usually well tolerated by patients sensitive to aspirin.

Dose: Adults: (Oral) 325 mg every 4 hours as necessary.
Children: (Oral) 60 to 120 mg four times daily.

Propoxyphene Hydrochloride, USP, BP (Darvon). Propoxyphene is a synthetic analgesic that is chemically related to the narcotics but has not been shown to be addicting. It has an analgesic activity similar to that of codeine and is administered orally for the relief of mild to moderate pain.

It is often combined with aspirin (Darvon with ASA) or with aspirin, phenacetin, and caffeine (Darvon Compound) for enhancement of its analgesic effect. In combination with acetaminophen it is called Darvocet-N.

Side effects are mild and are usually limited to mild allergic symptoms. Patients sensitive to aspirin should not be given the combination products. It is not recommended for children.

Dose: Adults: (Oral) 65 mg four times daily.

Sumatriptan Succinate (Imitrex). Sumatriptan succinate acts by binding to a specific type of serotonin receptor, 5-hydroxytryptamine (5-HT). It appears to constrict blood vessels in the carotid vascular bed and also blocks nerve fibers that conduct pain.

The agent is administered by self-injection for the treatment of vascular or migraine headaches.

At first hailed as "the most" effective drug in migraine therapy, it has proven disappointing in many cases, probably because many so-called migraines are not vascular headaches at all, but are tension, cluster, or muscular contraction types instead. It effectively causes vasospasm, thus relieving the vascular headache, but its side effects also relate to vasospasm; namely, angina pectoris, hypertension, and Raynaud's phenomenon have been reported.

Dose: 6 mg self-administered SC. A second dose may be given, but no more than 12 mg in 24 hours.

Alcohol

Alcoholic beverages have been prepared and used by humans as both beverages and medicinal agents since ancient times. At one time alcohol was thought to be a remedy for practically all diseases. During the past century therapeutic usefulness has diminished greatly because of the availability of more effective and efficient agents, but its abuse as a beverage has become both a medical and a sociological problem.

Ethyl alcohol (grain alcohol) is obtained by fermentation. It is formed by the growth of yeast in fruit and vegetable juices containing sugar or starch. Undistilled beverages such as wines and beers contain less than 14% alcohol; distilled liquors such as whiskey, brandy, rum, and gin contain about 50% alcohol.

When consumed, alcohol depresses the cells of the cerebral cortex. In large quantities, its depressant action extends to the cerebellum, the spinal cord, and the respiratory center of the medulla. Alcohol kills by paralyzing the respiratory center, which controls breathing.

One effect of alcohol on the cerebral cortex is depression of inhibitory behavior. Small amounts often produce a feeling of well-being, talkativeness, greater vivacity, and increased confidence in one's abilities. Large quantities may cause excitement and impulsive speech

and behavior. The special senses become dulled, and the person cannot hear normally and thus talks louder. This sense of freedom from inhibitions has given alcohol a false reputation as a stimulant. For this reason a sedative should not be given to an individual under the influence of alcohol, because it would add to the depression of the central nervous system.

Therapeutic uses of alcohol include the following:

Dilation of peripheral blood vessels in vascular disease
Improvement of appetite and digestion
Hypnotic effect in some individuals
Local antiseptic and astringent
Analgesic when injected in or around the sensory nerve trunks for pain relief

Anticonvulsants

The condition known as epilepsy is as old as the written pages of the history of humankind. It was the "royal illness" of Egyptian pharaohs. The convulsive seizure, the sinister cry, and the loss of consciousness can be traced back to the earliest medical records. Paracelsus described epilepsy as the "disease of lightning," for the individual was struck down as if by a bolt from the sky. Actually, the disease is characterized by an increase in electrical discharges from the brain, producing an irregular pattern. The brain wave patterns obtained by taking an electroencephalogram permit diagnosis of the disease.

There are several types of epilepsy.

Grand mal or *major motor seizures* are characterized by convulsions followed by coma. Before the seizure many patients have a warning, called an aura, which most commonly is a brief hallucination of sight, smell, odor, taste, or sense.

Jacksonian epilepsy is a special subdivision of the grand mal seizure in which the convulsions usually begin in a limited group of muscles on one side and then gradually spread over the rest of the body.

Petit mal or *absence attacks* are of short duration and are characterized by a dreamy state. The patient suddenly becomes helpless and stops talking; the eyes are fixed. In a few mo-ments consciousness returns. The patient may be unaware of what has happened and may resume conversation or activity as if nothing unusual had occurred.

Complex partial seizures are disturbances of consciousness without convulsive movements. The patient performs automatic purposeless or purposeful movements, such as chewing or scratching.

The first step taken to control epilepsy was in 1857, when Sir Charles Locock gave large doses of bromides to 14 epileptic patients. In nearly all of his cases the frequency of the seizures was diminished, as was their severity. Bromides produced many toxic effects when given over an extended period of time, however, which caused their use to be restricted to some extent.

In 1912, phenobarbital was found to be even more effective than bromides in producing depression of the motor cortex and reducing the number of seizures. Phenobarbital has the disadvantage of depressing the sensory areas of the brain along with the motor areas.

The next advance was made as recently as 1921, when one compound related to the barbiturates was found to depress the motor cortex only and not the sensory areas of the brain. This compound was diphenylhydantoin (now called phenytoin). Since that time, other analogues of this drug have been made and have brought epilepsy under excellent control. As yet there is no cure for epilepsy, but the disease may be controlled.

Some of the anticonvulsants available at present include the following.

Phenytoin, USP, BP (Dilantin). This drug causes depression of the motor cortex without depression of the sensory areas of the brain. It is used to a great extent for grand mal epilepsy and often is combined with phenobarbital for more effective therapy.

The principal untoward reactions to phenytoin are dizziness, muscular incoordination, gastric distress, weight loss, and skin rashes. None of these symptoms are severe, however, and they may be overcome by temporarily decreasing the dose or perhaps stopping the drug for a short period of time.

Dose: Adults: (Oral) 100 mg four times daily.

(IV) Rate of administration should not exceed 50 mg/min.
Children: (Oral) 5 mg/kg/day in three divided doses.

Mephenytoin, USP, BP (Methylphenylethyl Hydantoin) (Mesantoin). This drug is used to control grand mal seizures. Petit mal seizures are not improved with this agent.

Dose: Adults: (Oral) 100 to 200 mg three to four times daily.
Children: (Oral) 50 to 100 mg three times daily.

Carbamazepine, USP, BP (Tegretol). This agent is used in the management of psychomotor, major motor, and focal seizures. It is ineffective in petit mal seizures. In addition it may be useful in controlling the pain of trigeminal neuralgia and other forms of neuritis.

The side effects of this agent may be dangerous and include aplastic anemia, liver toxicity, congestive heart failure, acute urinary retention, nausea, vomiting, and gastric distress.

It should not be used for the control of seizures that respond to other less toxic agents.

Dose: Adults: (Oral) 200 to 400 mg four times daily.
Children: (Oral) 10 to 20 mg/kg/day in divided doses.

Clonazepam, USP, BP (Clonopin). Clonazepam is used in the management of petit mal and myoclonic seizures.

The most frequent side effects are drowsiness, ataxia, and behavioral disturbances. Tolerance to this drug may occur.

Dose: Adults: (Oral) 1.5 to 20 mg daily in three divided doses.
Children: (Oral) 0.1 to 0.5 mg/kg/day in three divided doses.

Ethosuximide, USP, BP (Zarontin). This agent is generally considered to be the drug of choice in the management of petit mal epilepsy.

The most common side effects are nausea, vomiting, gastric distress, anorexia, drowsiness, ataxia, and irritability. Very rarely blood disturbances, including aplastic anemia, have occurred.

Dose: Adults: (Oral) 20 mg/kg/day in a single dose. Dose should not exceed 1.5 gm daily.

Methsuximide, USP, BP (Celontin). Used in the control of petit mal, this agent is often combined with other antiepileptic agents, such as phenytoin or phenobarbital, for the management of combined types of epilepsy.

It has very rarely been associated with blood dyscrasias. Minor personality changes and fluid retention have been reported.

Dose: Adults: (Oral) Initially, 300 mg/day, then increased at weekly intervals until seizure control is obtained to a maximum dose of 1.2 gm daily in divided doses.
Children: Same as that for adults.

Paramethadione, USP, BP (Paradione). This agent is used in the management of petit mal seizures that have been found to be refractory to ethosuximide. It is not helpful in the control of other forms of epilepsy, except as an adjunct to other drugs in the treatment of combined types.

Severe blood dyscrasias have been reported. Skin rashes, drowsiness, visual disturbances, and alopecia have occurred.

Dose: Adults: (Oral) 900 mg to 2.4 gm/day in divided doses.
Children: (Oral) 300 to 900 mg/day in divided doses.

Phenacemide, USP, BP (Phenurone). Phenacemide is used in the control of severe seizure disorders that have not responded to other agents. It may be used with other agents to treat combined forms of epilepsy.

This drug is highly toxic, and its use must be monitored carefully. Aplastic anemia, fatal liver necrosis, and acute psychotic states have been observed. Anorexia and weight loss, drowsiness, paresthesias, skin rashes, and headaches are commonly observed.

Dose: Adults (Oral) 1.5 to 5 gm/day in divided doses.

Children older than 5 years: (Oral) 250 mg three times daily.

Phensuximide, USP, BP (Milontin). Phensuximide is used in the management of petit mal epilepsy, although its effects often decrease during long-term therapy.

Skin rashes, alopecia, and muscle weakness have occurred. No severe blood dyscrasias have been reported with this agent.

Dose: Adults: (Oral) 500 mg to 1 gm two to three times daily.
Children: Same as that for adults.

Primidone, USP, BP (Mysoline). This agent is used primarily in the treatment of psychomotor seizures, but it has been used in major motor seizures as well.

Mild toxic effects such as drowsiness, nausea, vomiting, ataxia, and dizziness are reported. Serious toxic effects are rare.

Dose: Adults: (Oral) 250 mg to 2 gm/day in two to four divided doses.
Children: (Oral) 125 to 750 mg/day in divided doses.

Trimethadione, USP, BP (Tridione). Trimethadione is used in the management of petit mal seizures refractory to ethosuximide and may be combined with other agents for the treatment of combined forms of epilepsy.

It has been associated with severe blood disorders, but these are rare. Skin rashes, drowsiness, visual disturbances, and alopecia have been reported.

Dose: Adults: (Oral) 300 mg three times daily. It may be increased to 2.4 gm daily in divided doses.
Children: (Oral) 100 to 300 mg three times daily.

Valproic Acid, USP, BP (Depakene). This agent has been shown to be extremely useful in the management of epilepsy. It may be used alone or with other agents in the management of petit mal, and it may be used with other agents for the control of multiple seizure types.

The most frequent side effects are nausea,

vomiting, and increased appetite with weight gain. Drowsiness, skin rashes, and decreased platelet counts have been observed.

Dose: Adults: (Oral) 15 mg/kg/day to a maximum dose of 30 mg/kg/day. It may be given once daily or in divided doses.

Phenobarbital, USP, BP. Its long duration of effect after oral administration makes phenobarbital useful in a once-daily dose for the management of all forms of epilepsy except petit mal. It may be given to prevent febrile seizures and to treat acute seizure states. It has a relatively slow onset of action even when administered intravenously, however. It is often combined with other agents for control of seizures.

The primary side effect is drowsiness. However, this is often minimized by a once-daily dose administered at bedtime. There is some rather alarming evidence that the sedation or lowering of intelligence may be cumulative and progressive when this agent is used for a long period of time. It seems to be reversible if phenobarbital is discontinued, however.

Dose: Adults: (Oral) 100 to 200 mg once daily.
(IV) For status epilepticus 200 to 600 mg slowly.
Children: (Oral) 3 to 5 mg/kg/day once daily.
(IV) 100 to 400 mg slowly.

Magnesium Sulfate, USP, BP. Although not generally used to treat epilepsy, this agent, when administered intravenously, is valuable in the treatment or prevention of seizures associated with eclampsia. It has an immediate onset of action, although the duration of action is only about 30 minutes. When administered intramuscularly, the onset of action is in 1 hour and the duration 3 to 4 hours.

Magnesium intoxication may occur after therapy, with side effects of flushing, sweating, hypotension, and circulatory collapse. The disappearance of the patellar reflex is a useful early sign of intoxication.

Dose: Adults: (IV) In diluted solution of 200 mg/mL at a rate of 150 mL/min. An initial dose of 4 gm may be used. (IM) 4 to 5 gm in alternate buttocks every 4 hours.

Diazepam, USP, BP (Valium). The injectable form of diazepam has been used intravenously with remarkable success for the control of convulsions from various causes. It may be administered to halt status epilepticus, convulsions secondary to brain damage, or tetany. Valium is of little value in the long-term control of epilepsy, however. Respiratory arrest may occur with intravenous infusion. Thus, resuscitation equipment should be available.

Its oral use is discussed in a later chapter.

Dose: Adults: (IV) 2 to 10 mg slowly.

Implications for the Student

1. Cental nervous system stimulants are generally given early in the day because they may interfere with the patient's sleep pattern.

2. Central nervous system stimulants may aggravate other medical conditions such as hypertension, cardiovascular disease, and hyperthyroidism.

3. An increase in blood pressure or heart rate is often a sign of untoward effects of central nervous system stimulants.

4. Central nervous system stimulants are often habit forming and should not be used to alleviate normal fatigue or induce undue wakefulness.

5. Hyperexcitability, insomnia, and irritability may be signs of untoward effects of the central stimulants.

6. Preanesthetic agents to promote sedation aid in the successful induction of general anesthetics. Efforts should be made to maintain the patient in a calm mental condition before surgery.

7. The nurse should be available to explain the actions of the preanesthetic medication and to answer any questions the patient may have about anesthetic induction.

8. Local anesthetics may have as a side effect central nervous system stimulation and irritability. In some cases stimulation may be severe enough to produce seizures.

9. Hypnotics are given to produce restful sleep in unfamiliar surroundings such as hospitals. Nursing measures such as a back rub and the maintenance of a quiet environment may be used to promote restful surroundings as well.

10. Hangovers or continued sedation the day after a hypnotic medication should be noted. Elderly persons are particularly susceptible to sedation from these agents and may need shorter acting hypnotics.

11. Guard rails are often used to prevent accidental injuries when a patient has been prescribed a sedative or hypnotic. The patient should be instructed not to get out of bed without assistance after administration of these agents.

12. When analgesics are prescribed as occasion requires, the nurse should give the medication within the prescribed time frame but ideally before the patient experiences severe recurrence of pain. Small, frequent doses are sometimes more effective than longer spacing of larger doses.

13. Addiction is generally not a problem when narcotics are prescribed for relief of a temporary painful situation, such as postoperatively.

CASE STUDIES

1. A 70-year-old man in his second postoperative day was observed to have slow, shallow respirations and "pinpoint" pupils. His hand shook when he reached for a magazine on his overbed table. What medications do you think he had received for pain? What steps should be taken to handle this situation? Should the physician be called?

2. Donny P., 9 months old, is brought to the pediatrician's office with a temperature of 104° F and a draining left ear. The mother states that she didn't have any aspirin to give the child to control the fever. The child had a convulsive seizure during the examination. What do you think caused the temperature elevation? What was the cause of the seizure? Are there any other measures that the mother could have taken to reduce the fever?

3. A 30-year-old single woman was brought to the emergency room after taking an overdose of phenobarbital. She is unconscious. What is the most important consideration in meeting this emergency situation?

4. It has been reported that a patient in your department has not been swallowing her sleeping pills. She is depressed and possibly suicidal. What is the nurse's responsibility when administering any medication? Does the nurse have other responsibilities for this patient? What would you do in this situation?

Review Questions

1. What are the symptoms of morphine overdose?

2. Codeine sulfate is a narcotic analgesic and an antitussive. What is the meaning of the word antitussive?

3. List side effects of Butazolidin.

4. What are important signs of severe blood disorders?

5. Differentiate between a hypnotic and a sedative and give an example of each.

6. What are the symptoms of barbiturate poisoning?

7. Why would you not give a sedative to an intoxicated person?

8. Which drug is most frequently used to treat status epilepticus?

9. What precautions should a nurse take when administering potent narcotics?

10. What facilities or agencies are available in your community to rehabilitate the drug-dependent person?

C H A P T E R | **23**

Tranquilizers and Antidepressants

Objectives for the Student

B E

A B L E

T O

■ 1. Distinguish between neurosis and psychosis.
■ 2. List drugs according to the following classifications by using a pharmacology book of student's choice:
    a. Minor tranquilizer
    b. Major tranquilizer
    c. Antidepressant drugs
        (1) Tricyclic type
        (2) Monoamine oxidase inhibitor type
    d. Psychomotor stimulants
■ 3. Distinguish between a minor tranquilizer and a major tranquilizer and give two examples of each type.
■ 4. Discuss adverse effects of phenothiazine type of antipsychotic drugs.
■ 5. Discuss important uses for phenothiazine type of antipsychotic agents.
■ 6. List indications for use of the minor tranquilizers.
■ 7. Summarize important responsibilities of the nurse related to administration of minor tranquilizers.
■ 8. Summarize important responsibilities of the nurse related to administration of major tranquilizers.

In recent years many new agents having useful sedative action applicable to emotional disorders have become available. The importance of mental illness in the United States is evident by the fact that approximately one half of hospital beds are occupied by patients with this class of illness. The most satisfactory management of this problem would, of course, be aimed at the prevention of emotional and mental disorders but this will take an unknown length of time,

161

for many and varied reasons. Until humankind provides a happy, peaceful environment for itself and its offspring, devoid of practices that lead to emotional trauma and instability, we will have man-made illnesses. The religious, sociological, educational, and political factors involved in rectifying the basic problems are so numerous and complicated that progress in the prevention campaign will undoubtedly be very slow. A much more practical solution would be to learn to adjust to our problems and difficulties rather than constantly seeking to be rid of them.

Mental illnesses fall into two main categories: *neurosis*—the individual, although still in contact with reality, does not adjust favorably to surroundings and situations; and *psychosis*—the individual is out of contact with reality and is unable to communicate satisfactorily. This is severe mental illness, and the individual should be hospitalized.

Psychotherapy and psychoanalysis have been used to help the patient uncover the underlying causes of his or her illness. Other methods are electroconvulsive shock therapy and insulin shock therapy as well as treatment with the various drugs that are now available.

Among the first drugs used for these illnesses were the simple sedatives, which served to calm the patient and sometimes induced sleep. The treatment was merely a symptomatic approach, however, for it did nothing to remove the conditions causing the illness in the first place, nor did it help the patient to adjust to the circumstances.

Alcohol is a self-treatment device of this type, and mental illness is largely responsible for the problem of alcoholism. The chronic alcoholic usually has such an emotional disturbance that he or she cannot or will not tolerate life when the mental faculties are alert. The problems the individual had before he or she adopted this escape measure are now multiplied by the additional problems of the chronic alcoholism. The narcotic addict is also an individual seeking to circumvent his or her inabilities and maladjustments.

The newer drugs are more selective in their action on the brain; they tranquilize or calm the patient without necessarily depressing the entire central nervous system, or they elevate the mood without notably stimulating the central nervous system.

TRANQUILIZERS

Reserpine, USP, BP (Serpasil). In addition to relieving hypertension, this drug tranquilizes agitated, anxious, hyperactive patients. It is capable of abolishing or at least reducing anguish, needless worry, or abnormal behavior and allows the person to return to a state close to normalcy.

Dose: Adults: (Oral) 5 to 10 mg daily.

Chlorpromazine Hydrochloride, USP, BP (Thorazine). The quieting, relaxing effect of this drug was quickly appreciated, and it has gained extensive use in recent years. It shows great tranquilizing effects in emotional upsets, such as anxiety and tension; in neuroses characterized by hyperactivity, agitation, and similar affects; and in certain types of schizophrenia. The important feature of this and similar agents is that they make the patient more amenable to psychotherapy. Treatment may have been all but impossible because of the inability even to communicate with the patient, much less reason with him or her, but upon administration of the drug the patient is able to discuss problems and fears in a calm and sensible manner. However, overuse of these agents can lead to continued dependence when the patient has reached a stage in which he or she should be able to adjust to problems without reliance upon drugs.

Chlorpromazine is useful in alleviating nausea and vomiting caused by certain conditions such as carcinoma, acute infections, radiation sickness, ingestion of certain drugs (e.g., nitrogen mustard), and postoperative effects.

Some of the side effects that may occur are tachycardia, hypothermia, dryness of the mouth, parkinsonism, jaundice, liver damage, blood dyscrasias, and rashes.

Dose: Adults: (Oral, IM, Rectal) 10 to 50 mg three or four times daily.

Children: (Oral, IM, Rectal) 0.55 mg/kg four times daily.

Prochlorperazine Maleate, USP, BP (Compazine). Although effective as a tranquilizing agent, prochlorperazine is rarely used for long-term therapy because of its high incidence of extrapyramidal symptoms, such as gait disturbances, restlessness, and aberrations in muscle contraction. Occasionally even on the first dose of this drug opisthotonos occurs, with arching of the back, inability to speak, and loss of muscle control. This reaction has been confused with a certain type of epileptic seizure but differs from it upon close observation. This drug is used primarily for its antinauseant effects, particularly postoperatively. It may be given orally or intramuscularly.

Dose: Adults: (Oral, IM, IV) 5 to 10 mg three to four times daily.
Children: (Oral, IM, IV) 0.1 mg/kg four times daily.

Trifluoperazine Hydrochloride, USP, BP (Stelazine). This drug is also chemically quite similar to chlorpromazine but is more potent; thus, it can be given in lower doses. Lower doses are given to outpatients; higher doses are usually reserved for hospitalized patients.

Dose: Adults: (Oral, IM) 1 to 10 mg two times daily.
Children over 6: (Oral) 1 to 10 mg daily in divided doses.

Thioridazine Hydrochloride, USP, BP (IM 1 mg twice daily. Mellaril). The wide range of doses and the relatively low incidence of side effects experienced with this compound make it very useful as a tranquilizer. It is used for the same purposes as chlorpromazine.

Dose: Adults: (Oral) 20 to 800 mg/day in divided doses.
Children: (Oral) 0.25 mg/kg four times daily.

Meprobamate, USP, BP (Equanil, Miltown). This drug has a depressant effect on the transmission of nerve impulses inside the spinal cord and possibly in certain areas of the brain. It has a relaxant action on the skeletal muscles owing to this depressant action. It is effective as a tranquilizer in moderately tense and anxious patients. Side effects are rare and of the minor type. They include skin eruptions, fever, chills, weakness of skeletal muscles, and, occasionally, a drop in blood pressure. There is a mild addiction with prolonged use of this drug, but withdrawal effects are minimal if the drug is tapered off rather than discontinued suddenly.

Dose: Adults: (Oral) 400 mg three to four times daily.
Children older than 6 years: (Oral) 100 to 200 mg two to three times daily.

Chlordiazepoxide Hydrochloride, USP, BP (Librium). Completely unrelated to other tranquilizers chemically and pharmacologically, this agent is indicated whenever fear, anxiety, and other emotional upsets complicate the medical picture. In low oral doses, it is effective in mild to moderate anxiety and tension. It is used for premenstrual tension, chronic alcoholism, and behavior disorders and in gastrointestinal, cardiovascular, gynecological, or dermatological disorders. It is controlled by the Dangerous Drug Act.

Drowsiness, confusion, and ataxia have been reported in some patients after administration of this drug, but such effects can be avoided in almost all instances by proper dosage control.

Dose: Adults: (Oral) 5 to 25 mg three to four times daily. (IM or IV) 50 to 100 mg every 2 to 4 hours.
Children older than 6 years: (Oral) 5 to 10 mg two to four times daily.

Hydroxyzine Hydrochloride, USP, BP (Atarax, Vistaril). This drug is used for mildly anxious and tense patients and in the treatment of dermatological conditions thought to be induced by a psychogenic component. It is quite effective as an antipruritic.

Dose: Adults: (Oral, IM) 25 to 100 mg three to four times daily.
Children: (Oral) 50 mg daily in divided doses. (IM) 0.5 mg/kg/6 hours.

Diazepam, USP, BP (Valium). Diazepam is useful in the treatment of anxiety reactions stemming from stressful circumstances or whenever illness is complicated by emotional factors. It may be given to patients in psychoneurotic states manifested by anxiety, tension, fear, and fatigue as well as in acute agitation resulting from alcohol withdrawal. It appears to be of some use in the alleviation of muscle spasms associated with cerebral palsy and athetosis. It is of little use in psychotic patients. Owing to its tendency to habituation, diazepam is controlled by the Dangerous Drug Act.

Side effects include drowsiness, nausea, dizziness, blurred vision, headache, incontinence, slurred speech, and skin rash. It is contraindicated for infants, patients with a history of convulsive disorders, and patients with glaucoma.

Dose: Adults: (Oral, IM, IV) 2 to 10 mg two to three times daily.
Children: (Oral, IM, IV) 1.0 to 2.5 mg three to four times daily.

Chlorprothixene, USP, BP (Taractan). This drug has approximately the same usefulness as diazepam. It produces a higher incidence of postural hypotension as a side effect, however. Other effects are constipation, dryness of the mouth, nervousness, insomnia, and slight edema. It is contraindicated in circulatory collapse.

Dose: Adults: (Oral or IM) 25 to 50 mg three to four times daily.
Children over 6: (Oral or IM) 10 to 25 mg three to four times daily.

Chlorazepate Dipotassium (Tranxene). Chlorazepate is used in the treatment of mild anxiety and tension states. It is not recommended for severely depressed or psychotic individuals.

Side effects include dizziness, nervousness, headache, ataxia, dry mouth, skin rashes, and decreases in blood pressure. It is not presently controlled by the Dangerous Drug Act, but the possibility of dependence must be considered when this agent is prescribed for a long period of time.

Dose: Adults: (Oral) 7.5 mg four times daily.

Children: No pediatric dose established.

Fluphenazine Hydrochloride, USP, BP (Permitil, Prolixin). This agent, a structural derivative of the phenothiazine agents, may be administered orally or intramuscularly to relieve the agitation associated with schizophrenia.

This agent has a slight increase in extrapyramidal side effects compared with the earlier phenothiazines. Sedation, nausea, polyuria, headache, glaucoma, and urinary and fecal retention occur with use.

Dose: Adults and children older than 12 years: (Oral) 0.5 mg to 10 mg daily in divided doses. (IM) 1.25 mg/6 to 8 hours.
Children: Not recommended for those younger than 12 years.

Haloperidol, USP, BP (Haldol). This phenothiazine derivative is used in the treatment of psychoses, the manic phase of manic-depressive conditions, and psychotic states associated with mental retardation or organic brain disease.

Side effects resemble those of fluphenazine.

Dose: Adults: (Oral) 0.5 to 1.5 mg two to three times daily. (IM) 3.0 to 5.0 mg. Additional doses may be administered every 30 to 60 minutes until control is obtained.
Children: No pediatric dose established.

Lithium Carbonate, USP, BP (Eskalith, Lithane, Lithonate). Lithium carbonate has been found to be highly effective in the control of the manic phase of manic-depressive psychoses. Although the exact mechanism of action is not known, it is believed to alter the metabolism of norepinephrine in the brain. The full effect of this drug is not seen until after 6 to 10 days of treatment; thus, other pharmacological agents with a more rapid onset of action are often prescribed with this drug in the early phase of treatment.

Serum lithium levels should be measured frequently to avoid toxic levels of this drug. Fine hand tremor, polyuria, thirst, nausea, and diarrhea are seen at therapeutic levels of this agent. At toxic levels serious neurological and cardiovascular effects are seen.

Dose: Adults and children older than 12 years: (Oral) Initially, 600 mg three times daily, then reduced to 300 mg three times daily.
Children: Not recommended for those younger than 12 years.

Other Agents in This Class

Droperidol, USP, BP (Inapsine)

Dose: Adults: (IM, IV) 2.5 to 10 mg 30 minutes before induction of general anesthesia.
Children: (IM, IV) 88 to 165 mg/kg 30 minutes before anesthesia.

Loxapine (Loxitane)

Dose: Adults: (Oral) 10 mg twice daily.

Mesoridazine Besylate, BP (Serentil)

Dose: Adults: (Oral) 10 mg three times daily. (IM) 25 mg; may be repeated in 30 to 60 minutes.

Molindone Hydrochloride (Moban)

Dose: Adults: (Oral) 5 to 15 mg three to four times daily.

Oxazepam, USP, BP (Serax)

Dose: Adults: (Oral) 10 to 15 mg three to four times daily.

Perphenazine, USP, BP (Trilafon)

Dose: Adults: (Oral) 6 to 24 mg/day in divided doses. (IM) 5 to 10 mg one or two times daily.

Piperacetazine, USP, BP (Quide)

Dose: Adults: (Oral) 10 mg two to four times daily.

Thiothixene, USP, BP (Navane)

Dose: Adults: (Oral) 2 mg three times daily to a total of 15 mg/day. (IM) 4 mg two to four times daily.

ANTIDEPRESSANTS

The discovery of agents that can reverse depression came by accident in the search for new antitubercular agents. One of these agents, iproniazide, when used in the treatment of tuberculosis, was found to have a persistent side effect of mood elevation. The use of this parent drug for its antidepressant activity has been discontinued because of side effects, but it led to the development of a new class of psychotherapeutic agents.

Clinical depression must be separated from despondency or sadness that is the result of life events. The latter is generally founded in difficult situations and is naturally reversed in time. New work with circulating hormones in the brain has shown that chemical changes occur in clinical depression.

Running can be used as a simple antidepressant. The production of natural endorphins after vigorous exercise has been shown to give an antidepressant or even euphoric effect. This is known as the runner's "high." Some institutions are now experimenting with vigorous physical exercise as an adjunct to the treatment of mental illness.

Generally, the antidepressants clinically alter the production of natural brain hormones. In this way they are distinct from the central nervous system stimulants.

The antidepressants, because they work indirectly on the brain, may take 2 to 3 weeks to exert their effect. These agents should be used with caution when other therapeutic agents are administered, because there are many drug interactions and untoward side effects in combination.

Nonpsychiatric Use of Antidepressants

In recent years it has become evident that the concomitant use of antidepressants may help many patients cope with pain. The mechanism of action of antidepressant drug action in chronic pain syndromes is unclear. The increased serotonin level that these drugs effect is somehow associated with increased analgesia, and decreased serotonin with hyperalgesia. Antidepressants can be only one component of a comprehensive therapeutic program, and it is essential that the chronic pain patient have other goals as well (i.e., returning to work, hobbies, or other daily activities).

Currently, there are insufficient data to choose one antidepressant over another for certain types of pain. Amitriptyline and doxepin have been studied most effectively.

The antidepressants have been used prophylactically to prevent migraine headaches. They do not seem effective during the headache. They are used in the treatment of other painful conditions such as shingles (varicella zoster), cancer, fibrositis, postherpetic neuralgia, and diabetic neuropathy.

Phenelzine Sulfate, USP, BP (Nardil). The best results obtained with this drug are seen when it is used for the true depressive states: patients who are sad, worried, and sleepless and who have gloomy thoughts and feel useless. This agent takes 1 to 2 weeks to attain the full therapeutic effect.

Because this drug is a monoamine oxidase inhibitor, it may not be taken with foods that are high in amines, such as Chianti wine, cheeses such as Swiss and cheddar, chicken liver, avocados, pickled herring, figs, and alcoholic beverages. If these are combined with phenelzine, a severe increase in blood pressure occurs. Optic damage, constipation, urinary retention, hypotension, liver damage, and skin rashes have been observed with the use of this agent.

Dose: Adults only: (Oral) 15 mg three times daily.

Tranylcypromine Sulfate, USP, BP (Parnate). This antidepressant, like phenelzine, is a monoamine oxidase inhibitor, and its actions, effects, and side effects are similar.

Dose: Adults only: (Oral) 20 to 30 mg/day in divided doses.

Imipramine Hydrochloride, USP, BP (Tofranil). Although similar in effect to phenelzine, this agent has the singular property of not stimulating the central nervous system unless the individual is actually depressed. It has very little or no effect on the normal individual. Because of this property, it has been used frequently for routine treatment of the aged. On days when the elderly individual is depressed, this agent has a mood-brightening effect; when the individual is not depressed, it does not produce overstimulation. It has been used with variable success in the treatment of enuresis.

Transient atropine-like effects, especially dryness of the mouth, are rather common during the initial phase of therapy, but they disappear with continued administration. Tachycardia, constipation, dizziness, and parkinsonism occasionally occur.

Improvement is often seen within 3 to 4 days, and the maximum effect is seen within 2 weeks.

Dose: Adults: (Oral) 75 to 300 mg daily in divided doses. (IM) 100 mg/day in divided doses.
Children older than 6 years for enuresis: (Oral) 25 to 50 mg once daily 1 hour before bedtime.

Amitriptyline Hydrochloride, USP, BP (Elavil). In addition to serving as a mood elevator, this agent has a tranquilizing component that helps alleviate the anxiety that often accompanies depression. Many physicians customarily treat anxious or agitated and depressed patients with a combination of an antidepressant and a tranquilizer. This is seldom necessary when this agent is used.

Side effects, when they occur, are usually mild. Dizziness, nausea, excitement, hypotension, tremors, headache, heartburn, dryness of the mouth, and blurring of vision have been reported.

Dose: Adults and children older than 12 years: (Oral) 25 to 300 mg/day in divided doses. (IM) 20 to 30 mg four times daily.
Children: Not recommended for those younger than 12 years.

Doxepin Hydrochloride, USP, BP (Sinequan, Adapin). Doxepin has been shown to be of benefit as an antidepressant and antianxiety agent and is recommended in the treatment of alcoholism, depression neuroses, anxiety associated with various organic diseases, and some forms of insomnia. The maximum effect may not occur for 2 weeks after therapy is begun.

Side effects are drowsiness, tachycardia, hypotension, extrapyramidal symptoms, nausea, vomiting, and paresthesias. It is administered orally.

Dose: Adults: (Oral) 25 to 50 mg three times daily, or the entire daily dose may be administered at bedtime.
Children: No pediatric dose established.

Desipramine Hydrochloride, USP, BP (Pertofrane). This antidepressant is useful in the treatment of mild to moderate depressive states.

Side effects include blurred vision, urinary retention, weakness, lethargy, nightmares, and euphoria.

Dose: Adults and children older than 12 years: (Oral) 75 to 300 mg/day in divided doses.

Nortriptyline Hydrochloride, USP, BP (Aventyl). Like desipramine, this agent is used in the treatment of mild to moderate depressive states.

Side effects resemble those of desipramine.

Dose: Adults and children older than 12 years: (Oral) 75 to 300 mg/day in divided doses.

Protriptyline Hydrochloride, USP, BP (Vivactil). The action and effects of this agent resemble those of desipramine.

Dose: Adults and children older than 12 years: (Oral) 15 to 30 mg/day in divided doses.

Fluoxetine Hydrochloride (Prozac). Fluoxetine acts as an antidepressant by preventing the uptake of serotonin, thus increasing the levels of serotonin at the neuronal membrane. It is used in the treatment of major depression and, because of its anorexic effect, has a limited use in the treatment of obesity.

Dose: Adults only: (Oral) 20 to 100 mg daily.

Sertraline Hydrochloride (Zoloft). This agent lifts depression and decreases symptoms of anxiety along with alleviating symptoms of insomnia. The most common side effects are gastrointestinal, with nausea and diarrhea being the most frequent. Dizziness and headaches have been occasionally reported.

Dose: 50 to 200 mg once daily.

Venlafaxine Hydrochloride (Effexor). The advantage of this drug is its relatively short onset of action, showing some antidepressant activity in about 4 days rather than the 14 to 21 days that are common with other agents. It is well tolerated by most patients, including the elderly; occasional headaches and dry mouth have been reported.

Dose: 75 to 375 mg orally daily in three divided doses.

ANXIOLYTIC AGENTS

~ a sedative or minor tranquilizer used primarily to treat episodes of anxiety

The anxiolytic agents are used primarily for disorders caused by anxiety. These agents are generally less sedating than the tranquilizer class of agents and lend themselves to more long-term treatment with fewer side effects.

Buspirone (Buspar). The principal pharmacologic effect of this drug is anxiolysis. It has no anticonvulsant or muscle-relaxing properties, does not significantly depress psychomotor function, and has little sedative effect. It is used for the management of anxiety disorders and has been shown to be useful for long-term therapy without losing its effectiveness. Dizziness, headache, nausea, and tachycardia have been reported in some patients. It has a slow onset of action, with three to four weeks before optimum clinical results are noted.

Dose: Adults only: (Oral) 10 to 30 mg daily in divided doses.

Implications for the Student

1. Psychotherapeutic agents are among the most overly prescribed medications.

2. Natural, temporary situations promoting sadness, anxiety, or restlessness need not always be treated by a psychotherapeutic agent.

3. Endogenous depression or a generalized sadness and listlessness without apparent cause may be alleviated by antidepressants.

4. A proper diet, vigorous physical exercise, and a pleasant environment are not to be ignored in the treatment of emotional disorders.

5. Anxiety that interferes with normal functioning may be effectively treated with a tranquilizer.

6. The nurse should be available to discuss the patient's anxiety about his or her condition or reason for hospitalization. Many times the patient's fears can be calmly discussed and alleviated. The patient may fear that the physician is not telling him or her everything and that the condition is worse than he or she is being told.

7. Elderly persons generally require lower doses of psychotherapeutic agents and may experience excessive sedation when these drugs are administered.

8. Guard rails and assistance in ambulation should be added to a patient's care when tranquilizers are first administered.

9. Self-administered medication such as antihistamines and cough preparations may cause excessive sedation when combined with tranquilizers.

10. Alcohol should not be combined with tranquilizers.

11. Antidepressants require several weeks to exert their therapeutic effect in most instances. The patient should be advised of this delay when these agents are administered.

12. The potential for abuse and addiction is high when tranquilizers are administered for an extended period of time.

13. The patient should not take more than the prescribed dose when these agents are administered. He or she should be counseled to this effect, particularly when ready for discharge from the hospital.

CASE STUDIES

1. Peter P., 32, has been hospitalized in the state mental hospital for 6 months and is considerably improved after therapy and treatment with Thorazine. He has begun to walk with an increased shuffle lately, and at rest his fingers have a pill-rolling movement. Is this serious? Does the medication need to be discontinued? What could help him?

2. Mrs. H. is crying and upset owing to the sudden death of her husband. She states that her fatigue is increasing daily, and many days she does not even get out of bed and dress. She doesn't feel like cooking for herself and usually just has tea and toast during the day. What medication could be of benefit? Any other suggestions?

3. Barry P., 52, recently lost his executive position owing to a company cutback. His wife brought him into the office today. In contrast to his previous appearance, he is now unshaven, his clothes are in some disarray, and he sits sullenly on the examining table, answering very few questions and then only in monosyllables. What medicine could be beneficial?

4. Helga H., 33, had the first appointment of the morning, and before the doctor could say the first word she broke down sobbing hysterically. She states that she and her husband are having trouble, her teenage son has been experimenting with drugs and is now at the Drug Abuse Center, and, in addition, her in-laws are coming to stay for 2 weeks. She feels if she could just get by the next few weeks, things may straighten themselves out. What medication might be of benefit here?

Review Questions

1. Which tranquilizer is frequently used effectively in treating fear, anxiety, and emotional upsets?

2. Explain the term *extrapyramidal effect.*

3. List side effects that may occur when Thorazine is given.

4. Give indications for the use of Librium.

5. What are some side effects experienced from the use of Librium?

6. What are the advantages of using Mellaril?

7. What is the primary use of Compazine?

Prostaglandins and Prostaglandin Inhibitors

Objectives for the Student

B E

A B L E

T O

■ 1. Recognize the drugs that are known as prostaglandins and understand their effects in the body.
■ 2. Recognize the effect a prostaglandin inhibitor will have on a given body tissue.
■ 3. Understand bodily functions that are carried out by prostaglandins.
■ 4. Recognize inflammation as a function of prostaglandins.

The drugs in this new class of pharmacological agents were at first believed to exert their effects through the central nervous system. Many of these agents exhibit analgesic and anti-inflammatory effects.

Early drugs, such as aspirin, long believed to be central nervous system analgesics, are known now to exert their effects through the prostaglandin system.

The first report of the prostaglandins was made in the 1930s when New York gynecologists Kurzrok and Lieb noted that human semen had an ability to produce strong contraction or relaxation of the uterus. It was soon found that this unknown substance, named prostaglandin because it was believed to be produced by the prostate gland, could affect other smooth muscle as well.

It was later found that the term prostaglandin was a misnomer because these substances were widely distributed in many tissues and body fluids. They are produced close to their sites of action and are rapidly metabolized when circulating through the body.

For simplicity, these agents are named alphabetically, prostaglandin A, B, C, and so forth, and simplified as PGA, PGB, and so on.

The known prostaglandins are discussed according to the body system that they affect.

THE REPRODUCTIVE TRACT

In men, prostaglandins are believed to assist in the emptying of the seminal vesicles, thus aiding in ejaculation.

In women, prostaglandin release is believed to aid in uterine contraction during menstruation. The commercial prostaglandins are used to induce uterine contractions in elective abortions. They do not seem to be effective in the induction of labor at the end of pregnancy, however.

Dinoprost Tromethamine, USP, BP (Prostaglandin F_2 Alpha). When administered by transabdominal intra-amniotic instillation, uterine contractions begin, and abortions generally occur within 48 hours. It is used for abortions as late as the end of the second trimester of pregnancy.

Dose: 40 mg via transabdominal catheter.

Dinoprostone (Prostaglandin E_2). This prostaglandin is generally administered intravaginally along with an infusion of oxytocin to induce uterine contractions and abortion.

Dose: (Vaginal) 20 mg by suppository every 2 to 3 hours.

Dinoprostone Cervical Gel (Prepidil Gel). When administered endocervically, this agent stimulates the gravid uterus to contract. It is indicated for ripening an unfavorable cervix at or near term when there is an obstetrical need for induction. Maternal gastrointestinal upset and headaches are common side effects.

Dose: 3-gm syringe applied to the cervix.

THE CIRCULATORY SYSTEM

Cardiac output is generally increased by prostaglandins E, F, and A, but the therapeutic use of these agents has not been perfected as yet.

The primary purpose of prostaglandin E has been to keep the ductus arteriosus open in infants with congenital heart disease. This enables the newborn to retain a function of fetal circulation and enhances oxygenation of blood in some instances. (Conversely, prostaglandin inhibitors such as indomethacin, discussed later in the chapter, are used to close the patent ductus arteriosus when natural processes fail to do so in an otherwise healthy infant. This has greatly reduced the necessity of surgery in many infants.)

Alprostadil Sterile Solution (Prostin VR Pediatric). This agent is administered by intravenous infusion to keep the ductus arteriosus open. Infants with certain congenital heart deformities rely on the patent ductus arteriosus to supply oxygenated blood until they are old enough or stable enough to undergo corrective heart surgery.

This agent should not be used in infants with respiratory distress syndrome. It has been noted to cause cortical proliferation of the long bones in long-term use.

Dose: As continuous IV infusion providing 0.1 µg/kg/min.

ALLERGY AND IMMUNOLOGY

It has been shown that prostaglandins prevent the release of histamine from sensitized cells. Very low doses of prostaglandins, however, provoke the opposite response and enhance histamine release. No therapeutic agents have yet been developed to exert a predictable response in this area.

PROSTAGLANDIN INHIBITORS

Although the exact action of the prostaglandins in many areas of the body remains uncertain, it was found that many therapeutic agents exert their effects through inhibition of the prostaglandin systems.

Because prostaglandins figure prominently in the process of inflammation and are found in inflammatory exudates, it was found that the mechanism of action of many of the anti-inflammatory agents was actually to prevent the synthesis of prostaglandins at the site of inflammation.

Many old and new agents are prostaglandin inhibitors.

Aspirin, USP, Acetylsalicylic Acid, BP. Although long used as an analgesic and an anti-inflammatory agent, it is only recently that aspirin's true mechanism of action was found, and it is now believed that aspirin inhibits the synthesis of prostaglandins.

Aspirin is used to relieve mild to moderate pain, treat headaches, act as an anti-inflammatory medication in arthritic conditions, and reduce platelet aggregation, thus preventing blood clot formation. For this use, low doses of aspirin are taken daily.

A relationship has been established between children who have taken aspirin and the development of Reye's syndrome, an often fatal condition characterized by encephalopathy and liver damage. It is now recommended that aspirin not be given to children for minor febrile conditions. It is still used in inflammatory conditions such as juvenile rheumatoid arthritis, however.

Dose: Adults: (Oral, Rectal) 325 to 650 mg every 4 hours.
Children: (Oral) 65 mg/kg/day for inflammatory conditions only.

Phenylbutazone, USP, BP (Butazolidin). This agent is used for many inflammatory conditions. Its side effect of bone marrow inhibition, however, prevents its use in minor conditions.

Dose: Adults only: (Oral) 100 mg three to four times daily.

Indomethacin, USP, BP (Indocin). Used orally in the treatment of arthritis, this agent is also injected into newborns to induce closing of the ductus arteriosus.

Dose: Adults: (Oral) 25 mg three times daily.
Newborns: 0.2 mg/kg; may be given up to six times.

Tolmetin Sodium, USP, BP (Tolectin). This agent is used for arthritis and more localized inflammatory conditions such as bursitis and tennis elbow.

Dose: Adults: (Oral) 400 mg three times daily, increased as necessary to 2 gm/day.
Children: (Oral) 10 to 30 mg/kg/day in divided doses.

Ibuprofen, USP, BP (Motrin). In addition to its use as an anti-inflammatory drug, this agent is frequently used in the treatment of menstrual cramps and ovulation pain.

Dose: Adults: (Oral) 200 to 600 mg four times daily.
Children: (Oral) 100 mg four times daily.

Piroxicam, USP, BP (Feldene). The main advantage of this agent is that it has a prolonged half-life in the body and can be taken in a once-daily dose for the treatment of inflammatory conditions.

Dose: Adults: (Oral) 20 mg once daily.

Ketorolac Tromethamine (Toradol). This agent can be used intramuscularly for the relief of acute pain. In pain management studies, the overall analgesic effect of 30 mg Toradol was equivalent to that of morphine between 6 and 12 mg or 100 mg meperidine. Intramuscularly it is very effective for postoperative pain, and the patient does not experience the sedation that accompanies narcotic analgesia.

Orally, the agent is effective in mild to moderate pain and has been used for headaches, dental, and other chronic recurrent pain disorders.

Dose: (IM) 30 to 60 mg as a loading dose; then 15 to 30 mg IM every 4 to 6 hours. Maximum daily dose: 150 mg. (Oral) 10 to 20 mg every 4 hours. Daily maximum of 40 mg.

OTHER PROSTAGLANDIN INHIBITORS

Naproxen, USP, BP (Naprosyn)

Dose: Adults: (Oral) 250 mg twice daily to a maximum of 740 mg daily.
Children: (Oral) 5 to 10 mg/kg/day.

Naproxen Sodium (Anaprox)

Dose: 275 to 500 mg orally twice daily.

Fenoprofen Calcium, USP, BP (Nalfon)

Dose: Adults: (Oral) 600 mg four times daily.
Children: No pediatric dose established.

Mefenamic Acid (Ponstel)

Dose: Adults: (Oral) 500 mg initially and then 250 mg every 6 hours.
Children: No pediatric dose established.

Sulindac, USP, BP (Clinoril)

Dose: Adults only: (Oral) 400 mg daily in two divided doses.

Diflunisal, USP, BP (Dolobid)

Dose: Adults only: (Oral) 1000 mg initially and then 500 mg every 12 hours.

Diclofenac (Voltaren)

Dose: 150 to 200 mg orally in two divided doses.

Meclofenamate (Meclomen)

Dose: 1200 to 2000 mg in three divided doses orally.

Flurbiprofen (Ansaid, Ocufen)

Dose: 200 to 300 mg orally daily in two to four divided doses.

Ketoprofen (Orudis)

Dose: 150 to 300 mg orally daily in three to four divided doses.

Etodolac (Lodine)

Dose: 800 to 1200 mg orally daily in two to three divided doses.

Implications for the Student

1. Aspirin and other prostaglandin agents have as their main side effect gastric irritation. The patient should be observed for signs of gastric distress when these agents are administered.

2. Routine use of aspirin and similar drugs should be discontinued before surgical procedures, because bleeding disorders occur with prolonged use. Surgical patients should be questioned about self-administration of aspirin-containing drugs.

3. Patients allergic to aspirin should be cautioned about aspirin-containing drugs such as Darvon Compound, Fiorinal, Robaxisal, and many combination and commercial antihistamine-analgesic combinations.

4. The patient should be cautioned about signs of bleeding disorders, such as bleeding gums, black stools, and petechiae, which are side effects of these medications.

5. Fluid retention and visual problems occur as side effects of the prostaglandin inhibitors. The patient should be observed for these problems.

6. Agents in this class are best taken about ½ hour before meals to allow sufficient time for drug dissolution; the coating effect that food provides will then prevent gastric irritation.

7. Tylenol is generally preferred to aspirin in children because of the association of aspirin intake with the development of Reye's syndrome. This is particularly im-

portant in seasons when influenza and chickenpox may occur, primarily winter and spring.

8. Certain of the prostaglandin inhibitors have a cross-sensitivity with aspirin. These should be avoided in aspirin-sensitive persons.

9. In addition to the anti-inflammatory medications, the application of warm compresses and physical therapy measures may increase joint mobility in the treatment of arthritic conditions.

10. Elevations in blood pressure may signify fluid retention, which may be observed as a side effect of these medications.

11. Parents should be advised to keep aspirin and other drugs safely out of the reach of children.

CASE STUDIES

1. Susan F., age 18, has been having considerable trouble with menstrual cramps. What agents may be prescribed to aid her? She states she has used many over-the-counter preparations without relief.

2. Mrs. J.S. has been using Tylenol tablets without relief for her arthritis. The doctor told her to get aspirin, but she states that aspirin irritates her stomach and she wants to take Tylenol instead. How could you explain her drug confusion to her?

Review Questions

1. Explain why a patient who had a myocardial infarction 6 months ago may benefit from two aspirin tablets a day.

2. Review Reye's syndrome and when it occurs.

3. What drugs may be used to do the following?
   a. Induce an abortion
   b. Close a patent ductus arteriosus
   c. Keep open the ductus arteriosus
   d. Treat menstrual cramps
   e. Treat bursitis
   f. Treat rheumatoid arthritis
   g. Treat osteoarthritis
   h. Treat tennis elbow

Drugs that Affect the Autonomic Nervous System

Objectives for the Student

B E

A B L E

T O

■ 1. Explain the major effects of drugs on the autonomic nervous system.
■ 2. Define the adrenergic effects.
■ 3. Give an example of an adrenergic drug.
■ 4. Give an example of an adrenergic blocking agent.
■ 5. Define cholinergic effects.
■ 6. Give an example of a cholinergic agent.
■ 7. Give an example of a cholinergic blocking agent.
■ 8. Identify specific drugs as antihypertensive agents.

The autonomic nervous system is composed of nerves leading from the central nervous system that innervate and control smooth muscle, cardiac muscle, and glands (Figure 25–1). The actions of this system ordinarily are not subject to voluntary control.

The system is divided into two parts: the sympathetic and the parasympathetic nervous systems. In general, if one system stimulates a function, the other inhibits it. The systems oppose one another in governing the functions of smooth muscle and glands in many parts of the body.

In both systems there are two nerve cells (neurons) in each unit that leave the central nervous system and go to control the muscle or gland. The junction of these two neurons is called a synapse; a group of synapses is called a ganglion (Figure 25–2).

There is evidence that the transfer of nerve impulses at the synapse is carried out by chemicals liberated at the junctions. Acetylcholine is liberated at the ganglia of both systems and at the postganglionic parasympathetic nerve endings. Epinephrine (or norepinephrine) is liberated at the postganglionic sympathetic nerve

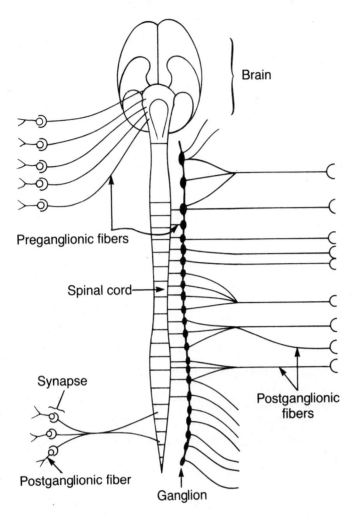

Brain

Preganglionic fibers

Spinal cord

Synapse

Postganglionic fiber

Ganglion

Postganglionic fibers

Figure 25–1. The autonomic nervous system.

endings. It is thought that these chemicals exist in the tissues and are activated or released by an impulse carried along the nerve.

Acetylcholine is rapidly inactivated by the enzyme acetylcholinesterase, and epinephrine is inactivated by the enzyme aminoxidase. The activity of these chemicals after they are liberated is short lived.

Drugs can act in four ways upon the autonomic nervous system. They may either stimulate or inhibit the sympathetic system, or they may stimulate or inhibit the parasympathetic system. Because the two systems oppose each other in action, it can be seen that, although a drug may actually act by inhibiting the action of one system (e.g., the parasympathetic system), it would actually have the same net effect as stimulation of the other system (i.e., the sympathetic system in this case).

Some of the major effects of the two systems may be compared as follows:

Sympathetic Effects

- Increase in cardiac rate and output*
- Constriction of blood vessels in skin and viscera*
- Elevation of blood pressure*
- Elevation of blood sugar*
- Relaxation of smooth muscle in bronchi
- Decrease in peristalsis
- Tightening of sphincters
- Promotion of urinary retention
- Dilation of pupils

*These are emergency reactions of the body.

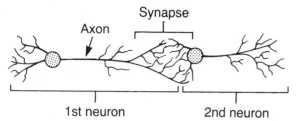

Figure 25–2. The junction of two neurons (nerve cells).

Parasympathetic Effects

- Decrease in cardiac rate and output
- Dilation of these blood vessels not pronounced
- Lowering of blood pressure
- No effect
- Constriction of smooth muscle in bronchi
- Increase in peristalsis
- Relaxation of sphincters
- Decrease in urinary retention
- Constriction of pupils

From the foregoing comparison, it can be seen that the sympathetic nervous system is the body's defense mechanism for emergency situations. The release of the sympathetic hormones is increased at these times, enabling the body to run, fight, or meet the situation at hand. The sympathetic hormones may be given to relieve an asthmatic attack because of the relaxing effect on the smooth muscle of the bronchi. The parasympathetic system is more concerned with maintaining the normal "status quo" of body operations.

SYMPATHOMIMETIC AGENTS (ADRENERGIC AGENTS)

These drugs produce or "mimic" the effects of stimulation of the sympathetic nervous system.

Epinephrine and Norepinephrine. These agents are normally produced by the adrenal medulla and at most sympathetic nerve endings. In stress situations the adrenal medulla secretes an increased amount of the hormone, accounting for the emergency reactions cited.

Therapeutically, epinephrine (Adrenalin) is used to constrict blood vessels in the eye and

nasal mucosa and to treat acute bronchial asthma and severe allergic reactions. It is perhaps the best heart stimulant in cases of heart block or acute heart failure.

These are very potent drugs, and care should be taken to be very accurate in the dosage given. When large doses are given, cardiac dilation, pulmonary edema, and cerebral accident may occur. Death may also result from ventricular fibrillation as a result of overstimulation of the myocardium.

Dose: Adults: (SC) 0.3 mg every 20 minutes or as necessary.

Levarterenol Bitartrate Injection, USP, BP (Levophed). Chemically related to epinephrine, this agent acts as an overall vasoconstrictor when given intravenously. It is used to treat hypotension and shock and may be given slowly in intravenous solutions for as long as it is needed for this purpose.

Care must be taken to prevent infiltration of the solution, because the powerful vasoconstriction produced in the skin of the surrounding areas will cause sloughing of the tissues. The best antidote for infiltration is Regitine, a sympatholytic agent, which is injected directly into the area of infiltration.

Dose: Adults: (IV) 5 µg/min.

Metaraminol Bitartrate, USP, BP (Aramine). Metaraminol is often preferred over levarterenol in the treatment of hypotension because it is not nearly as damaging to skin if it is accidentally extravasated into the surrounding tissues. If intravenous administration is not feasible in certain cases, it may even be given intramuscularly.

Dose: Adults: (IV, IM) 0.5 to 5 mg as necessary to control blood pressure.

Ephedrine Sulfate, USP, BP. In addition to the sympathomimetic actions, this agent stimulates the central nervous system. Its action is slower and weaker than that of epinephrine but more prolonged. This agent may be given orally, whereas epinephrine is usually injected.

The chief therapeutic uses of ephedrine are to

relieve nasal congestion, to dilate the pupils of the eye, and to relax hypertonic muscles in the bronchioles.

Dose: Adults: (Oral) 25 mg four times daily.

Phenylephrine Hydrochloride, USP, BP (Neo-Synephrine). Although this agent may be used parenterally for the sympathomimetic effects, its chief use is in nasal sprays and drops to relieve nasal congestion.

Dose: Adults: (Nasal) ½ to 1% solution in spray or drops 3 to 4 times/day.
Children: Same as adults.

SYMPATHOLYTIC AGENTS (ADRENERGIC BLOCKING AGENTS)

These drugs oppose or nullify the effect of stimulation of the sympathetic nervous system. The net result is similar to that obtained upon stimulation of the parasympathetic nervous system.

The adrenergic blocking agents are classified according to the receptor for which they are most specific. The two types, known as alpha and beta receptors, are found together in many types of tissue. For example, blood vessels have both alpha receptors, which cause vasoconstriction, and beta receptors, which cause vasodilation. In contrast, the heart has primarily beta receptors and almost no alpha receptors.

An alpha blocker, then, would block the alpha receptors, and a beta blocker the beta receptors. The therapeutic effects of the adrenergic blocking agents will therefore vary greatly.

Tolazoline Hydrochloride, USP, BP (Proscoline). This agent is used chiefly as a peripheral vasodilator.

Dose: Adults: (Oral) 50 mg three to four times daily.

Phentolamine Hydrochloride, USP, BP (Regitine). In addition to its use as an antidote for levarterenol infiltration, this agent has found considerable use as a diagnostic agent in the diagnosis of pheochromocytoma (tumor of the renal medulla). If a tumor exists, a significant lowering of blood pressure occurs when this drug is administered intravenously.

Dose: Adults: (IV) 5 mg.

Guanethidine Sulfate, USP, BP (Ismelin). By depressing the action of the postganglionic adrenergic nerve endings, this agent has proved effective in the treatment of hypertension. It is important that the dosage in the beginning of therapy be small because postural hypotension is often very marked when patients are treated with guanethidine. In some cases it has produced coronary or renal insufficiency, and it has been known to produce impotence. Administration is by the oral route.

Dose: Adults: (Oral) Initially 10 mg daily, then 10 to 25 mg daily, increased slowly.

Esimil. This commercial preparation is a combination of guanethidine monosulfate 10 mg and hydrochlorothiazide 25 mg. It is used to control moderately severe hypertension. It should be used with caution in patients with coronary or cerebrovascular insufficiency. Dizziness, weakness, diarrhea, impotence, vomiting, cramping, rash, urticaria, agranulocytosis, and postural hypotension have been noted on continued therapy.

Dose: Adults: (Oral) Regulated by individual needs, usually one to two combination tablets daily.

Methyldopa, USP, BP (Aldomet). Methyldopa is an antihypertensive drug that acts by interfering with the formation of the pressor amines norepinephrine and serotinin. It is used for patients with sustained moderately severe hypertension. It is not used in pheochromocytoma and is usually not used in the milder forms of hypertension that may be treated with sedatives and diuretics. It is administered by the oral route.

Side effects include hemolytic anemia, drug fever, drowsiness, weakness, aggravation of angina pectoris, dryness of the mouth, and nasal stuffiness. It should be used with caution in a patient with a history of liver disease.

Dose: Adults: (Oral) 500 mg to 2 gm daily.

Aldoril. This antihypertensive compound is available in two dosage sizes: Aldoril-15 contains in each tablet: 250 mg methyldopa, 15 mg hydrochlorothiazide; Aldoril-25 contains in each tablet: 250 mg methyldopa, 25 mg hydrochlorothiazide. The combination of the antihypertensive and a thiazide diuretic provides potentiation of effect toward the lowering of blood pressure.

Side effects are as described for the individual drugs.

Dose: Adults: (Oral) Two to four of the combination tablets daily, based on individual requirements.

Propranolol Hydrochloride, USP, BP (Inderal). This adrenergic blocking agent blocks the beta receptors in the heart and within the smooth muscles of the bronchi and blood vessels. Through its action on the heart, it decreases heart rate, decreases cardiac output, and increases cardiac volume.

The effect on the kidneys results in an increase in salt retention; thus, dietary salt must be restricted, and a diuretic is often prescribed.

This agent is useful in the treatment of hypertension because it inhibits vasoconstriction and decreases cardiac output. It is used alone or with other antihypertensive agents to control moderate to severe hypertension. In some patients it is used to manage angina pectoris resulting from coronary atherosclerosis, particularly when the patients do not respond to nitroglycerin.

Although it is not the drug of choice in the treatment of cardiac arrhythmias, propranolol has been used in the management of these patients. In some cases in which digitalis toxicity is present, this drug has been used to counteract the effects of digitalis excess.

The most common side effect is bradycardia, which may be accompanied by hypotension or shock. Severe bradycardia may be treated with atropine. It should be used with caution in patients with coronary disease, because congestive heart failure may be precipitated. Fluid reten-

tion, ataxia, dizziness, hearing loss, and visual disturbances have been noted as well as abdominal distress, rashes, and transient blood dyscrasias. It should be discontinued slowly when therapy is to be stopped to avoid rebound effects.

Dose: Adults: (Oral) Hypertension—initially, 80 mg/day in divided doses, then slowly increased to a maximum of 640 mg/day. Angina pectoris—10 to 20 mg three to four times daily, increased as necessary. Arrhythmias—10 to 30 mg three to four times daily. (IV) Arrhythmias—0.5 to 3 mg at a rate not exceeding 1 mg/min.
Children: (Oral) 0.2 to 4 mg/kg/day in divided doses. (IV) 10 to 20 µg/kg infused over 10 minutes.

Clonidine Hydrochloride, USP, BP (Catapres). After initial stimulation of adrenergic receptors, this agent then produces inhibition. It reduces blood pressure in both the supine and standing positions; thus, orthostatic hypotension upon arising is mild and infrequent. It is used in the treatment of hypertension alone or with other agents, such as diuretics.

Side effects include dry mouth, sedation, dizziness, headache, nightmares, and depression.

Dose: Adults: (Oral) 0.1 mg twice daily, increased as necessary to a maximum of 1.2 mg daily in divided doses.
Children: No pediatric dose established.

Diazoxide, USP, BP (Hyperstat). Effecting a direct vasodilation of the peripheral blood vessels, diazoxide is extremely valuable in the treatment of malignant hypertension or hypertensive crisis. It does cause salt and water retention; thus, a diuretic should be administered as well, particularly if repeated doses are to be used.

Mild hyperglycemia, orthostatic hypotension, and anginal pain, as well as gastrointestinal symptoms have been observed after administration. The patient should remain recumbent for 30 minutes after IV administration.

This agent is occasionally used orally for the treatment of hypoglycemia but is effective for hypertension in the intravenous form only.

Dose: Adults: (Oral) 3 mg/kg/day in three divided doses for treatment of hypoglycemia. (IV) 300 mg undiluted over 30 seconds.

Children: (Oral) 3 mg/kg/day in three divided doses for treatment of hypoglycemia. (IV) 5 mg/kg in one dose.

Prazosin Hydrochloride, USP, BP (Minipress). This oral agent is often used along with a diuretic in the treatment of hypertension. It may also be combined with other antihypertensive agents.

The most notable side effect of this drug is a sudden loss of consciousness or "drop attack." This may be minimized by administering low initial doses with subsequent gradual increases. Vomiting, diarrhea, nervousness, skin rashes, and insomnia have been reported.

Dose: Adults only: (Oral) 1 mg three times daily, gradually increased to a total of 20 mg/day in divided doses.

Metoprolol Tartrate, USP, BP (Lopressor). This blocking agent has a preferential effect on the beta receptors in the myocardium of the heart. It is given to reduce systolic blood pressure and has an effect on reducing the heart rate and cardiac output as well.

Dose: Adults only: (Oral) 100 mg daily in single or divided doses; may be increased to 450 mg daily.

Nadolol, USP, BP (Corgard). This agent is used to treat hypertension and angina pectoris. It is a beta-blocking agent.

Dose: Adults only: (Oral) 40 mg daily; may be increased to 320 mg daily.

Atenolol (Tenormin). This beta blocker is used in the treatment of hypertension, alone or with other agents. It reduces cardiac output and both the systolic and diastolic blood pressures.

Dose: Adults only: (Oral) 50 mg daily in one dose; may be increased to 100 mg daily.

Ergot Alkaloids. Although these agents do not lend themselves readily to classification as typical sympatholytic agents, they nevertheless do fall into this category. With the exception of ergotamine, the ergot alkaloids are used almost exclusively in obstetrics; thus, they will be discussed in Chapter 27.

Because of the similarity in the names of the ergot alkaloids, serious errors can occur if the drugs are confused.

Ergotamine Tartrate, USP, BP (Gynergen). Ergotamine is used to treat migraine headaches because of its ability to constrict the cerebral blood vessels. The periodic excruciating pain of migraine headaches is associated with factors such as stress and food allergies and is accompanied by dilation of the cerebral arterioles and later by edematous swelling of their walls. The pain is relieved by the vasoconstrictive effect of ergotamine.

Dangerous side effects can accompany too prolonged or too frequent use of this drug. Over a period of time the constriction of the blood vessels in the toes, fingers, hands, and feet causes death of the tissues, and the affected part may drop off. Constriction of the vessels in the retina of the eye may cause blindness.

Dose: Adults: (Oral) 2 mg at the onset of headache; may be repeated one or two times if necessary for relief.

Ergonovine Maleate, USP, BP (Ergotrate). This drug is used to cause contraction of the uterus and is valuable in treating postpartum hemorrhage. The dangerous similarity between the trade name for this drug, Ergotrate, and ergotamine is quite obvious.

Dose: Adults: (IM, IV) 0.2 mg repeated in 2 to 4 hours as necessary. (Oral) 0.2 to 0.4 mg two to four times daily.

Dihydroergotamine Mesylate, USP, BP (DHE 45). This synthetic drug is closely related to ergotamine, although it is less toxic and shows a lower incidence of side effects. It is very useful in the treatment of migraine headaches.

Dose: Adults: (Oral) 1 mg at onset of attack.

Methysergide Maleate, USP, BP (Sansert). Also a synthetic drug, this agent is used in the prophylactic treatment of migraine headaches. In this respect it differs from the other drugs used in the treatment of migraine headaches, because they are effective only during an attack.

Although the incidence of side effects is lower with methysergide maleate than with ergotamine, it should not be given when there is preexisting peripheral vascular disease or atherosclerosis.

Dose: Adults: (Oral) 2 mg three times daily.

PARASYMPATHOMIMETIC AGENTS (CHOLINERGIC AGENTS)

These agents "mimic" the effect of stimulation of the parasympathetic nervous system.

Because acetylcholine is so rapidly inactivated by the enzyme acetylcholinesterase, it is not used therapeutically. Instead, synthetic analogues of acetylcholine have been developed that, although they produce the parasympathomimetic effects of the natural hormone, are more resistant to the inactivating influence of the enzyme. Some drugs directly mimic the effects of acetylcholine, whereas others act by inhibiting the acetylcholinesterase and prolong the action of the natural acetylcholine.

Pilocarpine Nitrate, USP, BP (Pilocarpine Hydrochloride, USP). By stimulating the effector cells associated with the parasympathetic nerves, pilocarpine notably increases secretions, especially sweat, saliva, and nasal secretions. It is used mainly in the eye to produce miosis and to relieve pressure within the eye caused by glaucoma.

Dose: Adults: (Optic) Three to four drops of a 1 to 2% solution every 3 to 4 hours. Children: Same as that for adults.

Bethanechol Chloride, USP, BP (Urecholine). Bethanechol is similar in action to acetylcholine but is less active as well as less toxic. It is chiefly used in the treatment of postoperative abdominal distention, urinary retention, and gastric retention.

Dose: Adults only: (Oral) 10 to 30 mg three to four times daily. (SC) 2.5 to 5 mg at 15- to 30-minute intervals to a maximum of four doses.

Physostigmine Salicylate, USP, BP (Eserine). This drug inhibits acetylcholinesterase, the enzyme that breaks down acetylcholine; thus, it prolongs the effectiveness of the released acetylcholine at the nerve endings.

Although it is often used in the form of eyedrops for the treatment of glaucoma, this agent may be used whenever a parasympathomimetic drug is indicated systemically.

Dose: Adults: (Optic) One drop of a 0.02% solution several times daily. (Oral) 1 to 2 mg three to four times daily. Children: (Optic) One drop of a 0.02% solution several times daily.

Neostigmine Methylsulfate, USP, BP, Neostigmine Bromide, USP (Prostigmin). Like physostigmine, neostigmine inhibits acetylcholinesterase. It is not as potent as physostigmine but is often preferred when a drug to restore peristalsis or treat atony of the bladder is indicated. It may be used in the eye for the treatment of glaucoma also.

Dose: Adults: (Optic) One or two drops of a 5% solution. (Oral, IV) 0.25 to 0.5 mg three times daily. Children: (Optic) One to two drops of a 5% solution.

Edrophonium Chloride, USP, BP (Tensilon). The main use of this acetylcholinesterase inhibitor is as an antidote for curare and similar drugs. It increases the tone of skeletal muscles; thus, it overcomes the excessive relaxation produced by curariform agents.

Dose: Adults: (IM, IV) 10 mg.
   Children: (IM, IV) 1 to 5 mg.

Echothiophate Iodide, USP, BP (Phospholine Iodide). This drug, a so-called irreversible antiesterase, has a much more prolonged effect than physostigmine or neostigmine. It is chiefly employed in the treatment of glaucoma.

Dose: Adults: (Optic) One to two drops of 0.06 to 0.25% solution one to three times daily.
   Children: Same as adults.

PARASYMPATHOLYTIC AGENTS (CHOLINERGIC BLOCKING AGENTS)

These drugs oppose or nullify the effect of stimulation of the parasympathetic nervous system; hence, they have the same effect as stimulation of the sympathetic nervous system.

Belladonna. Three alkaloids are obtained from this plant drug: atropine, hyoscyamine, and scopolamine. Atropine is the one most often used, although there is not a great deal of difference among the actions of the three drugs.

Perhaps the most important action of the belladonna alkaloids is on the smooth muscles and the secretory glands. These drugs make tissues insensitive to acetylcholine, thus paralyzing the effects of the parasympathetic nerves. The gastrointestinal tract is relaxed and there is decreased peristalsis and muscle tone; hence, they are used as an antispasmodic in many of the various "colics." The smooth muscle of the bronchi is also relaxed, and this is accompanied by a decreased amount of secretion from the nose, pharynx, and bronchi.

Atropine Poisoning. Usually the first indications of atropine poisoning are headache, dryness of the throat and skin, dilated pupils, and dimness of vision. The skin is flushed and a rash may appear. The temperature rises because of decreased perspiration, and the pulse is rapid.

Antidote: Parasympathomimetic drugs, such as pilocarpine, gastric lavage, or tannic acid (tea). The patient should be catheterized to prevent reabsorption of the drug from the urine. The symptoms are then treated (e.g., cold sponging for fever, administration of respiratory stimulants).

Dose: Adults: (SC) Atropine 0.5 mg every 4 to 6 hours. (SC) Scopolamine 0.6 mg every 4 to 6 hours. (SC) Hyoscyamine 0.5 mg every 4 to 6 hours.

Anisotropine Methylbromide (Valpin). This oral anticholinergic drug is used as an adjunct in the treatment of peptic ulcer because it inhibits gastric acid secretion and reduces the motility of the gastrointestinal tract. For the same reasons it is frequently used in the treatment of spastic colitis.

It is contraindicated in glaucoma, obstructive disorders of the bladder or gastrointestinal tract, unstable cardiovascular disease, and myasthenia gravis. Side effects include diarrhea, drowsiness, blurred vision, tachycardia, nervousness, and skin rashes.

This agent is also available in combination form with phenobarbital (Valpin 50-PB), in which 15 mg phenobarbital is added to each tablet to provide a mild sedative effect.

Dose: Adults only: (Oral) 50 mg three times daily.

Librax. Each capsule contains 2.5 mg clidinium bromide and 5 mg chlordiazepoxide. This combination of the anticholinergic agent with chlordiazepoxide, a mild tranquilizer, is of benefit in the treatment of spastic colitis and as an adjunct in the treatment of peptic ulcer.

It is contraindicated in patients with glaucoma or bladder neck obstruction. Drowsiness, blurred vision, nausea, constipation, and blood dyscrasias have been reported as side effects. This drug should not be combined with alcohol or other sedative agents.

Dose: Adults only: (Oral) One capsule four
    times daily.

Methantheline Bromide, USP, BP (Banthine). This drug is used for patients with peptic ulcers, primarily because it decreases the motility of the gastrointestinal tract. It is also used as an antispasmodic for spastic conditions of the gastrointestinal tract. The toxic symptoms are atropine-like; urinary retention may be an undesirable side effect.

Dose: Adults: (Oral) 50 mg four times daily.

Propantheline Bromide, USP, BP (Pro-Banthine)

Dose: Adults: (Oral) 15 mg four times daily.

Oxyphencyclimine Hydrochloride, USP, BP (Daricon)

Dose: Adults: (Oral) 10 mg four times daily.

Tridihexethyl Chloride, USP, BP (Pathilon)

Dose: Adults: (Oral) 25 mg four times daily.

Combid. Each capsule of this combination drug contains 10 mg prochlorperazine maleate (Compazine) and 5 mg isopropamide iodide.

Also a combination of a tranquilizer and an antispasmodic, this agent is used to treat spastic colitis and is quite effective in controlling hyperemesis.

Dose: Adults only: (Oral) One capsule every
    12 hours.

GANGLIONIC BLOCKING AGENTS

These drugs prevent the transfer of impulses across the first ganglia of the autonomic nervous system. They are used primarily to relieve severe hypertension.

Mecamylamine Hydrochloride, USP, BP (Inversine). This agent blocks the transmission of impulses at both sympathetic and parasympathetic ganglia. It produces vasodilation, increased peripheral blood flow, and decreased blood pressure. It is used in the treatment of severe hypertension when the patient is refractory to other drugs.

Nausea, vomiting, dilated pupils, blurred vision, impotence, constipation, fatigue, and pulmonary edema have been observed.

Dose: Adults only: (Oral) 2.5 mg twice daily,
    increased gradually to a total daily
    dose of 25 mg in two to four divided
    doses.

Implications for the Student

1. The drugs that affect the autonomic nervous system are not very specific, and side effects may be observed frequently, according to which segment of the system is affected.

2. Assess the pulse and blood pressure for changes or irregularity when autonomic drugs are administered.

3. Weakness, nausea, vomiting, diarrhea, and abdominal cramps are frequent side effects of these agents. The patient should be carefully observed for these effects, which should be duly reported.

4. Blurred vision is a frequent side effect of these agents.

5. Nursing procedures may be used to alleviate certain side effects (e.g., dry mouth by the use of gum, hard candy, or lemon-glycerin mouth swabs).

6. Constipation as a side effect should be carefully monitored, and laxatives should be requested as necessary.

7. Patients who have glaucoma are unduly sensitive to the effects of anticholinergic drugs. In many cases these drugs are contraindicated in patients with glaucoma.

8. Eye discomfort or pain should be immediately reported if a patient is on anticholinergic drugs, because there may be underlying and unsuspected glaucoma.

9. Flushing and elevated temperature should be observed and reported to the physician as possible untoward effects of these agents.

10. When beta blockers are administered, bradycardia and congestive heart failure may be seen as serious toxic effects.

11. Beta blockers may increase blood sugar levels in diabetic patients on these medications.

12. When these drugs are given for the treatment of peripheral vascular diseases, signs of improvement in the patient's condition may be seen by decreased blanching of the extremities, decreased paresthesia, and improved nail bed color.

13. Postural hypotension is a common side effect of these agents. The patient should be out of bed with assistance only, particularly in the early days of treatment.

14. The patient should be observed carefully for any signs of urinary retention when on these agents.

CASE STUDIES

1. Mr. P.J., 57, has been feeling tired lately with morning headaches. He hasn't been to a doctor for 10 years, works hard, drinks somewhat excessively at times, is 30 lb overweight, but otherwise has no significant medical history. His blood pressure is noted to be 160/110. As he leaves the office, he comments that he hopes his blood pressure gets cured fast because he surely doesn't want to be on medicine when he goes to Europe this fall. Would you have any suggestions as to how he should be counseled regarding his medication?

2. Mrs. H.H., 35, has just been diagnosed as having a duodenal ulcer, as found on her upper gastrointestinal series. Her doctor prescribed a bland diet, Maalox, and Librax. She expresses to you her annoyance with her uninteresting diet (she is a gourmet cook) and secretly worries that she will become a drug addict, because a friend told her that Librax has a tranquilizer or "some kind of dope" in it. How would you help her understand her treatment?

3. Miss Grace S., a retired teacher, has had headaches for years with only minimal relief using analgesics, such as Darvon and aspirin. During this hospital admission, her physician placed her on Gynergen, which is giving her excellent results. When you take her vital signs on the evening shift you notice her massaging her hands continually. What questions should you ask? Should her physician be called?

Review Questions

1. Discuss the ways drugs act upon the autonomic nervous system.

2. What complications might result from large doses of Adrenalin?

3. Which division of the autonomic nervous system is the body's defense mechanism for emergency situations?

4. How is Aldomet classified?

5. What side effects are associated with Aldomet?

6. What is the most common side effect of Inderal?

7. What are the symptoms of atropine poisoning?

8. Differentiate between adrenergic drugs and cholinergic drugs, and give an example of each.

26

Drugs that Affect the Digestive System

Objectives for the Student

B E

A B L E

T O

- ■ 1. Identify the drug groups that affect the digestive system and give an example of one drug belonging to each group.
- ■ 2. List the various types of cathartics, and give an example of each one.
- ■ 3. Explain how fecal softeners achieve their effects.
- ■ 4. Discuss nursing responsibilities related to use of antacids and laxatives.

The digestive system is composed of organs or structures that enable food to be ingested (introduced into the system), digested (broken down into the basic components of the food), and absorbed (passed into the blood stream). The blood stream then transports the nutrients to various sites for utilization in growing tissue or producing energy.

Very simply stated, the digestive system consists of a tube within the head and trunk of the body with two external openings. Only after food is digested and has left this tube and its constituents have passed through a membrane into the blood stream may it actually be considered to have entered the body (Figure 26–1).

The tube is not of one size throughout. There are enlargements and constrictions in some areas as well as characteristic qualities at differ-

ent places. From the cells of its glands come enzymes and various chemical reagents that transform crude masses of food into simpler compounds suited for use by the body.

The intestinal part of the tract is in almost continual movement and carries on its functions without the knowledge of the individual, except in the appreciation of the strength and well-being gained from food or the periodic removal of residue from the tract.

When food is taken into the mouth, it is cut and ground by the teeth and thoroughly mixed with saliva. The saliva performs three functions: it acts as a solvent (thus making taste possible), it initiates digestion, and it lubricates the food so that it can be swallowed. Saliva contains the enzyme ptyalin, which reduces the more complex carbohydrates to simpler forms.

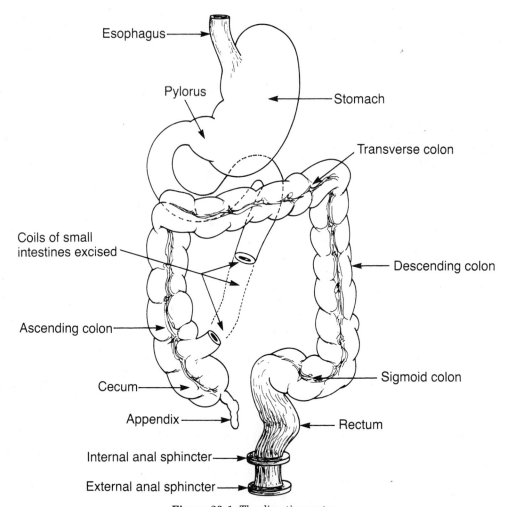

Figure 26–1. The digestive system.

In some cases saliva also contains maltase, which breaks maltose down into glucose.

The gastric juice normally contains mucin, hydrochloric acid, and the enzymes pepsin, rennin, and lipase. Mucin is a viscous fluid that tends to cling to the surface of the mucosa, serving to protect it from injury by coarse particles of food and, to a certain extent, from the action of the enzymes and hydrochloric acid. The enzymes pepsin and lipase act on protein and fat, respectively, to break these molecules into smaller, usable fractions. Rennin coagulates milk, producing a flocculent mass called the curd and clear fluid called whey. (Rennin obtained from calves' stomachs is used in making cheese because of its ability to coagulate milk.) Hydrochloric acid is necessary to provide an acid medium for the action of pepsin as well as to kill or inhibit many of the microorganisms that find their way into the stomach via food or other ingested materials.

Sometimes, however, the acid becomes so strong that it can actually erode an area of the stomach by its dissolving action. Ordinarily, the stomach is peculiarly resistant to this digestive action because of a protective coat of mucus, but under certain conditions, such as excessive or prolonged secretion of hydrochloric acid during periods of worry or stress, a small area of the surface membrane breaks down. The underlying connective tissue of the wall of the stomach is not nearly as resistant to acid as the lining membrane. The gastric juice may then eat away at the tissue and cause an open ulcer, termed a "peptic ulcer."

It is necessary to neutralize the hydrochloric acid over a period of weeks to allow the ulcer to heal. The goal of this therapy is the re-establishment of the completely intact lining membrane with its natural immunity to the action of the acid.

HELICOBACTER PYLORI AND PEPTIC ULCER DISEASE

Peptic ulcer disease has long been believed to be caused by high gastric secretion, in some cases aggravated by stress or drug therapy with gastric irritants such as nonsteroidal anti-inflammatory drugs (NSAIDs).

An infectious agent, *Helicobacter pylori,* has been found in 90% of duodenal ulcers. It has been a matter of dispute and considerable research whether there is a cause-and-effect relationship with this organism as related to peptic ulcer disease. It is believed by some that this is just an opportunistic infection of already ulcerated tissue.

In chronic peptic ulcer disease, however, it has been found that eradication of the microorganism prevents ulcer relapse in about 95% of the cases. In addition, the relationship between *Helicobacter* infection and adenocarcinoma of the stomach continues to strengthen. In some cases, eradication of the microorganism has apparently cured some malignancies.

Treatment for *Helicobacter* includes the following:

1. Bismuth products
2. Metronidazole (Flagyl)
3. Antibiotics such as doxycycline, tinidazole, amoxicillin, norfloxin, penicillin, trimethoprim-sulfamethoxazole (Septra), dicloxacillin
4. Triple therapy with all the agents listed previously
5. Antisecretory agents

Further research will undoubtedly provide better diagnostic ability and potentially the best type of treatment.

ANTISECRETORY AGENTS

Although most of the anticholinergic agents currently used as adjuncts in the treatment of peptic ulcer inhibit gastric secretion indirectly, direct inhibition of gastric secretion, particularly hydrochloric acid inhibition, is now possible.

Cimetidine, USP, BP (Tagamet). This agent inhibits the effect of histamine on the parietal cells that produce hydrochloric acid; thus, it greatly reduces acid output in the stomach.

It is used in the treatment of peptic ulcers and in Zollinger-Ellison syndrome (a combination of peptic ulcer and pancreatic tumors). Antacids may be used as well to reduce pain. Treatment with this agent is usually continued for 4 to 6 weeks. It is usually administered orally; however, intravenous therapy may be used in certain instances.

> Dose: Adults and children older than 12 years: (Oral) 300 mg four times daily with meals and at bedtime. (IV) 300 mg in diluted solution every 6 hours.

Ranitidine, USP, BP (Zantac). The primary use of this agent is to inhibit gastric acid secretion. It is used to assist in the healing of peptic ulcers and associated conditions. Ulcers are generally healed in 2 weeks.

> Dose: Adults and children older than 12 years: (Oral) 150 mg twice daily for 2 to 4 weeks.

Nizatidine (Axid). Nizatidine is a histamine H_2-receptor antagonist. It is used to inhibit the acid secretion of the parietal cells. It is indicated for treatment of active duodenal ulcer for up to 8 weeks and may be used for maintenance therapy at a reduced dose. Sweating, urticaria, and somnolence are infrequent side effects.

> Dose: 300 mg orally daily in one or two divided doses. 150 mg orally at bedtime or maintenance dose.

Misoprostol (Cytotec). This agent has both antisecretory and mucosal protective properties.

It is particularly effective in counteracting the gastric effects of NSAIDs. The NSAIDs are anti-prostaglandin agents, and, as such, they diminish bicarbonate and mucous secretion in the intestine, contributing to mucosal damage. Misoprostol counteracts these effects.

The most frequent side effects are diarrhea and abdominal pain.

Dose: 200 μg orally four times daily with food.

ANTACIDS

These agents destroy the acid either wholly or in part by neutralizing or adsorbing it and rendering it inactive.

Sodium Bicarbonate, USP, BP (Baking Soda). This is the home remedy used most often for gastric hyperacidity and heartburn. Heartburn is a burning sensation caused when some of the acid from the stomach is regurgitated into the esophagus.

Sodium bicarbonate has been greatly overused by the general public, and far too many people feel justified in using it for any number of ailments. There are many disadvantages to the use of sodium bicarbonate as an antacid. Because of its solubility it rapidly neutralizes all the acid present in the stomach and, just as rapidly, passes out of the stomach into the intestines. This frequently results in "acid rebound," or a very high secretion of acid after the rapid neutralization and alkalinization of the stomach. This may cause considerable distress shortly after the administration of the antacid. Unknowing, and thinking this distress is a recurrence of the indigestion, the individual may consume more sodium bicarbonate, thus causing the whole cycle to repeat itself. The alkaline reaction produced in the stomach also inhibits the action of pepsin because hydrochloric acid is needed to activate this enzyme.

Another undesirable effect is caused by the absorption of the sodium bicarbonate from the intestine, which produces a disturbance in the acid-base balance in the blood known as alkalosis. Alkalosis results in stress on the kidneys as they attempt to maintain the blood in stable

acid-base reaction. Renal failure may occur if the disturbance is prolonged.

A further disadvantage is the production of gas in the stomach as a result of the neutralization reaction.

$$HCl + NaHCO_3 \rightarrow NACl + H_2O + CO_2$$

The carbon dioxide thus produced causes distention of the stomach, a symptom that is quite uncomfortable and may be quite dangerous, particularly if the patient has an ulcer near the perforation point. Oral use is not recommended.

Dose: Adult: (IV) 1 ImEq/kg/dose, then titrated as necessary. Repeated doses of 0.5 mEq/kg as necessary.
Children: (IV) 1 to 5 mEq/kg/dose, then titrated as necessary.

Aluminum Hydroxide Gel, USP, BP (Amphojel, Creamalin). This gel is formed when aluminum oxide is added to water. It is insoluble and colloidal in nature and, therefore, does not have some of the undesirable effects of sodium bicarbonate. Because it is insoluble and not absorbed, it does not interfere with the acid-base balance of the blood. Because of its insolubility, its neutralization reaction is slower; thus, it eliminates the "acid rebound" caused by the faster-acting baking soda. Carbon dioxide is not produced; therefore, no abdominal distention is observed.

The colloidal particles possess absorptive properties; thus, hydrochloric acid adheres to the surface of these particles and is inactivated in this way in addition to the chemical neutralization that takes place.

Aluminum hydroxide gel is a mild astringent and demulcent. These qualities are helpful for local action in protecting and soothing the ulcer. The main disadvantage of this drug is the constipation produced, and it may actually produce a bowel obstruction in persons prone to constipation.

Dose: Adults: (Oral) 8 ml three to six times daily.

Precipitated Calcium Carbonate, USP, BP (Precipitated Chalk). This compound is given as a powder because it is insoluble in water. In the stomach it neutralizes the acid and protects the ulcer. It also has a tendency to cause constipation; therefore, commercially it is usually combined with a magnesium compound.

Marblen liquid consists of calcium carbonate, magnesium carbonate, magnesium trisilicate, and aluminum hydroxide. Andercid wafers contain calcium carbonate, magnesium trisilicate, and milk solids. These are combined in an over-baked wafer with a much more agreeable taste and texture than is found in most antacid preparations.

Dose: Adults: (Oral) 1 gm three to four times daily.

Magnesium Oxide, USP, BP. This is used quite frequently in powder form for its protective and antacid properties. In small doses it is an antacid; in large doses it is a laxative.

Dose: Adults: (Oral) (as an antacid) 250 mg three to four times daily; (as a laxative) 500 mg to 1 gm daily.

Sucralfate (Carafate). This complex of sucrose and aluminum hydroxide is used to aid in the healing of ulcers by its topical, soothing effect. It adheres to the ulcer itself, thus acting as a mechanical protectant against the action of acid and digestive enzymes.

Dose: Adults only: (Oral) 1 gm four times daily.

DIGESTANTS

Digestants are drugs that promote the process of digestion in the gastrointestinal tract and constitute a type of replacement therapy in deficiency states.

Hydrochloric Acid, USP, BP (Diluted). A deficiency of hydrochloric acid in the stomach can result from (1) a deficient secretion of the acid; (2) excess secretion of mucus, which neutralizes the acid; (3) regurgitation of alkaline substances from the intestine; (4) pernicious anemia; or (5) carcinoma of the stomach. If there is decreased secretion of hydrochloric acid from the stomach gland, the condition is known

as hypochlorhydria. If there is no secretion, it is known as achlorhydria. Achlorhydria is common in carcinoma and is also observed in pernicious anemia, infections, renal disease, and diabetes. Occasionally, it occurs in individuals apparently otherwise normal in every respect.

Dilute hydrochloric acid may be given to combat these conditions and is taken in water through a glass straw to protect the enamel of the teeth.

Dose: Adults: (Oral) 4 cc of the dilute acid.

Malt Extract. A mixture prepared from germinated barley, this extract contains dextrin, amylolytic enzymes, maltose, and glucose. It is used to aid carbohydrate digestion.

Pepsin. A proteolytic enzyme obtained from the glandular layer of a hog's stomach, this agent is given orally, often in the form of elixir of lactated pepsin, to aid protein digestion.

Dose: Adults: (Oral) 8 mL elixir three times daily.

Pancreatin, USP, BP (Enzypan, Viokase, Panteric Granules). This commercial preparation of the pancreas tissue of hogs and oxen contains all the pancreatic digestive enzymes. It is used to replace pancreatic enzymes in such conditions as cystic fibrosis and various malabsorption syndromes.

Dose: Adults: (Oral) 500 mg three times daily with meals.
Children: Same as that for adults.

Pancrelipase, USP, BP (Cotazym, Ilozyme, Pancrease, Ku-Zyme). This standardized pancreas enzyme replacement is made from hog pancreas. It has more digestive enzymes on a weight basis than does the cruder product pancreatin. It is used in cystic fibrosis and other disorders of pancreatic dysfunction.

Dose: Adults: (Oral) 900 mg with each meal and 300 mg with each snack.

Bile and Bile Salts. These agents aid in the normal digestion of fats and the absorption of fatty acids and fat-soluble vitamins. In addition, they also promote normal peristaltic activity in the intestine and restore muscle tone, producing a laxative effect.

Dose: Adults: (Oral) 150 mg three times daily.

CARMINATIVES

These agents aid in the expulsion of gas from the stomach and intestine. For the most part, they are aromatic substances that have volatile oils as the active ingredients.

In the mouth the aromatic oils increase the flow of saliva, in the stomach they promote a feeling of warmth and relaxation, and in the intestine they help relieve gaseous distention. Whiskey or brandy in hot water or a few drops of peppermint in hot water are frequently used home remedies for elderly patients.

EMETICS

These drugs produce vomiting. They are used today primarily as a first aid measure when prompt emptying of the stomach is essential. Large amounts of tepid water will distend the stomach and produce this effect, and 2 teaspoonfuls of salt or mustard in the tepid water will hasten emesis. Mild soap suds solution is also used.

The use of emetics should be avoided in cases of corrosive poisoning, because tissue damage to the mouth, pharynx, and esophagus is increased by the second passage of the material over these structures.

The use of emetics at present is limited because to a great extent they have been replaced by gastric lavage using a stomach tube.

Ipecac Syrup, USP, BP. This syrup is administered orally to produce vomiting when indicated in the management of acute poisonings. After oral administration almost all patients will vomit within 30 minutes. It is important to give additional fluids after the dose of ipecac to increase the effectiveness of the drug.

Emesis should not be produced when caustic substances, such as lye, have been ingested nor for petroleum distillate ingestion, such as gasoline, fuel oil, or paint thinners. If the second dose does not produce emesis within 30 minutes, gastric lavage should be performed.

Ipecac syrup is available without a prescription.

Dose: Children younger than 1 year: (Oral) 5 to 10 mL.
Children 1 year of age and older: (Oral) 15 mL.

Apomorphine Hydrochloride, USP, BP. This central emetic acts by direct stimulation of the vomiting center in the brain. Vomiting usually occurs within a few minutes of the injection. Large doses produce depression, however, so it should not be used for patients who are already depressed.

Dose: Adults: (SC) 5 mg.

ANTIEMETICS

These drugs relieve nausea and vomiting. Numerous preparations have been used, but ordinarily the most effective treatment must be chosen with due respect to the cause of the nausea. Vomiting may be attributed to irritation of the gastric mucosa, stimulation of the vomiting center in the brain, or possibly a combination of both.

Antiemetics readily available for home use are carbonated drinks and hot tea.

Certain types of vomiting are relieved by administering central depressants such as the bromides or barbiturates. Other agents used include the following:

Dimenhydrinate, USP, BP (Dramamine). This agent inhibits vomiting and causes sedation. It is frequently used to relieve motion sickness and control the nausea, vomiting, and vertigo associated with other conditions, such as electric shock therapy, radiation sickness, and hypertension.

Dose: Adults: (Oral) 50 mg three times daily.
Children older than 8 years: (Oral, IM) 25 mg three times daily.

Meclizine Hydrochloride, USP, BP (Bonine). This drug prevents the nausea and vomiting of motion sickness and sometimes the morning sickness of the first months of pregnancy. It is similar in action to dimenhydrinate.

Dose: Adults: (Oral) 25 mg three times daily. Children: Not recommended.

Prochlorperazine Maleate, USP, BP (Compazine). In addition to its tranquilizing effect, this agent is very effective in controlling vomiting. It is used postoperatively for this purpose, and it may also be given orally in tablet or liquid form.

Dose: Adults: (Oral, Rectal, IM, IV) 5 to 10 mg three to four times daily.
Children: (Oral) 2.5 to 5 mg two times daily.

Emetrol. A commercial preparation containing phosphorated carbohydrate solution, it acts directly on the smooth muscle of the stomach to decrease the contractions. Emetrol should not be taken with water because the local effect is greatly decreased when it is diluted.

Dose: Adults: (Oral) 8 mL as needed.

Trimethobenzamide Hydrochloride, USP, BP (Tigan). Effective orally, rectally, or parenterally, this agent is closely related to the antihistamines. It acts centrally on the vomiting center to decrease nausea and vomiting.

Dose: Adults: (Oral, IM, Rectal) 100 to 250 mg one to four times daily.
Children: (Oral) 100 mg three times daily. (Rectal) 100 mg every 8 hours.

CATHARTICS

These drugs relieve constipation, which is the condition that occurs when fecal material remains too long in the large intestine and too much water is absorbed from it. It becomes hardened, and the lower bowel becomes distended. Constipation usually results from one or more of the following causes: (1) an improper diet that leaves too little residue in the intestinal tract, (2) insufficient fluid intake, (3) nervous tension and worry, (4) lack of exercise (an important factor in hospitalized patients), or (5)

failure to respond to the normal defecation impulses. In most cases correction of one or more of these simple health rules will take care of the constipation problem. In other cases, however, laxatives should be given as an adjunct.

It is important to remember that there is no set time limit between bowel movements. Many parents become extremely upset when the child does not develop a regular habit of once every 24 hours. Continual expounding on this point can create an emotional problem in the child as well as constipation. As long as the stool is of normal consistency and as long as there is no discomfort resulting from distention after elimination, there is no constipation. Many perfectly healthy individuals may have normal eliminations no more often than every 3 or 4 days.

The administration of laxatives or cathartics of any kind must be absolutely avoided in the presence of abdominal pain, nausea, vomiting, or similar symptoms that may indicate the presence of appendicitis.

Bulk-Increasing Laxatives

These agents act by swelling when in the presence of water and mechanically stimulate the intestine to contract because of the increased volume. They usually take 24 to 48 hours for action.

Agar. This is a hydrophilic colloid obtained from seaweed. In water it swells to form a mucilaginous mass that is soothing to the gastric mucosa. It increases the bulk and keeps the intestinal contents moist and soft. It is contained in the commercial preparation Agoral.

Dose: Adults: (Oral) 4 gm.

Psyllium Seed. The powdered mucilaginous portion of these seeds swells in water to form a gel. It has a soothing effect on the mucosa and produces a soft, moist stool. It can be found in the commercial preparations Metamucil and Casyllium.

Methylcellulose, USP, BP. This compound is made synthetically from cellulose. In water it swells to form a gel. It is available in tablet or liquid form and is found in the commercial preparations Cellothyl, Cologel, and Hydrolose.

Dose: Adults: (Oral) 1 gm.

Lubricant Laxatives

These laxatives act by mixing with and softening the fecal mass but do not increase the bulk. They take 12 to 18 hours for action.

Mineral Oil, USP, BP. A mixture of hydrocarbons obtained from petroleum, it is indigestible and not absorbed. It is purely a mechanical lubricant. One disadvantage to its continued use, however, is that it prevents absorption of the oil-soluble vitamins and carries them through the intestinal tract. Mineral oil is contained in the commercial preparations Parasyllium, Petrogalar, and Agoral.

Dose: Adults: (Oral) 15 mL.

Olive Oil. This is a digestible oil that is absorbed, but when large amounts are administered, some of the oil is retained in the intestine and acts as a bulk lubricant.

Dose: Adults: (Oral) 15 mL.

Corn Oil. This is also a digestible oil with a mode of action that is very similar to that of olive oil.

Dose: Adults: (Oral) 15 mL.

Saline Cathartics

These are highly water-soluble substances that are poorly absorbed from the gastrointestinal tract. Because of their high osmotic pressure, they hold water in the tract and cause more water to be absorbed into the tract from other tissues. This greatly increases the bulk in the intestine and promotes contraction of the smooth muscle.

In addition to their use as laxatives, these agents may also be used to treat edematous conditions as well as food poisoning in which the most rapid evacuation possible is desired. They act in 1 to 4 hours, but considerable griping may be produced.

Osmotic pressure may be best explained by citing an example. An aqueous solution of sugar or salt is placed in a small, closed semipermeable (permeable to water; impermeable to the dissolved molecules) sac made of cellophane, parchment, or sausage skin and immersed in a container of water. Water from the container is drawn into the sac, but the sugar or salt solution does not pass out. The pressure within the sac increases because of the increased volume of water; the walls of the sac become distended and may rupture. The force created in this way is spoken of as the osmotic pressure.

Osmosis is the passage of water through a semipermeable membrane from a less concentrated to a higher concentrated area; this tends to dilute the more highly concentrated solution and to equalize the concentrations of the solutions on either side of the semipermeable membrane.

Magnesia Magma, USP, BP (Milk of Magnesia). The mildest of the saline cathartics, it is the agent preferred for children. In addition to its use as a laxative, if it is given in smaller doses it is an effective antacid.

Dose: Adults and children: (Oral) (as an antacid) 4 cc every few hours; (as a laxative) 15 cc at bedtime.

Magnesium Citrate Solution, USP, BP (Citrate of Magnesia). This is a fast-acting saline cathartic in liquid form. Because the solution contains a considerable amount of sugar, it should not be given to a diabetic unless this sugar is taken into consideration.

Dose: Adults: (Oral) 6 to 12 oz.

Sal Hepatica
Mineral Water
Crazy Water Crystals

Irritant Cathartics

These agents act by irritating the mucosa of the intestinal tract; thus, they produce contraction of the muscle and elimination.

Castor Oil, USP, BP. This oil is broken down

in the intestine, like any other digestible fat, to glycerin and a fatty acid. It is this fatty acid that is responsible for the irritation and the laxative effect of the oil. It is given in larger doses than are strictly needed for laxation because as soon as enough oil is hydrolyzed, laxation is produced, and the remainder of the unhydrolyzed oil gives a soothing effect to the mucosa as the mass moves through the tract.

Dose: Adults: (Oral) 15 cc.

Aromatic Cascara Fluidextract, USP, BP (cascara sagrada). One of the most extensively used cathartics, its action is comparatively mild and is less likely to produce griping than some of the other irritant cathartics. Cascara is incorporated in the commercial preparations Hinkle's Pills, Cascara Tablets, and Fluidextract of Cascara.

Dose: Adults: (Oral) 5 mL of fluidextract.

Phenolphthalein Tablets, USP, BP. An odorless, tasteless powder, this agent is conveniently incorporated in many of the candy laxatives. It has a mild irritant action unaccompanied by griping. Repeated use may cause nausea in some individuals, and a skin rash may appear. It is contained in the commercial preparations Ex-Lax and Feen-a-Mint Gum.

Dose: Adults: (Oral) 60 mg.

Dulcolax. This commercial irritant laxative is used either in tablet or suppository form.

Dose: Adults: (Oral, Rectal) 10 mg.

Fecal Softeners

Relatively new in laxative therapy, these agents are surface active agents or detergents. Their action is accomplished by mixing with the fecal material, causing it to be "wetted" by the water in the gastrointestinal tract, thereby emulsifying and softening it for easier elimination. These agents gain the desired effect without irritating the gastric mucosa and without increasing the bulk content of the intestine. For these reasons they are the agents of choice for cardiac patients.

The fecal softeners take 1 to 3 days for action; thus, they cannot be used when a faster elimination is desired. Commercial preparations containing these fecal softeners are Colace and Doxinate.

Occasionally, the surface active agent is combined with one or more of the other laxatives for a faster effect. Commercial preparations having a combination of this type are Noloc, Doxan, and Pericolace.

Dose: Adults: (Oral) One or two capsules daily.

ANTIDIARRHEALS

These agents are used to treat diarrhea, which is a symptom of a disorder of the bowel associated with too rapid passage of intestinal content, griping action, and frequent, watery stools. Some of the causes of diarrhea are (1) contaminated or partially decomposed food; (2) intestinal infection; (3) nervous disorders; (4) circulatory disturbances; and (5) inflammatory conditions of the adjacent viscera. In view of these numerous causes, the treatment of diarrhea varies greatly. In some cases even a cathartic that brings about emptying of the entire bowel may be a means of relieving the diarrhea because it removes the irritating material. If the condition is caused by an infection, the treatment must be directed toward killing the invading organisms.

Agents used for the treatment of simple diarrhea fall into two classes.

Demulcents. These agents have a soothing effect on the irritated membrane of the gastrointestinal tract. Boiled starch and boiled milk are convenient home remedies of this type. Others are acacia, glycyrrhiza, and glycerin.

Adsorbents. These agents act by adsorbing the irritating material on the surface and thereby removing it. Examples of this type are activated charcoal, kaolin, and kaolin mixture with pectin (Kaopectate). This last mixture combines the adsorbing properties of kaolin with the demulcent effect of pectin. Sometimes an agent that decreases peristalsis is added to these preparations, such as paregoric or belladonna alkaloids. Antibiotics may be combined with the adsorbents also.

Implications for the Student

1. Antacids interfere with the absorption of many drugs, particularly antibiotics. The ideal time for administration of antacids is 2 hours after a meal when the acid rebound occurs. They should be given alone, not at the time when other drugs are administered.

2. Many drugs that affect the gastrointestinal tract are liquids. They should be shaken well before administration.

3. Observe the patient for symptomatic relief when gastrointestinal drugs are being administered. This is generally noted in gastric pain and abdominal distention.

4. Dietary habits should be discussed with the patient. A bland diet that eliminates fried or spicy foods and beverages that contain alcohol or caffeine should be encouraged.

5. Liquid antacids may cause either constipation or diarrhea, depending on their composition. The patient should be observed for these effects.

6. Antiemetic drugs have as their usual side effects dry mouth, blurred vision, and urinary retention. The patient should be observed for these effects.

7. Injectable antiemetics should be administered into a large muscle mass because they are often irritating to tissues.

8. Antiemetic agents have as a primary side effect central nervous system depression. The patient should be cautioned about this effect. Concurrent administration with other depressants such as alcohol and sedative or hypnotic agents should be avoided if possible.

9. The nurse can often instruct the patient in improvement of dietary habits to include substances such as bran and fiber to eliminate the need for routine laxative therapy.

10. Laxatives are often necessary in hospitalized patients because inactivity and bed rest alter normal bowel function.

11. Laxatives are generally given to hospitalized patients at bedtime to promote effects the following morning.

12. Antidiarrheal preparations that contain paregoric or its analogues may be habit forming.

CASE STUDIES

1. Sally L., 12 years old, is brought to the physician by her mother, who reports that in spite of every laxative and food program she could think of, Sally is "constantly constipated," having a bowel movement only every 3 or 4 days. There never seems to be any problem or pain associated with the stools, but the mother is concerned that she become "regulated." What is your advice?

2. John K., 58, had a heart attack 2 months ago but is now doing well except that he is constipated. He calls the office to speak to you because he doesn't want to bother the doctor. He is just about to take a big dose of Epsom salts to "flush out his system," but his wife made him call to check with you first. What is your advice?

3. Mrs. P.F. calls the physician's office nearly frantic because her 2-year-old has eaten half a bottle of baby aspirin. The doctor is not back from lunch yet. What would you advise?

Review Questions

1. A patient is prescribed 4 mL of dilute hydrochloric acid. How will you administer it?
2. List the most common causes of constipation.
3. List and give an example of each type of laxative.
4. What are the contraindications for using baking soda as an antacid?
5. What is the main disadvantage in using Amphojel?
6. Define and give an example of the following:
   a. Emetic
   b. Carminative
   c. Digestant
   d. Antinauseant
   e. Demulcent
   f. Adsorbent

27

The Endocrine Glands and Hormones

Objectives for the Student

BE ABLE TO

- 1. Name the glands that are included in the endocrine system.
- 2. State the function of each endocrine gland.
- 3. Identify conditions caused by abnormal functioning of each endocrine gland.
- 4. Identify contraceptives that are commonly available.
- 5. Discuss side effects of the oral contraceptives.
- 6. Identify oxytocic agents and discuss precautions to be observed when these are administered.

The endocrine glands do not possess ducts or any openings to the exterior. Their secretions, called hormones, pass into the blood stream and are carried to the various tissues of the body, upon which they exert their action.

A hormone may be defined as any substance formed by a tissue of the body and carried in the blood to some tissue or organ upon which it acts.

The organs of the endocrine system, although separated physically, are unified and well integrated. The main organs belonging to this group of structures that furnish internal secretions to the body are the pituitary, the thyroid, the parathyroids, the adrenals, the gonads, and the pancreatic islets of Langerhans. The endocrine glands as well as the mammary glands and the growth of the body's skeletal system are under the control of the anterior lobe of the pituitary gland, sometimes called the "master gland."

THE PITUITARY GLAND

The anterior lobe of the pituitary, a small gland located at the base of the brain, secretes regulating hormones to other endocrine glands of the body. These regulating hormones are called the tropic hormones and are surnamed

201

according to the gland they affect (e.g., the thyrotropic hormone, the adrenocorticotropic hormone). These regulating hormones cause the endocrine glands to secrete their respective hormones into the blood stream (Figure 27–1).

THE THYROID GLAND

This gland is composed of two lobes located on either side of the larynx. The thyrotropic hormone from the anterior pituitary stimulates the thyroid gland to secrete the thyroid hormone. The exact mechanism of action of this hormone, thyroxin, is not known, but it apparently causes all cells to accelerate their rate of metabolism.

Hypothyroidism means a reduced activity of the thyroid gland. If the thyroid gland of a growing child does not function adequately, the child fails to develop normally. There are pronounced mental retardation and slow sexual development, and the skin is thickened, dry, and wrinkled. The tongue is thick and protrudes from the mouth, the abdomen protrudes, the legs are short, the hands and feet are poorly developed, and the body musculature is weak. Such a child

is called a cretin; the disorder is called cretinism.

Cretinism develops whenever the thyroid gland fails to function properly during the formative years of a child's development. For the most part, it occurs in regions having a deficiency of iodine in the drinking water and food. Cretinism may be corrected if thyroid hormone therapy is given in early infancy. If therapy is not begun until later, permanent mental retardation results.

Hypothyroidism in the adult, called myxedema, is characterized by a gradual slowing of mental and physical functions. The hands and feet are puffy, the skin is thick and leathery, and the patient is hypersensitive to cold. Good results are usually obtained by treatment with thyroid hormone, because full mental and physical development have already been achieved.

Goiter is the term applied to an enlarged thyroid gland. This increase in size may be caused by hyperthyroidism (overactivity of the gland), or it may be caused by hypothyroidism, the growth resulting then from a body "reflex" to compensate for the inefficiency of the gland. It is, therefore, impossible to predict thyroid abnormalities from the appearance of the gland.

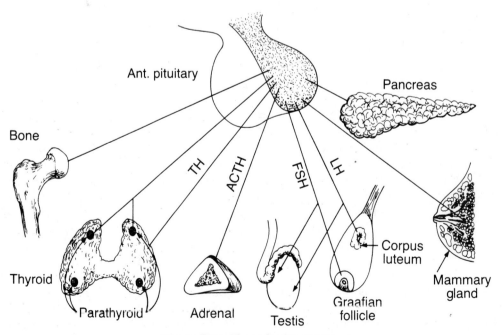

Figure 27–1. The endocrine system.

Hyperthyroidism, the condition caused by an overproduction of the thyroid hormone, is characterized by an enlargement of the thyroid gland, protruding eyes, elevation of the basal metabolic rate (BMR), disturbance of carbohydrate metabolism, nervousness, and hyperactivity. The condition is also known as Graves' disease. Hyperthyroidism may be treated with an antithyroid drug such as propylthiouracil (dose: 100 mg), methimazole (dose: 10 mg), or radioactive iodine, or else part of the gland may be removed surgically.

Thyroid Preparations

Thyroid, USP, BP. Thyroid is the cleaned and dried thyroid gland obtained primarily from hogs. It may be used in varied doses as necessary to attain thyroid function in the normal range.

The T_4 level is often used to evaluate thyroid function and therapy. The normal range is 5 to 12 μg%, with most effective range from 7 to 10 μg%.

Full thyroid replacement of normal function is 180 mg per day. Partial hypothyroidism requires smaller doses.

Dose: Adults: (Oral) Up to 180 mg daily.
Children: Same as that for adults.

Synthetic Thyroid Preparations

There is obvious natural variability in the pulverized crude gland when used for therapy; thus, the more accurate form of thyroid replacement is found in synthetic preparations. They have various potencies; a comparative dose scale follows.

Thyroid Agent	Equivalent Dose
Thyroid	60 mg (1 grain)
Levothyroxine (Levoxine, Synthroid)	100 μg
Liothyronine (Cytomel)	25 μg
Thyroglobulin (Proloid)	65 mg

Calcitonin-Salmon (Calcimar). Calcitonin is a polypeptide secreted by the parafollicular cells of the thyroid gland in mammals, birds, and fish. It is synthesized to mimic the calcitonin of salmon origin. The salmon calcitonin has greater potency and a longer duration of action than human derivatives.

Calcitonin is used to prevent bone resorption and thus is helpful in the treatment of osteoporosis, Paget's disease of the bone, and hypercalcemia.

Allergic reactions may occur with administration, as may nausea and skin rashes.

Dose: 50 to 200 IU SC daily.

THE ADRENAL GLANDS

The adrenal glands are located directly above the kidneys and are composed of two parts: an outer portion, the cortex, and an inner part, the medulla. The medullary portion secretes epinephrine and norepinephrine. The cortex secretes a number of hormones that are essential to life. Death results when this cortex is removed or severely impaired.

Some of the hormones secreted by the adrenal cortex are cortisone, hydrocortisone, aldosterone, and deoxycorticosterone. These hormones are secreted when the gland is activated by the adrenocorticotropic hormone from the anterior pituitary. The most important functions of these hormones in the body are (1) regulation of water and salt metabolism in the body; (2) regulation of carbohydrate metabolism; and (3) production of anti-inflammatory effects.

A destructive disease of the adrenal cortex in humans is known as Addison's disease. If untreated, it is gradually progressive, and death occurs within 2 or 3 years. This condition is characterized by weight loss, weakness, and disturbed carbohydrate and mineral metabolism; in addition, there is increased bronzing pigmentation of the skin. The skin may be mottled with areas of depigmentation adjacent to areas of overpigmentation. Addison's disease may be treated by administering deoxycorticosterone along with a diet high in sodium and low in potassium.

Cortisone and hydrocortisone are potent anti-inflammatory drugs. When irritation or inflammation is present anywhere in the body, there is an increase in the production of these hormones by the adrenal cortex. If the inflammation is very severe, the adrenals may be unable to secrete an adequate supply to overcome the effects. Additional hormones may be administered to the patient from another source, thus increasing the level in the circulation and affording relief from the symptoms. Cortisone and hydrocortisone are useful in the suppression of the symptoms of rheumatoid arthritis, bursitis, and various types of skin diseases.

Neither cortisone nor hydrocortisone nor any of their derivatives will cure the disease or cause any real improvement. They merely suppress the symptoms; upon withdrawal of the drug symptoms recur.

Upon continued use of these agents many side effects will occur. These are primarily salt and water retention, "moon face," muscular weakness, hirsutism, acne, and occasionally mental disturbances. Because their action is to suppress the inflammatory response of the body, this suppression occurs also when it is not desired; hence, ulcers may be perforated before the patient is aware of them and tuberculosis may advance at an alarming rate. These drugs should be used with caution in patients with peptic ulcers, and they are contraindicated for individuals suffering from tuberculosis or other severe infectious diseases.

The newer synthetic compounds are similar in action to cortisone and hydrocortisone, but to a great extent they have lessened the number and severity of the side effects produced.

Cortisone Acetate, USP, BP (Cortogen, Cortone)

Dose: Adults: (Oral) 25 mg.

Hydrocortisone, USP, BP (Hydrocortone, Cortef, Cortril)

Dose: Adults: (Oral) 25 mg.

Prednisone, USP, BP (Deltasone, Deltra, Meticorten, Paracort)

Dose: Adults: (Oral) 5 mg.

Prednisolone, USP, BP (Delta-Cortef, Hydeltra, Meticortelone, Paracortol, Sterane)

Dose: Adults: (Oral) 5 mg.

Methylprednisolone, USP, BP (Medrol)

Dose: Adults: (Oral) 4 mg.

Triamcinolone Acetonide, USP, BP (Aristocort, Kenacort)

Dose: Adults: (Oral) 4 mg.

Paramethasone Acetate, USP, BP (Haldrone)

Dose: Adults: (Oral) 2 mg.

Dexamethasone, USP, BP (Decadron, Deronil, Gammacorten)

Dose: Adults: (Oral) 0.75 mg.

Betamethasone, USP, BP (Celestone)

Dose: Adults: (Oral) 0.6 mg.

Fluocinolone A, USP, BP (Synalar)

Dose: Adults: (Topical) 0.025%.

Flurandrenolide Ointment, USP, BP (Cordran)

Dose: Adults: (Topical) 0.05%.

THE PANCREAS

Clusters of cells known as the islets of Langerhans are found on the pancreas and are the sources of the hormone known as insulin. In a normal individual insulin serves three purposes: (1) it aids in the utilization of glucose as energy; (2) it stores excess glucose as glycogen in the liver; and (3) it is responsible for the conversion of glucose to fat. However, when the pancreas does not secrete sufficient insulin to carry out these reactions, the glucose level in the blood becomes quite high after the ingestion of carbohydrates. This condition is known as diabetes mellitus.

If diabetes is not treated, sugar spills over into the urine, acidosis and ketosis occur owing to utilization of fat as energy, and the patient eventually becomes comatose and dies. The dose of insulin required to treat this condition varies from individual to individual. It is determined

Table 27-1. SYMPTOMS OF HYPERGLYCEMIC AND HYPOGLYCEMIC REACTIONS

Diabetic Coma	Regular Insulin Reaction	Protamine Zinc or NPH Insulin Reaction
Onset: Slow (days) in adults Fairly rapid in children	Sudden, rapid (minutes) Reaction occurs in daytime	Insidious, slow (hours) Reaction occurs in evening

Symptoms: Weakness, mental
    dullness
	Trembling, mental confusion,
	    weakness, drowsiness, nervousness
		Weakness, drowsiness, nervousness,
		    trembling, irritability

Frequently:
  Nausea, vomiting
  No appetite
  Thirst
  Hot, dry skin
  Abdominal pain
  Dim vision
  Deep, labored breathing
  Air hunger
  Loss of consciousness
  Fruity odor on breath
	Frequently:
	  No nausea
	  Hunger
	  No abdominal pain
	  Cold, clammy skin
	  Double vision
	  Normal or shallow breathing
	  Loss of consciousness
		Occasionally:
		  Nausea, vomiting
		
		Frequently:
		  Headache
		  Hunger
		  No abdominal pain
		  Cold, clammy skin
		  Double vision
		  Normal or shallow breathing
		  Loss of consciousness

Treatment: Check urine—high sugar
    Call doctor, who will
    prescribe REGULAR
    INSULIN
	Check urine—will contain sugar
	Keep awake: give sugar or orange
	    juice
	Call doctor
		Check urine—most likely will be sugar-
		    free
		Give sugar or orange juice for fast effect,
		    and milk, crackers, or bread for
		    prolonged effect
		Call doctor

by four factors: (1) weight of the patient; (2) metabolic rate; (3) physical activity; and (4) degree of diabetes. It is obviously very important to be accurate in the dosage of insulin because an overdose can lead to insulin shock, and too small a dose can result in diabetic coma (Table 27–1). For mild cases, diet therapy alone may be sufficient, along with regulated exercises to maintain the blood sugar level. In more severe cases, however, insulin must be given.

There are several different types of insulin (Table 27–2).

Insulin Injection, USP, BP (Regular Insulin). This is a clear, aqueous solution of insulin.

When injected, it takes effect rapidly (within 1 hour), but the disadvantage is that it is short acting; to maintain the diabetic, injections would have to be given every 3 to 4 hours. This is the type of insulin used in psychiatric insulin shock therapy (IST) and when the patient is in a diabetic coma.

Isophane Insulin Suspension, USP, BP (NPH Insulin). This is a cloudy suspension of fine crystals and is prepared to have a long-lasting effect. There is a 2-hour delay in onset after the dose is given, but the effect lasts for 28 hours. There is a more uniform blood level

Table 27-2. A COMPARISON OF THE TYPES OF INSULIN

Insulin Type	Onset (hr)	Peak (hr)	Duration (hr)
Rapid-Acting			
Regular insulin	1/2–1	2–3	5–7
Prompt insulin zinc (Semilente)	1/2–1	4–7	12–16
Intermediate-Acting			
Insulin zinc (Lente)	1–2	8–12	18–24
Isophane (NPH)	1–2	8–12	18–24
Long-Acting			
Extended insulin zinc (Ultralente)	4–8	16–18	36
Protamine zinc insulin (PZI)	4–8	14–20	36

obtained with this long-lasting form, which is safer as well as more convenient to the patient.

Protamine Zinc Insulin Suspension, USP, BP. Another long-acting insulin, this form is quite similar to NPH insulin. However, it requires 6 to 8 hours for onset after the dose is given and lasts for 28 hours. Usually the individual can be maintained on one injection daily, for the previous dose will cover the time span necessary for onset of action.

Insulin Zinc Suspension, USP, BP, Extended Insulin Zinc Suspension, USP, BP, Prompt Insulin Zinc Suspension, USP, BP. The action of zinc on insulin under specific chemical conditions gives us three forms of this delayed-action insulin. The product formed from the reaction is relatively insoluble at the pH of blood. The prompt form has the smallest particle size and, hence, has the shortest duration of action, lasting from 12 to 16 hours. The extended form has the largest particle size and a duration of action of 36 hours or more. Insulin zinc suspension is a mixture of the first two and has a duration of 24 to 48 hours. This form is used for the same purposes as NPH insulin.

Human Insulin (Humulin). Human insulin is structurally identical to endogenous insulin secreted by the human pancreas. It is not extracted from human donors but is prepared by using microorganisms and DNA recombinant technology. It may be used for the control of diabetes mellitus and does not have the allergic tendencies that insulin derived from animal sources has.

The forms of human insulin are similar to those from animal products (i.e., Regular, Isophane or NPH, Lente, and Ultralente).

Dose: (Subcutaneous) No standard dose is used. The individual requirements range from 10 to 100 units per dose and may be given one to six times a day.

Oral Hypoglycemic Agents

More recent developments have produced oral hypoglycemic agents. These are not insulin derivatives but agents that lower the glucose level in the blood.

Chlorpropamide, USP, BP (Diabinese). Although a potent oral hypoglycemic agent, this is not a routine insulin substitute. It acts on the pancreatic cells to cause them to release residual insulin. Not all patients with diabetes are suitable candidates for chlorpropamide therapy. It is essential that the patients be carefully selected by the physician because the drug would be of little value if the pancreatic cells contained little or no residual insulin to release. This drug should not be used alone in the juvenile type of diabetes or when the disease is complicated by acidosis, coma, infection, surgical procedures, or severe trauma. In these cases insulin is indispensable. Any physician using chlorpropamide should insist that the patient report at least once weekly for the first month of therapy because the initial test period should be carefully controlled. The main indication for the use of this agent is uncomplicated diabetes of the stable, mild, or moderately severe maturity onset or adult type. It may, however, be used in other types of the disease to decrease insulin requirements.

Dose: Adults: (Oral) 100 mg.

Tolbutamide, USP, BP (Orinase). Because of suspected cardiovascular difficulties with tolbutamide dosage, its recommended use has been restricted to those cases in which diet and insulin are ineffective. Its effect is similar to that of chlorpropamide.

Dose: Adults: (Oral) 500 mg.

Tolazamide, USP, BP (Tolinase). Tolazamide, another hypoglycemic agent that acts by stimulating the release of insulin from the beta cells of the pancreas, has the advantage of a longer half-life in the body; thus, in most cases patients can be maintained on once-daily oral doses. There is a low incidence of hypoglycemia with this agent, and when it occurs, it usually means that the dose is too high for the patient's needs. Nausea, vomiting, rash, pruritus, dizziness, weakness, malaise, and headache have been noted in a few cases.

Dose: Adults: (Oral) 100 to 250 mg once daily.

Acetohexamide, USP, BP (Dymelor). Another of the agents that promote the release of endogenous insulin from pancreatic beta cells is acetohexamide, which is used in the control of diabetes with onset in adulthood. Usually 7 to 10 days of oral therapy is required before a satisfactory response can be obtained.

Severe and prolonged hypoglycemia has been noted to occur with excessive dosage of this drug; thus, careful control during initial therapy is essential. It should be used with caution in patients with liver or kidney damage. Other side effects noted are nausea, gastritis, skin eruptions, headache, paresthesias, jaundice, and pancytopenia.

Dose: Adults: (Oral) 250 mg to 1.5 gm daily according to needs.

Glipizide (Glucotrol). Like the other sulfonylurea agents, glipizide lowers blood glucose levels in diabetic and nondiabetic patients. On the weight basis, it is the most potent drug in this class. It is used as an adjunct to dietary control in the management of noninsulin-dependent (Type II) diabetes.

Dose: Adults only: (Oral) 2.5 to 40 mg daily in divided doses.

Glyburide (Diabeta, Micronase). In addition to lowering blood sugar, this agent produces a mild diuresis. It is used along with dietary management to control noninsulin-dependent diabetes.

Dose: Adults only: (Oral) 1.25 to 20 mg daily in divided doses.

THE GONADS

The gonads (sex glands) of the female are the ovaries and of the male the testes. These gonads, under the stimulation of the gonadotropic hormones from the anterior pituitary gland, release the sex hormones. The same gonadotropic hormones are produced in both the male and the female, but they naturally act on different organs, and the sex hormones released by the respective glands are different. The gonadotropic hormones from the anterior pituitary are the follicle stimulating hormone (FSH) and the luteinizing hormone (LH).

Female Hormones

Figure 27–2 is a cross-section of the female reproductive organs. At maturity, FSH stimulates the maturation of the graafian follicles in the ovaries. These follicles are developed from the germinal epithelial cells that cover the surface of the ovary. Small groups of cells separate from the columns and become arranged with a large cell in the center and others in a single layer around it. These primary graafian follicles are found in great numbers in fetal ovaries and in the ovaries of children. The central, somewhat large, cell is called a primitive ovum. Under the influence of FSH the cells around the ovum produce the female hormone estradiol, which is responsible for (1) the changes in the accessory organs of reproduction during the first part of the menstrual cycle; and (2) the development of the secondary sex characteristics.

The removal of the ovaries of a young female animal prevents it from becoming sexually mature. The accessory organs fail to develop, menstruation does not occur, secondary sex characteristics do not appear, and the sex instinct is never manifested. Injection of the female sex hormone into such an animal corrects all the effects of ovariectomy.

As the follicle matures or ripens, it becomes distended by the accumulation of fluid and moves outward to the surface of the ovary. It projects from the surface of the ovary as a small cyst-like swelling that eventually bursts and discharges the ovum. In women this process is known as ovulation and occurs about every 28 days (Figure 27–3).

The cavity of the ruptured follicle becomes filled with a clot of blood that is soon replaced by a mass of cells filled with a yellow, fat-like material called lutein. The body is now called the corpus luteum, and under the developmental stimulation of LH the corpus luteum produces progesterone, which prepares the uterus for the reception of the ovum.

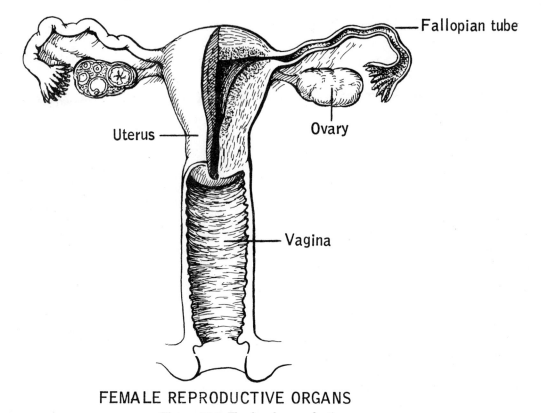

FEMALE REPRODUCTIVE ORGANS

Figure 27–2. The female reproductive organs.

Progesterone is responsible for (1) the uterine changes characteristic of the first half of the menstrual cycle (e.g., thickening of the uterine wall, increased supply of blood vessels); (2) the development of the placenta (the organ that enables the embryo to receive nourishment from the mother during pregnancy; after the birth of a child, the placenta is expelled from the uterus as the "afterbirth"); (3) the maturation of the mammary glands during pregnancy; (4) the multiplication of the uterine muscle fibers; and (5) the inhibition of uterine contraction. In

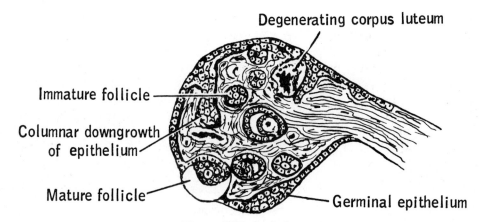

Figure 27–3. Ovulation.

short, progesterone induces favorable conditions for the growth and development of the fetus.

If fertilization occurs, the corpus luteum continues to increase in size until the later months of pregnancy, and its hormone continues to exert an influence on the growth and functional integrity of the placenta and uterus.

As the termination of pregnancy approaches, the corpus luteum disintegrates, the uterus contracts because the inhibiting influence of progesterone is no longer present, and parturition (birth) occurs.

Progesterone may be given parenterally in cases of threatened abortion. If the corpus luteum disintegrates early or if progesterone is not produced naturally because of an accident, full-term pregnancy can be brought about by administration of the deficient hormone.

If fertilization does not occur, the corpus luteum disintegrates, and the unfertilized ovum as well as the thickened uterine lining passes off in the menstrual flow.

Figure 27–4 is a diagrammatic illustration of the menstrual cycle, showing the fluctuations in hormone concentrations in the blood, the growth of the follicle and corpus luteum, and the changes in the uterine lining during the menstrual cycle.

If fertilization occurs, the placenta produces hormones that are similar to the gonadotropins produced by the anterior pituitary gland. These hormones are called the anterior pituitary-like hormones (APLH) or the chorionic gonadotropins, named after the chorion, which is the part of the placenta that develops around the fetus. The presence of these hormones in the urine is the basis for the pregnancy test.

It is necessary to give female sex hormone therapy in cases in which a deficiency of this hormone is known, because therapy brings about a normal physiological state. It is used to treat conditions such as sexual infantilism and senile vaginitis in elderly women and to provide a smooth transition during menopause.

Contrary to popular opinion, 85 percent of women have almost no symptoms at meno-

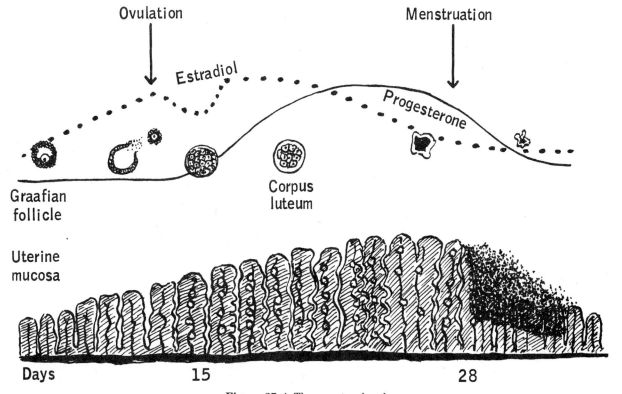

Figure 27–4. The menstrual cycle.

pause. Only one third of the remaining 15 percent have symptoms that are severe enough to warrant treatment. Although formerly hormones were used during the transition phase only, now longer term hormone therapy appears to have benefit in preventing osteoporosis and other tissue changes in postmenopausal women and is often routinely prescribed during and after the menopause. An increased risk of uterine cancer has been observed after hormone use, however.

It has also been found that estrogens in high concentration in the blood tend to inhibit the female organs; thus, estrogenic preparations may be given postpartum to inhibit lactation if the mother does not choose to nurse the infant. Commercial preparations used to suppress lactation include the following.

Chlorotrianisene, USP, BP (TACE)

Dose: Adults: (Oral) 12 mg four times daily for 7 days.

Estradiol Suspension, USP, BP

Dose: Adults: (IM) 1.66 mg daily until symptoms are controlled.

Estrone, USP, BP (Theelin)

Dose: Adults: (IM) 4.5 mg every 4 hours for five doses.

Estrogens, Conjugated, USP, BP (Premarin)

Dose: Adults: (Oral) 0.625 to 2.5 mg daily.
(IV) 25 mg daily.
(Vaginal) As cream.

Oral Contraceptives

Oral contraceptives are agents that prevent pregnancy by virtue of their estrogen content. Estrogens act to prevent ovulation by repressing the release of FSH from the anterior pituitary. The estrogens are administered in combination with progesterone to prevent the side effects of estrogen administration (i.e., breakthrough bleeding and prolonged menses).

Side effects of oral contraceptives include breast changes, loss of scalp hair, dermatoses, headache, nervousness, thromboembolic disorders, and emotional instability. Oral contraceptives accelerate the growth of preexisting uterine fibroids and cervical polyps and will accelerate the growth of preexisting breast and uterine carcinomas. They are contraindicated in patients with a history of breast or genital cancer or thrombophlebitis, myocardial infarction, or coronary artery disease or preexisting liver, kidney, or heart dysfunction. They should be used with extreme caution in patients with epilepsy.

Some of the commercially available oral contraceptives include the following.

Triphasil. This oral contraceptive consists of three different drug combinations to be taken at appropriate times during the month. It more nearly replicates the natural hormone variations.

Phase 1. (six tablets): Each tablet contains levonorgestrel 0.05 mg; ethinyl estradiol 0.03 mg.
Phase 2. (five tablets): Each tablet contains levonorgestrel 0.075 mg; ethinyl estradiol 0.04 mg.
Phase 3. (ten tablets): Each tablet contains levonorgestrel 0.125 mg; ethinyl estradiol 0.03 mg.

For other oral contraceptives, see Table 27–3.

Medroxyprogesterone Acetate, USP, BP (Depo-Provera). Medroxyprogesterone is administered intramuscularly every 3 months for contraception. The level of this progesterone-like hormone is sufficient to prevent ovulation.

Menses may cease entirely or become irregular with the administration of this agent.

Statistically, it is 99 percent effective in preventing pregnancies and is useful for women who do not wish to take oral contraceptives for any reason.

Dose: 150 mg IM every 3 months.

Levonorgestrel Implants (Norplant). This product is intended for long-term contraception and is useful for up to 5 years. It consists of a set of six flexible closed capsules that are in-

Table 27-3. ORAL CONTRACEPTIVES

Brand	Generic	Dose		
Enovid	Norethynodrel Mestranol	5 mg 0.075 mg		
Enovid-E	Norethynodrel Mestranol	2.5 mg 0.1 mg		
Ortho Novum (three strengths)	Norethindrone Mestranol	2 mg 2 mg 0.1 mg	$\dfrac{1/50}{1\text{ mg}}$ 0.05 mg	$\dfrac{1/80}{1\text{ mg}}$ 0.08 mg
Ovulen	Ethynodiol diacetate Mestranol	1 mg 0.1 mg		
Demulen	Ethinyl estradiol Ethynodiol diacetate	50 µg 1 mg		
Norlestrin (two strengths)	Ethinyl estradiol Norethindrone acetate	50 µg 1 mg	or	50 µg 2.5 mg
Ovral	Ethinyl estradiol Norgestrel	50 µg 500 µg		
Lo/Ovral	Ethinyl estradiol Norgestrel	0.03 mg 0.3 mg		

serted subcutaneously often in the upper arm. Slow release of the hormone prevents ovulation.

Most women experience bleeding irregularities after insertion of the implants.

Dose: 6 Silastic capsules each containing 36 mg of levonorgestrel, or a total of 216 mg implantation, every 5 years subcutaneously.

Agents to Promote Ovulation

Agents to promote ovulation are occasionally used as a last resort in an attempt to promote pregnancy in a woman previously unable to conceive. Only one agent is acceptable for use in the United States at this time.

Clomiphene Citrate, USP, BP (Clomid). Clomiphene is a synthetic, nonsteroidal compound that may be administered orally to promote ovulation in women who have been anovulatory. It is believed to act by promoting the release of pituitary gonadotropins, which in turn promote ovulation. Multiple pregnancies (including triplets, quadruplets, quintuplets, and sextuplets) increase 10-fold when this drug is used. Infant mortality is very high in the multiple pregnancies often because of premature delivery.

This drug is contraindicated in patients with a history of liver disease and those with abnormal uterine bleeding. Other side effects include blurred vision, hot flashes, abdominal discomfort, nausea, vomiting, breast engorgement, headache, dizziness, and skin reactions.

Dose: Adults: (Oral) 50 mg daily for 5 days.

OXYTOCIC AGENTS

Although many drugs may be used during the course of pregnancy and delivery and immediately postpartum, the drugs specifically related to obstetrics are the oxytocic agents.

Oxytocic drugs are so named because they resemble the action of oxytocin, a hormone secreted from the posterior pituitary gland.

Oxytocin Injection, USP, BP (Pitocin, Syntocinon). Oxytocin stimulates the uterine muscles and produces rhythmical contractions. Sensitivity to this drug increases as the pregnancy progresses. It is contraindicated in the first stage of labor because, if used when the cervix is undilated and rigid, severe laceration and trauma are likely. This drug is administered in small doses as an intravenous drip to induce labor, but this procedure must be carried out under close medical supervision.

Overdose of oxytocin may produce uterine tetany. The drug must be given with great caution to patients with cardiovascular disease, to those who have previously had a cesarean section, when there is a malpresentation of the fetus, or when rupture of the uterus threatens for any reason.

Dose: Adults: (IM) 3 to 10 units.
(IV) 10 units slowly in diluted solution.

Ergonovine Maleate, USP, BP (Ergotrate). The dangerous similarity in names between this ergot alkaloid and ergotamine, a drug used to treat migraine headaches, has been discussed in Chapter 25.

Like oxytocin, this drug has a constricting effect on uterine muscles, although it appears to have a greater selective action on the uterus, causing less peripheral vasoconstriction, and it acts more quickly than oxytocin. It is used for the treatment of postpartum and postabortion hemorrhage.

Chronic use of this drug may produce ergotism, a prolonged constriction of the blood vessels in other parts of the body, and may lead to gangrene and loss of the affected parts of the body.

Dose: Adults: (IM, IV, Oral) 0.2 mg every 2 to 4 hours for a total of five doses.

Methylergonovine Maleate, USP, BP (Methergine). This synthetic drug may be administered orally or parenterally to effect constriction of the uterus. Its action is similar to that of ergonovine, but it is more potent and has a more prolonged duration of action. In addition, it has less tendency to cause an elevation in blood pressure; thus, it is preferred for patients with threatened eclampsia.

Dose: Adults: (IM, IV, Oral) 0.2 mg every 2 to 4 hours for a total of five doses.

Sodium Chloride 20% Injection. Injected directly into the amniotic fluid, this concentrated sodium chloride solution is useful in the induction of second trimester abortions.

When performed correctly, there is little sodium chloride absorbed by the mother. However, it is recommended that at least 2 L of water be given to the mother before the abortion is induced. Side effects include a sensation of heat, thirst, and mental confusion, and there have been reported maternal deaths as a result of hypernatremia.

Dose: Adults: (IV) 200 to 250 mL by transabdominal intra-amniotic catheter.

Urea 40% to 50% Injection (Carbamide). Hypertonic urea, especially in conjunction with intravenous oxytocin, induces abortion and fetal death.

When the procedure is performed correctly there is little risk. However, the patient should take fluids during the procedure to facilitate urea excretion. Monitoring for signs of fluid and electrolyte imbalance should be performed throughout the procedure.

Dose: Adults: (IV) 200 to 250 ML by transabdominal intra-amniotic catheter.

Male Hormones

In the human male, as already stated, the same two gonadotropic hormones are produced by the anterior pituitary as are found in the female. In the male, however, FSH causes production of spermatozoa, whereas LH causes development of the interstitial cells that produce testosterone, the male hormone.

Testosterone is responsible for normal development of the male reproductive tract and maintains the secondary sex characteristics. It plays a role in the development of the penis, the seminal vesicles, the prostate gland, and the descent of the testes from the abdominal cavity.

The accessory sexual characteristics affected by testosterone are the depth of the voice, the distribution of facial and body hair, and the development of the masculine skeletal muscles. Muscular strength and endurance are increased immeasurably by the administration of the male hormone.

Testosterone confers a sense of "well-being" and restores mental equilibrium and energy. It can also increase the resistance of the central nervous system to fatigue. It may be used therapeutically in the following instances: (1) when a deficiency of the hormone is known; (2) in females to treat certain ovarian dysfunctions such as menorrhagia and dysmenorrhea; and (3) in females to treat breast engorgement and suppress lactation. (Some commercial preparations, e.g., Deladumone, contain a combination of estrogen and androgen for this purpose.)

Certain protein anabolic agents, for example, Nilevar (dose: 25 mg) and Dianabol (dose: 10 mg), are used to promote weight gain. These agents have a low androgenic activity but improve the appetite, develop muscle tissue, and increase the sense of well-being. They are used most often in elderly, debilitated patients.

Implications for the Student

1. When preparing the vial of insulin before giving an injection, rotate the bottle in the palm. Vigorous shaking produces bubbles, which interfere with accurate dosage.

2. Carefully measure the exact dose of insulin to be administered using a calibrated insulin syringe or a tuberculin syringe.

3. The sites of injection are to be rotated. Chart the site of injection for effective rotation.

4. Insulin may be ordered by sliding scale, depending on the glucose in the previous urine sample. It should be remembered that the glucose in the urine represents the blood level of a few hours previously. Blood samples of glucose are more accurate than urine levels.

5. It is necessary for a diabetic to follow his or her diet closely. The nurse should be familiar with dietary requirements and be available to answer any questions that the patient may have regarding the diet.

6. Vigorous exercise alters the diabetic's requirements for insulin and dietary requirements.

7. The patient who is vomiting or who has missed a meal should have the insulin requirements reduced to prevent insulin shock.

8. Infection, surgery, and physical and emotional stresses alter the requirements for insulin.

9. The diabetic patient should become familiar with the Medic-Alert tag and wear it at all times.

10. Thyroid tablets deteriorate with excessive exposure to light and moisture. The patient should be instructed in their proper storage.

11. Excessive thyroid medication will produce symptoms of hyperthyroidism, including hypertension, tachycardia, chest pain, and heat intolerance.

12. The symptoms of Cushing's syndrome are similar to the side effects experienced when a patient is administered adrenocorticoid drugs.

13. Patients should be instructed about taking oral contraceptives daily as prescribed. Pregnancy can result if pills are missed during the month. If a period does not occur at the end of the cycle, the patient should be instructed not to resume the oral contraceptive and to consult her physician.

14. Symptoms of breakthrough bleeding midcycle are seen with some of the oral contraceptives. This can often be corrected by increasing the strength of the contraceptive.

CASE STUDIES

1. Mrs. S.L., 53, is brought to the office for a checkup by her daughter. Mrs. S.L. is afraid of doctors and hasn't seen one since her last child was born 25 years ago. She is noted to speak slowly, has dry hair that is thinning in the central scalp, and has an edematous appearance to her skin. What may be her problem?

2. Mr. D.H., 57, has received Decadron for his rheumatoid arthritis for 6 months now. He is noted to have a rounder face than previously and has gained 8 pounds, although he claims he has not changed his eating habits. His arthritis is improved, but he is afraid the doctor will stop the medication because of his "side effects." What would you tell him?

3. John H., 7, was diagnosed as having diabetes mellitus 1 year ago. Since yesterday he has been vomiting and is unable to eat. This morning his mother gave him his regular insulin dose. Now, 3 hours later he is sweaty, stuporous, trembling, and nervous. What is the most likely diagnosis?

What should the mother do before she brings John to the office?

After John is recovered, the mother wants to know if John's medication can be changed to the diabetic "pills" that she has heard about so he won't have all this trouble with insulin anymore. What is your answer?

4. Jenni J., 23, has been married 1 month and comes to the office with her husband, who states that she cries all the time, although they are "deliriously happy." Jenni has been on oral contraceptives for 4 months now and takes no other medication. She also states she doesn't know why she acts this way and wants a mood elevator. What other steps might be taken?

5. Mrs. S.L., 32, has had recurrent problems with varicose veins for 8 years. Her surgeon is now speaking about vein stripping in the near future. She wants to know if she can be placed on oral contraceptives because a pregnancy would be inconvenient now that surgery is a possibility. May she?

Review Questions

1. Which type of insulin can be given intravenously?

2. Distinguish between hypoglycemic and hyperglycemic reactions.

3. What are the symptoms of hyperthyroidism, and what are some of the methods used to treat this condition?

4. What are the functions of the adrenal glands?

5. Discuss the therapeutic use of male hormones.

6. List side effects that may occur when Clomid is being taken.

7. Name the abnormalities of the thyroid gland.

8. What are the functions of the female hormones?

9. Which type of insulin is given for hyperglycemia?

10. Name three oral antidiabetic agents.

11. What are contraindications for use of "the pill"?

12. Define oxytocics.

13. What is the danger caused by prolonged use of Ergotrate?

14. Why is oxytocin not given during the first stage of labor?

15. What other precautions must be taken in the use of oxytocin?

16. What is the nurse's responsibility when oxytocics are administered?

17. For what purpose are prostaglandins used?

Diuretics and Drugs that Affect the Urinary System

Objectives for the Student

■ 1. Give an example of each type of diuretic.
■ 2. Discuss the ability of the kidney to regulate output.
■ 3. Explain the importance of antidiuretic hormone for the excretion of urine.
■ 4. Discuss nursing responsibilities for the administration of diuretics.
■ 5. Name three drugs that are used to treat enuresis.

The kidney is the principal organ of the body involved with water balance. If the output of water from the body exceeds the water intake, the body is said to be in a negative water balance. This imbalance leads to dehydration of the body. In the other extreme, a positive water balance occurs when the intake of water exceeds the output. Ordinarily, however, the body maintains a balance between the water ingested and the water excreted.

In addition to excretion via the kidney, water may also be lost by diffusion through the skin, by insensible perspiration, or by sensible perspiration that involves the sweat glands. Sweat, or sensible perspiration, consists of a weak solution of sodium chloride and a few other substances. It is possible to lose 3000 mL of water through the skin in 24 hours when both sensible and insensible perspiration routes are active.

The kidney has the ability to regulate its output according to the amount of fluid ingested and the amounts lost by other routes from the body. Thus, in very warm weather the output from the kidneys is considerably less than it is in cool weather.

The kidney consists of more than 1 million functional units, or nephrons (Figure 28–1). The nephron is composed of a tuft of capillaries, called a glomerulus, which is encapsulated in a cup-like structure, the Bowman's capsule. Wa-

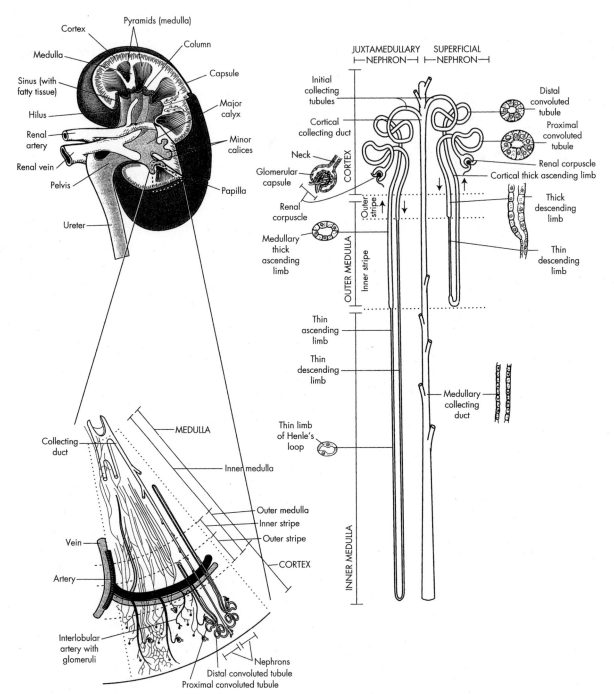

Figure 28–1. The structure of the kidney. (Reprinted with permission from Dorland's Illustrated Medical Dictionary, 28th ed. Philadelphia, W. B. Saunders Co., 1994.)

ter, salts, and waste products can filter through the thin walls of the capillaries into the Bowman's capsule and through the series of collecting tubules to the pelvis of the kidney. The renal pelvis opens into the ureter, the ureter leads to the bladder, and from the bladder excretion is accomplished via the urethra.

A great deal more fluid is filtered into the Bowman's capsule than is excreted in the urine, however. This is because much of the fluid is reabsorbed where the collecting tubule from the Bowman's capsule circles back through another capillary bed on its way to the renal pelvis. It is estimated that for every 125 mL of fluid filtered through the glomerulus, only 1 mL is eventually secreted.

Reabsorption of the filtered fluid is largely due to the influence of the antidiuretic hormone from the posterior pituitary gland. Diabetes insipidus is a disease in which this hormone is missing or present in inadequate amounts. This disease is characterized by the excretion of copious amounts of urine—sometimes 10 to 12 L a day. This condition is treated by the administration of posterior pituitary hormone.

DIURETICS

A diuretic is a drug that increases the flow of urine. These drugs are often used to rid the body of sodium as well because it causes edema if it is retained in the body fluids in excessive amounts.

We consider diuretics under the following headings: (1) osmotic diuretics, (2) acid-forming diuretics, (3) xanthine diuretics, (4) carbonic anhydrase inhibitors, (5) thiazide diuretics, (6) steroid antagonists, and (7) miscellaneous diuretics.

Osmotic Diuretics

Potassium Salts. Potassium salts, such as potassium chloride and potassium nitrate, may be used to replace a potassium deficit in the body, but if given in sufficient quantities they act as diuretics because the kidney tends to excrete excessive amounts of this salt when it is present in the blood. No salt can be excreted without an accompanying amount of water; thus, potassium effectively pulls water along to increase urine flow.

Potassium salts should be given with caution to avoid the toxic effects of excessive amounts of potassium. They should not be given if there is evidence of renal disease, in Addison's disease, or on the first postoperative day unless the serum potassium is low.

Dose: Adults: Potassium chloride: (IV) 1.5 to 3 gm daily. (20 to 40 mEq). (Oral) 2 to 10 gm daily.
Adults: Potassium nitrate: (Oral) 2 to 10 gm daily.

Urea, USP, BP (Urevert, Carbamide). Although it is a normal constituent of body fluids, urea serves as an osmotic diuretic when administered in sufficiently large doses. Most of the urea administered remains in the glomerular filtrate and is not reabsorbed; thus, it also holds water in the tubule and increases the urine output.

Urea should not be administered when there is evidence of renal disease characterized by nitrogen retention.

Dose: Adults: (IV) 8 to 20 gm three times daily.

Glucose, USP, BP. Ordinarily, all the glucose secreted into the Bowman's capsule is reabsorbed before the filtered fluid reaches the pelvis of the kidney. When excessive amounts are present in the blood, however, the amount of glucose exceeds the renal threshold (the maximum amount that can be reabsorbed by the kidney), and glucose spills over into the urine. This happens regularly in the uncorrected diabetic and will also occur if large doses of glucose are administered. Glucose then acts as an osmotic diuretic and holds water in the tubules as well; thus, it increases the amount of urine secreted.

Large or repeated doses of glucose may cause renal damage; therefore, the use of glucose as a diuretic has largely been replaced by newer and safer diuretics.

Dose: Adults: (IV) 50 mL of a 50% solution.

Acid-Forming Diuretics

Because one of the functions of the kidney is to maintain a proper acid-base balance in the body, the use of drugs that increase the acidity of the blood plasma will tend to cause secretion of the acid-forming substance with an appropriate amount of water.

Ammonium Chloride, USP, BP. After ammonium chloride is absorbed, it is converted to urea in the liver, and consequently chloride and hydrogen ions are released. The buffering mechanisms of the body are put into action, and eventually the chloride ions are excreted in the urine in increased amounts with an accompanying amount of water. Compensatory mechanisms of the body are soon brought into play, however, and the diuresis brought about by ammonium chloride lasts for only a few days; then the urine volume returns to normal. The ammonium chloride should be discontinued for a few days and then administered again for a diuretic effect.

Ammonium chloride should not be given unless the kidney function is normal, because there is a danger that uncompensated acidosis may occur.

Dose: Adults: (Oral) 4 to 12 gm daily.

Xanthine Diuretics

Xanthine diuretics are so named because of their basic chemical structure. Caffeine, theobromine, and theophylline all have this basic xanthine structure and all act as diuretics, but theophylline is the most potent—it is the only one used clinically for its diuretic effect.

Theophylline Ethylenediamine, USP, BP (Aminophylline). Theophylline is combined with ethylenediamine to increase its solubility and usefulness in the body. This drug has other uses in the body in addition to its use as a diuretic. It is quite effective in relaxing the smooth muscle of the bronchi and is administered for the relief of asthma. It is used as a diuretic and myocardial stimulant for the relief of edema and dyspnea that accompany congestive heart failure.

When given orally, theophylline may cause nausea, vomiting, and gastric discomfort. Other side effects include headache, restlessness, dizziness, anxiety, delirium, and even convulsions. If it is administered intravenously, care must be taken to administer the drug very slowly because it can cause cardiac arrest or ventricular fibrillation. For this reason the more concentrated intramuscular preparation may never be given intravenously.

Dose: Adults: (Oral, IM, IV) 100 to 500 mg several times daily.

Carbonic Anhydrase Inhibitors

Carbonic anhydrase is an enzyme that causes the formation of carbonic acid from carbon dioxide and water in the blood. When the enzyme is inhibited, as by one of these drugs, carbonic acid is not formed in any considerable amount.

Carbonic acid is needed to have a supply of the bicarbonate ion in the blood. Because the bicarbonate ion ordinarily combines with sodium, which is filtered out into the Bowman's capsule, and assists in its reabsorption into the blood stream, in the absence of this ion, sodium is excreted in excessive amounts and is accompanied by water to increase the urine volume.

$$H_2O + CO_2 \underset{\text{anhydrase}}{\overset{\text{carbonic}}{\rightleftharpoons}} H_2CO_3 \rightleftharpoons H^+ + HCO_3^-$$

In addition in their diuretic effects, carbonic anhydrase inhibitors exert a beneficial effect in glaucoma. This enzyme is needed for the formation of the intraocular fluid aqueous humor; thus when this enzyme is inhibited, the formation of the fluid is greatly slowed. For this reason, carbonic anhydrase inhibitors are often prescribed with topical ophthalmic drops for the management of glaucoma.

Acetazolamide, USP, BP (Diamox). Acetazolamide is useful in the treatment of edema resulting from congestive heart failure, in obstetrical and gynecological conditions, for premenstrual distress associated with fluid retention, and in glaucoma. It is not useful in patients with nephritis.

Because of a self-limiting effect of this drug, it is not effective as a diuretic for more than 2 or 3 days. After a resting period of a few days, however, it is again effective as a diuretic.

Dose: Adults: (Oral) 250 mg two to four times daily. (IV or IM) 500 mg; may be repeated in 2 to 4 hours.
Children: (Oral) 3 to 10 mg/kg three times daily. (IM) 5 mg/kg once daily.

Thiazide Diuretics (Benzothiadiazine Diuretics)

Thiazide diuretics, although they act in part by inhibiting carbonic anhydrase, also exert action directly on the collecting tubules of the kidney and promote the excretion of sodium, potassium, chloride, and bicarbonate along with the necessary excretion of water. Potassium depletion often is a problem when the thiazide diuretics are used over a prolonged period of time; thus, a potassium supplement or foods high in potassium, such as oranges and bananas, are often added to the diet.

In addition to their activity as diuretics, the thiazides have an additional effect as antihypertensive drugs. This action is separate from their effect on diuresis, but it is not completely understood as yet. When used by themselves, their action in lowering the blood pressure is mild; but when combined with other drugs such as reserpine, hydralazine, or ganglionic blocking agents, they are a useful adjunct in the treatment of hypertensive patients because they greatly increase the activity of these drugs.

Side effects of these drugs include alterations in the body chemistry such as hypochloremic alkalosis, hypotension, tachycardia, aplastic anemia, jaundice, hyperuricemia, glycosuria, muscle cramps, and weakness. They should be used with caution in patients known to have gout or liver or kidney disorders.

Chlorothiazide, USP, BP (Diuril). Chlorothiazide was the first diuretic to be synthesized in the thiazide group. It is used as a diuretic in heart failure, during pregnancy, in premenstrual fluid retention, or as an adjunct in the treatment of hypertension.

Dose: Adults: (Oral) 500 mg one to two times daily.
Children: (Oral) 10 mg/kg two times daily.

Hydrochlorothiazide, USP, BP (Hydro-Diuril, Esidrix, Oretic). A small alteration in the chemical structure of chlorothiazide greatly increases the potency of this compound. Greatly decreased doses of this drug will give diuretic effects comparable to those of chlorothiazide.

Dose: Adults: (Oral) 50 to 100 mg one to two times daily.
Children: (Oral) 1 mg/kg twice daily.

Bendroflumethiazide, USP, BP (Naturetin). This compound is also prepared by making a small chemical alteration in the structure of chlorothiazide and is even more potent than hydrochlorothiazide. It has the same uses and effects as those of its parent compound but may be administered in smaller doses.

Dose: Adults: (Oral) 2.5 to 5 mg daily.
Children: (Oral) 50 to 100 μg/kg once daily.

Methylclothiazide, USP, BP (Enduron). Although this compound is as effective as bendroflumethiazide, the incidence of side effects is higher; thus, it has not found as great an acceptance clinically as the previously mentioned compounds.

Dose: Adults: (Oral) 2.5 to 10 mg daily.
Children: (Oral) 50 to 200 μg/kg once daily.

Trichlormethiazide, USP, BP (Metahydrin, Naqua). In all respects the action of this compound is similar to that of bendroflumethiazide.

Dose: Adults: (Oral) 2 to 4 mg daily.
Children: (Oral) 70 μg/kg once daily.

Polythiazide, USP, BP (Renese). Polythiazide is said to conserve more serum potassium than other drugs while still promoting excretion of an effective amount of sodium. Its uses and diuretic effects are comparable to those of the other diuretics in this class.

Dose: Adults: (Oral) 1 to 4 mg daily.
Children: (Oral) 20 to 80 µg/kg once daily.

Steroid Antagonists

The steroid antagonists act by inhibiting aldosterone, an adrenal hormone that promotes the retention of sodium and the excretion of potassium. The excretion of sodium and chloride is accompanied by an appropriate amount of water.

Spironolactone, USP, BP (Aldactone). Spironolactone is useful in the treatment of edema associated with congestive heart failure, hepatic cirrhosis with ascites and nephritis, and edema of unknown origin.

Side effects observed with the use of this drug include mild headache, confusion, dermatitis, drowsiness, ataxia, and mild abdominal pain.

Dose: Adults: (Oral) 50 to 400 mg daily.
Children: (Oral) 3.3 mg/kg daily in divided doses.

Aldactazide. Aldactazide is a combination of 25 mg hydrochlorothiazide and 25 mg spironolactone per tablet. The combined form of the two drugs is more effective as a diuretic than either of the two used singly, because the reabsorption of fluids and electrolytes in the kidney is blocked by two methods.

Dose: Adults: (Oral) 1 tablet four times daily (25 mg of each drug).
Children: (Oral) 1.65 to 3.3 mg/kg of each drug daily in divided doses.

Miscellaneous Diuretics

Chlorthalidone, USP, BP (Hygroton). The diuretic effect of chlorthalidone closely parallels that of hydrochlorothiazide. It is useful for both its diuretic and antihypertensive effects.

The most noticeable side effects observed with

the administration of this drug are dizziness, lightheadedness, nausea, vomiting, and weakness. Occasionally, gastrointestinal distress is noted.

Dose: Adults: (Oral) 50 to 200 mg daily.
Children: (Oral) 2 mg/kg three times a week.

Quinethazone, USP, BP (Hydromox). The action and side effects of this drug closely resemble those of chlorthalidone.

Dose: Adults: (Oral) 50 to 100 mg daily.
Children: No pediatric dose established.

Triamterene, USP, BP (Dyrenium). This drug is often combined with hydrochlorothiazide because the diuretic and hypotensive effects are increased by the combination.

Nausea, vomiting, headache, and weakness occur occasionally with the use of this drug.

Dose: Adults: (Oral) 100 mg one to two times daily.
Children: (Oral) 1 to 2 mg/kg one or two times daily.

Furosemide, USP, BP (Lasix). Furosemide is a diuretic that has been shown to act throughout the collecting tubules of the nephron, particularly on the ascending limb of the loop of Henle, to prevent the reabsorption, and hence cause the excretion of, sodium and chloride. Unlike the thiazides, this drug does not cause the loss of a disproportionate amount of potassium. It may be used in congestive heart failure associated with liver or kidney disease. It is of particular value when other less potent diuretics have failed to decrease edema.

Side effects are electrolyte depletion, dizziness, weakness, jaundice, leg cramps, vomiting, and confusion.

Although usually administered orally, it may be administered intramuscularly or intravenously.

Dose: Adults: (Oral) 20 to 80 mg once daily.
(IM, IV) 20 mg to 1 gm daily.
Children: No pediatric dose established.

Ethacrynic Acid, USP, BP (Edecrin). Like furosemide, this agent works throughout the nephron tubules to prevent the reabsorption of sodium and water. The potency of the two drugs is approximately equal. Ethacrynic acid is available in oral form only.

Dose: Adults: (Oral) 50 to 400 mg daily.
Children: (Oral) Initially 25 mg, then stepwise increments until results are achieved.

URINARY ANTISEPTICS

Bacterial infections of the urinary tract are the causative agents of various symptomatic conditions that may be described as cystitis, pyelitis, or pyelonephritis. These terms merely refer to the location of the infection or the source of the symptoms indicating an infection in the urinary tract.

Many patients who have had a single urinary tract infection have recurrences after asymptomatic periods. For this reason, they are often placed on long-term drug therapy.

Most of the sulfonamides as well as antibiotics, such as the tetracyclines, chloramphenicol, erythromycin, streptomycin, kanamycin, and cephalothin, may be used to treat these conditions. Because these drugs have previously been discussed in other chapters, this section is reserved for drugs used more exclusively as urinary antiseptics.

Nitrofurantoin, USP, BP (Furadantin). This synthetic drug has a spectrum of activity that encompasses the majority of urinary tract infective agents. After oral administration, approximately 45 percent of the dose is excreted in the urine—imparting to it a brown color. The administration of the drug should be continued for at least 3 days after sterility of the urine has been attained to minimize the possibility of recurrent infections.

Nausea, vomiting, or sensitivity reactions may occur with administration of this drug. The gastrointestinal symptoms may be minimized if the dose is given with food or milk.

Dose: Adults: (Oral) 50 to 100 mg four times daily.

Children: (Oral) 1.25 to 1.75 mg/kg four times daily.

Methenamine Mandelate, USP, BP (Mandelamine). This combination of methenamine and mandelic acid is a well-tolerated urinary antiseptic and is particularly useful for chronic, resistant, or recurrent infections. It is effective against almost all strains of microorganisms that are causative agents in urinary infections and may be effective even against strains resistant to antibiotics or sulfonamides. It may be given alone or in combination with other drugs.

Sensitization in the form of allergic reactions rarely occurs with this drug, but it is contraindicated in patients with severe hepatitis or renal insufficiency.

Dose: Adults: (Oral) 1 gm four times daily.
Children younger than 6 years: (Oral) 18 mg/kg four times daily.
Children older than 6 years: (Oral) 34 mg/kg four times daily.

Nalidixic Acid, USP, BP (NegGram). Nalidixic acid is a synthetic drug that is chemically unrelated to the sulfonamides, antibiotics, or nitrofurantoin. It is highly effective against gram-negative bacteria and also is effective in some infections caused by gram-positive microorganisms. It is compatible with other antibacterial agents and may be administered concurrently with them.

Although prolonged therapy with nalidixic acid has been generally well tolerated, it should be used with caution in patients with liver disease or severely impaired kidney function. Skin disorders, blood dyscrasias, and transient neurological disorders have occasionally been noted during therapy with nalidixic acid.

Dose: Adults: (Oral) 0.5 to 1 gm four times daily.
Children: (Oral) 55 mg/kg daily in four divided doses.

Urised. Each tablet of this preparation contains:

Atropine sulfate 0.03 mg
Hyoscyamine 0.03 mg

Methenamine 40.8 mg
Methylene blue 5.4 mg
Phenyl salicylate 18.1 mg
Benzoic acid 4.5 mg

The action of the urinary antiseptics methenamine and methylene blue along with the antispasmodic effects of atropine and hyoscyamine makes this preparation relatively effective in treating mild urinary infections.

Patients should be warned that the methylene blue in the tablet will turn the urine blue.

Dryness of the mouth, dizziness, rapid pulse, and blurring of the vision occur occasionally. It is contraindicated in myasthenia gravis and glaucoma.

> Dose: Adults: (Oral) 2 tablets four times daily.
> Children older than 6 years: Dose reduced by proportionate body weight.
> Children younger than 6 years: No dose established.

Ethoxazene Hydrochloride (Serenium). Ethoxazene is used to relieve pain associated with acute or chronic infections of the urinary tract. It is often administered with urinary antiseptics for this purpose.

> Dose: Adults: (Oral) 100 mg three times daily.
> Children: No pediatric dose established.

Phenazopyridine Hydrochloride, USP, BP (Pyridium). Like ethoxazene, this drug acts promptly to produce an analgesic effect on the urinary tract mucosa. It usually acts within 30 minutes to relieve the symptoms of pain, burning, urgency, and frequency associated with urinary infections. This drug is compatible with any antibacterial or with other corrective therapy for infections of this nature. The patient should be informed that the urine will turn a reddish color.

> Dose: Adults: (Oral) 200 mg three times daily.
> Children: No pediatric dose established.

Pyridium is often combined with urinary antiseptics in tablet form. The following are examples of such combinations:

Azo Gantrisin
Azo Gantanol

In addition to the symptomatic relief of the discomfort associated with urinary infections that is afforded by the phenylazodiaminopyridine (Pyridium), the hyoscyamine acts to reduce the smooth muscle spasm, and butabarbital acts as a sedative. It is often prescribed with urinary antiseptics. The use of this drug results in urine that is red-orange in color.

> Dose: Adults: (Oral) 1 tablet four times daily.
> Children: No pediatric established dose.

Bactrim, Septra. The commercial preparations of Bactrim and Septra contain identical formulations, with tablets consisting of a combination of 80 mg trimethoprim and 400 mg sulfamethoxazole. Each company also produces a double-strength tablet labeled DS (Bactrim DS, Septra DS).

The combination of a sulfonamide with the synthetic antibacterial compound trimethoprim has been shown to be very effective against chronic urinary tract infections, primarily pyelonephritis, pyelitis, and cystitis. Its use should be reserved for chronic infections, however, because untoward effects do occur from this drug. These agents are discussed in Chapter 20 for their use in upper respiratory infections and in Chapter 17 (sulfonamides).

The patient should be warned to report sore throat, fever, pallor, purpura, or jaundice to the physician immediately because these may be early signs of blood dyscrasias noted with this drug. Adequate fluid intake should be maintained during therapy to prevent the formation of renal calculi. The drug should be used with caution in patients with impaired renal or liver function. It is contraindicated in pregnant women.

> Dose: Adults: (Oral) 2 tablets every 12 hours for 10 to 14 days (or 1 tablet of the double-strength form every 12 hours).

Children: (Oral) 8 mg/kg trimethoprim and 40 mg/kg sulfamethoxazole daily in two divided doses.

DRUGS USED FOR THE TREATMENT OF ENURESIS

Enuresis, or nighttime bedwetting, is a fairly common problem in children. Without treatment, the percentage of bedwetters gradually decreases to the age of 21 years, but a small percentage are still wetting at that age.

It is well established that withholding fluids in the evening, many nightly awakenings by the parent, and other behavioral techniques may give temporary improvement, but 100% relapse as soon as the awakenings cease. Various alarms and early warnings of wetting have been devised again without real improvement.

The problem seems to be a small or spastic bladder that is stimulated to empty automatically when a certain volume of urine is present, much as an infantile bladder will empty.

Various drugs are in use for this problem.

Imipramine Hydrochloride (Tofranil). This agent, an antidepressant as well, may improve the symptoms of enuresis in some children. The mechanism of action in the improvement of enuresis is thought to be apart from its antidepressant effect.

Dose: Children 6 years or older 25 mg orally at bedtime.
Children older than 12 years 75 mg at bedtime.

Oxybutynin Chloride (Ditropan). This agent has a direct antispasmodic effect on the smooth muscle and relaxes bladder smooth muscle in patients with involuntary bladder symptoms. It may be used for day and night wetting. Side effects include drowsiness, decreased tearing, dry mouth, constipation, and palpitations.

Dose: Children 12 years and older: 5 mg three times daily orally.
Children 5 to 12 years: 5 mg orally twice daily.

Desmopressin Acetate (DDAVP Nasal Spray). This is an antidiuretic hormone that affects renal water conservation. It is an analogue of vasopressin. It is used as a nasal spray in children 6 years of age and older. Side effects include headache, rise in blood pressure, nosebleed, and sore throat.

Dose: 10 to 40 µg by nasal spray pump at bedtime.

Implications for the Student

1. Diuretics are generally administered in the morning so that diuresis does not interfere with sleep.

2. The patient should be observed for the intended effects of diuretic medication. This will be seen in the increased urine volume, lessening of edema about the face and extremities, and weight loss.

3. The patient receiving a diuretic should be instructed in the importance of a low-sodium diet. Sodium promotes fluid retention and counteracts the desired effect of the diuretic.

4. Potassium loss is an untoward effect of many diuretics. The patient may receive potassium supplements or be instructed to consume foods that are high in potassium, such as raisins, oranges, and bananas.

5. Fluid and electrolyte changes that occur with diuretics may cause postural hypoten-

sion. The patient should be instructed to be observant if he or she experiences dizziness on arising or in ambulation.

6. Diuretics are often given to aid in the management of hypertension and to diminish the fluid and sodium content of the body.

7. Diuretics are of great value in the treatment of congestive heart failure when the weakened heart cannot mobilize excessive bodily fluids.

8. When a patient is receiving urinary antiseptics, it is often advisable to maintain an acid urine to aid the drug in its intended effect. Large doses of vitamin C and cranberries and prunes promote an acid urine. Carbonated beverages and citrus fruits produce an alkaline urine.

9. Certain agents given for urinary tract infections, such as Urised and Pyridium, cause blue or red-orange discolorations of the urine. The patient should be counseled to expect this effect.

10. An adequate fluid volume intake should be encouraged when the patient is being treated for a urinary tract infection.

11. The most common side effect of the urinary tract antiseptics is a skin rash. The patient should be observed for this effect. Other untoward reactions include headache, nervousness, and drug fever. An elevation of temperature may be a drug reaction, not a worsening of the infection.

12. The patient should be observed for signs of improvement of the urinary tract infection (i.e., less dysuria, frequency, and hesitancy on urination). The urine volume often increases as the infection is eradicated.

13. Withholding fluids before bedtime is not effective in treating enuresis.

CASE STUDIES

1. After taking HydroDiuril for hypertension for 1 year, Mrs. S.P., 48, now comes to the office with complaints of fatigue and weakness and many somatic complaints that include nonspecific malaise. Her blood pressure is 130/80, and the doctor orders serum electrolyte determinations. The results are sodium, 145; potassium, 2.8; chloride, 110; and carbon dioxide, 28. Should her medicine be discontinued? What is her problem? How can it be helped?

2. Glen F. has noted nausea and vomiting since he has been taking Furadantin for a urinary tract infection. He is now concerned that he is coming down with an intestinal virus and asks you to see if the doctor will give him some Tigan, which he says usually works for him. Would you have any other recommendations?

Review Questions

1. Name the two most potent diuretics.

2. Explain the important nursing responsibilities for patients on diuretic therapy.

3. List the most frequent side effects of diuretic therapy.

4. What foods could be given to supplement potassium in the diet?

5. What instructions would you give a patient who is taking Pyridium?

6. Name the various types of diuretics and give an example of each.

7. What does insensible fluid loss mean?

29

Antineoplastic Drugs

Objectives for the Student

B E

A B L E

T O

- 1. Identify antineoplastic drugs and give an example of each type.
- 2. Explain the use of drugs as an adjunct to therapy.
- 3. Discuss nursing measures that provide supportive therapy.

Neoplastic diseases, or cancer, are caused by uncontrolled cell division. These abnormal, rapidly dividing cells invade surrounding healthy tissues or organs and interfere with their function, ultimately causing the death of the entire organism.

Surgery and irradiation are still the primary tools in the fight against malignant diseases, but antineoplastic drugs have come into use in the past few years as a very important adjunct to therapy. Drugs are important particularly when cancer is widespread throughout the body or when the organ or tissue involved cannot be removed, and in some cases they are used prophylactically along with surgery or irradiation in an attempt to destroy undiscovered nests of malignant cells.

Because the malignant cell is dividing more rapidly than normal cells, it has a higher metabolic rate; thus, it is more sensitive than normal cells to products that interfere with cell growth or metabolism. This difference is only relative, however, and the main disadvantage of the cancer drugs is that they serve as a metabolic toxin

to normal cells as well. The more rapidly dividing healthy tissues (such as the gastrointestinal epithelium, oral mucosa, bone marrow, lymphoid tissue, and gonads) are often the first affected by the antineoplastic drugs, and too much tissue destruction in these areas often necessitates withdrawal of the antineoplastic drug before the disease is brought under control. Antineoplastic drugs may be classified as follows:

1. Alkylating agents, which attach "alkyl groups" or organic side chains to the proteins within the cancer cell, thus poisoning it
2. Antimetabolites, which interfere with some phase of normal cellular metabolism
3. Hormones, which may antagonize certain tumors of the reproductive tract and accessory sex organs by altering normal hormonal balance
4. Antibiotics, which act usually by interfering with DNA or RNA synthesis
5. Radioisotopes, which destroy certain cellular components by emission of radioactive particles

229

6. Immunotherapy in cancer
7. Miscellaneous drugs, which are a heterogeneous group of drugs having various mechanisms of action

ALKYLATING AGENTS

As just stated, this group of drugs alters the chemical composition of proteins, probably the nucleoproteins, of the cell. The cell cannot function normally in the presence of these aberrant molecules. The alkylating agents were one of the first forms of antineoplastic therapy and have remained in use because of their undisputed effectiveness in the palliation of certain types of cancer. They are all highly toxic compounds, however, and produce many unpleasant as well as dangerous side effects upon continued use.

Mechlorethamine Hydrochloride, USP, BP (Nitrogen Mustard, Mustargen). This drug was produced as a result of experiments with the poisonous mustard gas of World War I. It is particularly useful for lymphosarcoma, Hodgkin's disease, polycythemia vera, and mycosis fungoides.

Nitrogen mustard is very irritating to the skin; thus, extreme caution should be used when the drug is mixed. It may be administered intravenously, intra-arterially, or as an intracavitary instillation.

Side effects include nausea, vomiting, diarrhea, bone marrow depression, and dermatitis. Chlorpromazine or a similar antiemetic may be given 1/2 hour before administration of this drug to minimize vomiting.

Dose: Adults: (IV) 0.1 to 0.4 mg/kg daily.
Children: Same as that for adults.

Chlorambucil, USP, BP (Leukeran). Chlorambucil has its greatest effect on the blood-forming tissues; thus, it is used primarily in the treatment of leukemias and malignancies of the lymphatic system. It has the advantage over mechlorethamine in that it can be administered orally. Side effects are similar to those of mechlorethamine.

Dose: Adults: (Oral) 0.1 to 0.2 mg/kg daily.
Children: Same as that for adults.

Busulfan, USP, BP (Myleran). Like chlorambucil, this drug is administered orally and is used primarily for malignancies of the blood-forming organs.

Dose: Adults: (Oral) 4 to 8 mg daily.
Children: (Oral) 0.06 mg/kg daily.

Cyclophosphamide, USP, BP (Cytoxan). Cyclophosphamide may be administered orally, intramuscularly, intravenously, or as an intracavitary infusion. It is used occasionally in leukemias when the patient has become resistant to other drugs. In addition, it has been useful in the treatment of Hodgkin's disease, multiple myeloma, and carcinoma of the reproductive tract and as an immunosuppressive agent.

Side effects are similar to those of nitrogen mustard with the exception that cyclophosphamide is not as irritating to tissues.

Dose: Adults: (Oral) 1 to 5 mg/kg daily. (IV) 10 to 20 mg/kg daily for 2 to 5 days, then 10 to 15 mg/kg every 7 to 10 days.
Children: (Oral) 2 to 8 mg/kg daily. (IV) 2 to 8 mg/kg daily.

Thiotepa, USP, BP. Thiotepa is administered topically or as an intracavitary infusion as well as intravenously, intra-arterially, or intramuscularly. It is primarily used in the treatment of cancer of the reproductive tract, lymphomas, leukemias, and cancer of the bladder. It is often instilled into the pleural space to decrease pulmonary effusions that occur with local neoplastic diseases. It is occasionally instilled into the bladder to aid in the treatment of small bladder tumors by topical action. Side effects are similar to those of the other drugs within this group.

Dose: Adults: (IV, IM, Intra-arterial) Up to 200 μg/kg daily for 5 days, then once weekly. (Topical) 15 mg diluted with a small amount of water.
Children: Same as that for adults.

Carmustine (BiCNU). This alkylating agent

is a derivative of nitrosourea. It is used in the treatment of malignant brain tumors and in combination with other agents for the treatment of multiple myeloma and Hodgkin's disease.

The most serious and frequent side effect is a cumulative and delayed bone marrow toxicity that usually occurs 4 to 6 weeks after therapy. Nausea, vomiting, and renal and hepatic toxicity as well as skin rashes occur.

Dose: Adults: (IV) 200 mg/M² body surface every 6 weeks.

Dacarbazine, USP, BP (DTIC-Dome). The exact mechanism of action of this agent is not known, but it is presumed to be an alkylating agent. It is used in the treatment of malignant melanoma and with other agents in the treatment of Hodgkin's disease, soft tissue sarcomas, and neuroblastomas.

Bone marrow suppression, nausea, vomiting, and a flu-like syndrome of fever, myalgia, and malaise frequently occur with therapy.

Dose: Adults: (IV) 2.5 to 4.5 mg/kg daily for 10 days. This regimen may be repeated at 4-week intervals.

Lomustine (CCNU, CeeNU). This agent is well absorbed from the gastrointestinal tract and is generally administered orally, although it may be used as a topical application in certain cases. It is used in the treatment of brain tumors and tumors of the gastrointestinal tract and kidney. It has been used topically in the treatment of mycosis fungoides and psoriasis.

Delayed bone marrow toxicity, nausea, vomiting, alopecia, liver and kidney toxicity, and skin reactions occur with therapy.

Dose: Adults: (Oral) 130 mg/M² body surface as a single dose. It is given in intervals of at least 6 weeks.
Children: Same as that for adults.

Uracil Mustard, USP, BP. This derivative of nitrogen mustard is used in the treatment of lymphocytic leukemia and lymphomas including Hodgkin's disease and in the palliative treatment of mycosis fungoides and polycythemia vera.

Bone marrow suppression, nausea, vomiting, pruritus, dermatoses, and hyperuricemia are seen with uracil mustard therapy.

Dose: Adults only: (Oral) 1 to 2 mg daily until improvement or toxicity occurs.

Melphalan, USP, BP (Alkeran). This drug may be given orally for the treatment of multiple myeloma. It is of limited value in this disease, however. Melphalan has not proven effective against other forms of malignant diseases. Side effects are similar to those of other drugs in the group.

Dose: Adults: (Oral) Initially 6 mg daily, then 2 mg daily for maintenance.
Children: No pediatric dose established.

ANTIMETABOLITES

Antimetabolites are a group of antineoplastic drugs that act by interfering in a specific phase of cell metabolism. Because neoplastic cells are more rapidly growing cells, they are theoretically affected by these drugs at dosage levels that cause only minimal interruption in the metabolism of normal cells. Unfortunately, this does not always prove to be true, and severe bone marrow depression in particular will very often occur, necessitating withdrawal of the drug. Denuding of the gastrointestinal epithelium and ulcers of the oral mucosa are also frequent side effects of the antimetabolites.

Methotrexate, USP, BP (Amethopterin). Methotrexate is a folic acid antagonist that exerts its action by interfering with the formation of the reduced, or active, form of folic acid in the body. It is administered orally and is particularly useful in acute lymphocytic leukemias of childhood. The disease eventually becomes resistant to this compound, but often remissions lasting months or even years may be obtained. In addition, it has been used effectively in uterine choriocarcinoma and in lymphosarcoma as well as in the treatment of psoriasis.

It is also available in a parenteral form that may be given intramuscularly, intravenously, intra-arterially, or intrathecally. Because the oral form is highly effective, parenteral administration is largely limited, with the exception of the intrathecal route, which is used in the treatment of leukemic meningitis. Other forms of administration do not allow sufficient concentrations of the drug to cross the blood-brain barrier.

Dose: Adults: (Oral, IV, IM) As antineoplastic 2.5 to 30 mg daily. (Oral) As antipsoriatic 10 to 25 mg once a week.
Children: (Oral, IV, IM) As antineoplastic 0.12 mg/kg daily.

Mercaptopurine, USP (Purinethol, 6-MP). Mercaptopurine is an antimetabolite that inhibits the synthesis of purines (components of DNA). It is administered orally with some effectiveness in the treatment of acute lymphocytic leukemias, Hodgkin's disease, and other tumors of the lymphatic system.

Dose: Adults: (Oral) 2.5 mg/kg daily.
Children: Same as that for adults.

Fluorouracil, USP (5-FU). Fluorouracil is a chemical analogue of uracil, a component of DNA. When incorporated into the DNA molecule, it interferes with normal growth and metabolism of the cell. It is administered intravenously or intra-arterially for the treatment of carcinomas of the reproductive tract, liver, pancreas, and gastrointestinal tract. It may also be applied topically to treat actinic keratoses.

Dose: Adults: (IV) 12 mg/kg once daily for 4 days, then 6 mg/kg every other day for four doses. Maintenance dose ranges from 10 to 15 mg/kg once a week. (Topical) 1 to 5% cream applied twice daily to the lesion.

Cytarabine, USP, BP (Cytosar). The antimetabolic effect of this drug appears to occur by interference with DNA formation. It is used primarily in the treatment of acute myelocytic leukemia in adults, although it has been used in the treatment of other adult and childhood leukemias.

The primary side effects are suppression of bone marrow and gastrointestinal symptoms. Fever, rash, cellulitis, pain at the injection site, sore throat, conjunctivitis, and alopecia also occur frequently.

Dose: Adults: (IV) 2 mg/kg daily for 10 days, then increased to 4 mg/kg daily, maintained until beneficial effects or toxicity occurs.

Floxuridine, USP, BP (FUDR). By interfering with the synthesis of DNA, floxuridine has been found to be beneficial in certain malignancies. It is recommended only for intra-arterial infusion and is used primarily for tumors of the head, neck, brain, liver, gallbladder, and bile ducts.

Side effects are generally related to the drug-infused area and include oral stomatitis, esophagopharyngitis, duodenal ulcer, and gastrointestinal bleeding. Localized erythema, ataxia, blurred vision, and vertigo have also been described.

Dose: Adults: (Intra-arterial) 100 to 600 μg/kg in diluted solution daily. Therapy is generally continued until toxicity occurs.

HORMONES

Hormones have varied uses in the treatment of malignant diseases.

Corticosteroids have long been shown to be of value in producing remissions of certain malignancies, notably acute lymphocytic leukemia of childhood, and they are used either alone or in combination with other drugs. The mechanism of action here is not fully understood. They have been used with less effectiveness in Hodgkin's disease and lymphosarcoma. Side effects are those of excessive administration of corticosteroids (i.e., salt and water retention, moon facies, edema, and striae). In many cases dietary salt may have to be strictly curtailed during administration. Prednisone is the corticosteroid that perhaps is used more than any other in treating malignancies, but other compounds would be similarly effective.

Sex hormones have been used to palliate carcinomas of the reproductive tract. Estrogens may be administered to males with carcinoma of the prostate and have also been found to be of value in the treatment of postmenopausal women with breast cancer. Androgens are administered to premenopausal women with breast cancer. These agents are only palliative, not curative. Side effects are as expected: masculinization when androgens are given to a female and feminization when estrogens are given to a male.

Testolactone Suspension, USP, BP (Teslac). This analogue of testosterone is a hormone derivative that is used exclusively in the treatment of malignancies. It has been used as palliative therapy for metastatic breast carcinoma in the premenopausal woman when surgery is not feasible. There are definite advantages to the use of this compound for the treatment of carcinoma in preference to the regularly used testosterone preparations, but the mechanism of action of this drug is not yet fully understood. It is administered intramuscularly or orally.

Side effects include neurological symptoms, nausea, vomiting, and alopecia.

Dose: Adults: (IM) 100 mg three times weekly. (Oral) 50 mg three times daily.

Calusterone (Methosarb). This hormone, structurally related to testosterone, is used in the treatment of carcinoma of the breast, primarily in postmenopausal women.

This agent produces more virilization than testolactone. Hirsutism occurs frequently, and approximately one fourth of the patients report deepening of the voice, acne, and facial hair growth. Enlargement of the clitoris, nausea, and vomiting have also been reported.

Dose: Adults: (Oral) 150 to 300 mg daily in divided doses.

Megestrol Acetate (Megace). Chemically related to progesterone, megestrol is used in the treatment of endometrial carcinoma, breast cancer, endometriosis, and prostatic hypertrophy.

Very few side effects occur with this agent. It should be used with caution in patients with a history of thrombophlebitis.

Dose: Adults: (Oral) 40 mg daily in divided doses.

Tamoxifen Citrate (Nolvadex). This antiestrogenic compound is similar to clomiphene. It competes with estradiol for receptor sites in tumors of the breast, uterus, and vagina and other tumors with estrogen receptors. Its primary use is in the treatment of advanced breast cancer in postmenopausal women.

Dose: Adults: (Oral) 20 to 40 mg daily in two divided doses.

ANTITUMOR ANTIBIOTICS

Dactinomycin, USP, BP (Actinomycin D, Cosmegen). Dactinomycin is an antibiotic that exerts its effect as an antineoplastic agent by interfering with RNA synthesis. It is used in the treatment of Wilms' tumor of the kidney and for control of the metastases of this tumor. It has been used in combination with other agents in the treatment of metastatic tumors of the testes, choriocarcinoma, and certain lymphomas.

Toxic effects include bone marrow suppression and liver and kidney toxicity as well as nausea, vomiting, oral stomatitis, anorexia, and various skin eruptions.

Dose: Adults: (IV) 500 μg daily for 5 days.
Children: (IV) 15 μg/kg for 5 days.

Bleomycin Sulfate, USP, BP (Blenoxane). The antibiotic action of this agent appears to occur by causing a splitting of the DNA chain. It is used in the treatment of Hodgkin's disease and squamous cell carcinomas of the skin, penis, vulva, head, neck, and larynx.

Unlike most antineoplastic agents, this drug has a very low incidence of bone marrow toxicity. The most serious toxic effect is interstitial pneumonitis. Skin or mucocutaneous lesions, alopecia, fever, chills, and hypotension have been reported.

Dose: (IV, IM, SC, Intra-arterial, Intrapleural injection) 0.25 to 0.5 U/kg weekly.

Doxorubicin Hydrochloride, USP, BP (Adriamycin). Doxorubicin is an antibiotic produced by a strain of *Streptomyces*. As with the other antibiotics in this group, it has anti-infective properties but is generally considered to be too toxic to be utilized in this way. It is used in the treatment of solid tumors of the breast, ovaries, bladder, lung, thyroid gland, and bone. It is also of value in the treatment of neuroblastoma; Wilms' tumor; Hodgkin's disease; Ewing's tumor; squamous cell tumors of the head, neck, cervix, and vagina; and carcinomas of the testes, prostate, and uterus.

The major side effects are on the bone marrow and gastrointestinal tract. Cardiotoxicity as manifested by electrocardiographic changes should be monitored. Facial flushing, edema, alopecia, fever, chills, and skin rashes also occur.

Dose: Adults: (IV) 60 to 75 mg/M^2 body surface as a single dose at 21-day intervals.

Mithramycin, USP, BP (Mithracin). Also produced by a strain of *Streptomyces,* mithramycin is used primarily in the treatment of testicular tumors. It has been noted to lower serum calcium levels; thus, it is also used in the treatment of hypercalcemia associated with a variety of neoplasms.

The primary side effects are on bone marrow and the intestinal tract. Facial flushing, malaise, depression, phlebitis, and skin rashes have also been noted.

Dose: Adults: (IV) 25 to 30 μg/kg daily for 8 to 10 days or until toxicity occurs.

Mitomycin, USP, BP (Mutamycin). This antibiotic is used in the treatment of adenocarcinoma of the stomach, pancreas, colon, and rectum; squamous cell carcinomas of the lungs, cervix, head, and neck; and malignant melanoma.

Bone marrow depression, mouth ulcers, nausea, vomiting, and renal toxicity are among the side effects seen after administration.

Dose: Adults: (IV) 50 μg/kg daily for 5 days. The schedule may be repeated in 2 to 3 weeks.

Daunorubicin Hydrochloride (Cerubidine). This antibiotic functions as an antineoplastic agent because of its effect as an inhibitor of DNA synthesis. It is used primarily to treat acute myelogenous leukemia. It has also been used in the treatment of lymphocytic leukemias and in disseminated neuroblastoma.

Dose: Adults: (IV) Infusion in a daily dose of 30 to 60 mg/M^2 for 3 to 5 days.
Children: Same as that for adults.

RADIOACTIVE ISOTOPES

Radioactive isotopes may be used in the treatment of many forms of cancer. They may be inserted locally in the form of radioactive pellets, used in radiotherapy, or administered systemically to be picked up and concentrated in the malignant tissue.

The following are some of the more commonly used radioisotopes.

Radium (^{226}Ra). Radioactive radium needles are often used for intrauterine carcinoma. They are inserted within the uterine cavity and are quite effective in delivering a high dose of radiation to a small circumscribed area. They may be used before surgical removal of the tumor to facilitate the operative procedure by shrinking the tumor.

Cobalt (^{60}Co). The use of cobalt irradiation is one of the more important clinical advances in the treatment of carcinoma. Radiation can be administered to a very localized area by use of the teletherapy machine and rotation of the patient. In this way the maximum amount of radiation can be delivered to the tumor from several directions. It is used for a wide variety of tumors.

Gold (^{198}Au). Radioactive gold is used primarily for intracavitary administration, particularly for pleural and peritoneal effusions that are due to malignant processes.

Iridium (^{192}Ir). Iridium-containing needles have been used in place of radium pellets for insertion into malignant organs. They are used particularly in intrauterine carcinoma.

IMMUNOTHERAPY IN CANCER

In the 1950s when it was discovered that there was an interference phenomenon between viruses, subsequently labeled "virus-inhibitory factor," there was no recognition that the scientists had stumbled upon one of the arsenals of the body's own defense mechanism. This interference substance, then called interferon, was found to be produced by white blood cells, and it demonstrated antitumor effects in tissue cultures and animal experiments. The current development of interferons via recombinant DNA techniques has paved the way for a new form of cancer treatment.

Interferon exerts a variety of effects on tumor cells. It has an antiproliferative action and can work with antineoplastic drugs to increase their efficacy. Whereas tumor cells generally are useless blobs of cells that do not mature and become functional, interferon in some cases causes differentiation and maturity in these cells. Interferon also augments the cell-mediated cytotoxicity.

Interferon has been used in the treatment of leukemias, Kaposi's sarcoma (often seen in AIDS patients), gynecological tumors, Hodgkin's lymphomas, and a variety of other malignant conditions.

Cancer research is concentrating heavily in this field, and immunotherapy for cancer holds much promise for the future.

MISCELLANEOUS DRUGS

Vincristine Sulfate, USP, BP (Oncovin). Vincristine acts by interfering with normal cellular division. It must be administered intravenously and is used especially in the treatment of acute leukemias when the disease has become resistant to other orally administered drugs.

Side effects include bone marrow depression, neurologic symptoms, vomiting, diarrhea, and abdominal pain.

Dose: Adults: (IV) 0.5 to 0.15 mg/kg weekly.
Children: Same as that for adults.

Vinblastine Sulfate, USP, BP (Velban). Like vincristine, this drug acts primarily by in-

terfering with cell division. It is also administered intravenously and has been used with limited success in the treatment of Hodgkin's disease, lymphosarcoma, and choriocarcinoma. It is of no practical value in the treatment of leukemias.

Side effects are similar to those of vincristine.

Dose: Adults: (IV) 0.1 to 0.5 mg/kg weekly.
Children: (IV) 0.1 to 0.2 mg/kg weekly.

Procarbazine Hydrochloride, USP, BP (Matulane). This drug has been shown to be somewhat effective in the oral treatment of Hodgkin's disease but has no clinical effect in other types of malignancies.

Side effects include leukopenia, nausea, vomiting, muscle and joint pain, and neurological symptoms. This drug accentuates the central nervous system depressant action of sedatives, tranquilizers, narcotics, and antihistamines; thus, it should not be given simultaneously with these drugs. It should be used with caution in patients with kidney or liver damage.

Dose: Adults: (Oral) 100 to 300 mg daily.
Children: (Oral) 50 mg daily.

Pipobroman, USP, BP (Vercyte). Pipobroman has been used in the oral treatment of polycythemia vera and chronic granulocytic leukemia. It has not been proven to be effective in the treatment of childhood leukemias.

Side effects include nausea, vomiting, diarrhea, abdominal pain, and restlessness. It is a very toxic bone marrow suppressant.

Dose: Adults: (Oral) 1.5 to 3 mg/kg daily.
Children: No pediatric dose established.

Hydroxyurea, USP, BP (Hydrea). This derivative of urea is an antineoplastic drug believed to act by interfering in the formation of DNA. It is used orally in the treatment of malignant melanoma, ovarian carcinoma, and chronic granulocytic leukemia when the patient is resistant to other forms of therapy.

Side effects are bone marrow depression, nausea, vomiting, diarrhea, ulceration of the buccal mucosa and gastrointestinal epithelium, neurological symptoms, alopecia, and dermatoses.

Dose: Adults: (Oral) 20 to 30 mg/kg daily.
Children: No pediatric dose established.

Azathioprine, USP, BP (Imuran). Although the exact mechanism of action of this drug is not known, it is believed to inhibit RNA and DNA synthesis. It is administered orally primarily at this time to prevent the rejection of kidney transplants.

Bone marrow depression, nausea, vomiting, jaundice, mucous membrane ulcers, a persistent negative nitrogen balance, and muscle wasting have been observed after administration.

Dose: Children and Adults: (Oral) 5mg/kg/day.

Mitotane, USP, BP (Lysodren). This agent is believed to suppress the adrenal cortex and alter the utilization of steroids. It is used in the treatment of adrenocortical carcinoma.

Gastrointestinal disturbances, somnolence, dizziness, anorexia, nausea, vomiting, and diarrhea have occurred following administration.

Dose: Adults only: (Oral) 9 to 10 gm daily in three or four divided doses.

Quinacrine Hydrochloride Injection, USP, BP (Atabrine). Used initially as an anthelmintic and plasmodicidal drug, quinacrine has been used more recently as an intracavitary instillation to treat pleural and peritoneal infusions, generally from neoplastic diseases.

Fever, hyperthermia, nausea, vomiting, respiratory depression, hypotension, and decreased cardiac output have been reported as side effects.

Dose: Adults only: (Intracavitary) 50 mg to 1 gm daily as infusion.

Implications for the Student

1. The patient receiving antineoplastic agents is often anxious and upset. Efforts should be made to provide emotional support to the patient and family.

2. The patient should be instructed in the importance of good nutrition. The nurse should instruct the patient about his or her nutritional requirements.

3. Assess the patient's understanding of his or her illness and the possible side effects of medication.

4. Nursing procedures, such as an ice cap placed on the scalp before the administration of intravenous antineoplastic, may decrease hair loss. The patient should be advised that the hair will grow back in time, even if total alopecia results from the treatments.

5. Oral lesions and bleeding from the gums may result from antineoplastic agents. Good oral hygiene should be promoted, such as the use of lemon-glycerin swabs and the avoidance of irritating foods or acidic juices.

6. Common side effects of these agents are fever, sore throat, blood dyscrasias, and infections. The patient should be monitored for these effects.

7. The patient on antineoplastic medication is susceptible to untoward effects from minor illnesses. The patient and family should be counseled in the avoidance of contact with possibly infected persons.

8. Sedation or antiemetic medication before the administration of intravenous agents may minimize the nausea and vomiting produced as side effects. Administration in

the evening may allow remission of the nausea before the next morning. The patient should be encouraged to eat small, frequent meals.

9. The site of injection should be observed carefully for signs of extravasation, because these agents may produce sloughing of tissues.

10. Observe the patient for therapeutic effects, such as reduction in tumor size and weight gain.

CASE STUDIES

1. Janie C., 5, is undergoing treatment for acute lymphocytic leukemia and is receiving methotrexate presently. She has now noticed that her long hair is falling out rapidly. What would you say to her?

2. Mrs. T.L., 43, is receiving multiple antineoplastic therapy for metastatic breast carcinoma. She has been resisting all attempts to brush her teeth because of extreme soreness in her mouth and throat. What nursing procedures may make her more comfortable?

3. John H., 32, is undergoing treatment for Hodgkin's disease with uracil mustard. This morning when you made his bed you noticed a deep purple rash on his back and thighs. Should you report this to the physician or merely assure the patient that this, like his recent hair loss and mouth ulcers, is a side effect to be expected and tolerated?

Review Questions

1. What are some of the side effects caused by antineoplastic drugs?

2. Which agent is used to treat acute lymphocytic leukemia of childhood?

3. Discuss important responsibilities of the nurse in the care of patients on antineoplastic drugs.

4. What special precautions must be observed during use of radioactive isotopes?

Immunizing Agents and Immunosuppressives

Objectives for the Student

B E

A B L E

T O

■ 1. Become familiar with immunization schedules for children.
■ 2. Be aware of side effects of the immunizing agents.
■ 3. Know the uses for immunosuppressive agents.
■ 4. Know the general action and effects of immunosuppressives.

IMMUNIZING AGENTS

Immunity to an infectious disease may be brought about by actual contact with the disease or by the administration of a vaccine that provides immunity with an altered microorganism. In the latter case, immunity may be gained without the attendant deleterious effects of the disease itself.

Active immunity is achieved when the antigen, or attenuated microorganism, is injected into the body, and natural antibodies are produced against the antigen.

Passive immunity is obtained when the previously formed antibodies are injected into the body. This provides a faster immunity; however, it is short lived and will last only a few weeks or months.

Because of the proven success of the vaccines against infectious diseases, childhood immunization is now required by law, generally before admission to school (Table 30–1). There are usually only minor complications to childhood vaccines. Rare serious effects do occur, but considering the infant morbidity and mortality previously associated with these diseases, there can be no doubt that the vaccines provide a safe and effective way to ensure the health of the population.

Agents that Provide Active Immunity

Absorbed Diphtheria, Pertussis Vaccine, and Tetanus Toxoid, USP, Diphtheria, Pertussis, and Tetanus Vaccine, BP (DPT). The

Table 30-1. SCHEDULE FOR IMMUNIZATION

Age	Vaccine
2 months	DPT, trivalent oral polio vaccine
4 months	DPT, trivalent oral polio vaccine
6 months	DPT, trivalent oral polio vaccine
9 months	Tuberculin skin test
15 months	MMR vaccine
18 months	DPT, oral polio, tuberculin skin test, HIB vaccine
24 months*	b-Capsa I Vaccine (*Haemophilus influenzae*)
4–5 years	DPT, oral polio, tuberculin skin test
12–14 years	DT, oral polio, tuberculin skin test
Every 10 years thereafter	DT, or at least tetanus toxoid

*Haemophilus influenzae vaccine has been introduced to be given to children from 24 months through 6 years of age. At this time it is not a required vaccine.

DPT = diphtheria, pertussis, tetanus; MMR = measles, mumps, rubella; HIB = *haemophilus influenzae* type B; DT = diphtheria, tetanus.

combination of the toxoids, or altered bacterial products of *Corynebacterium diphtheriae* (the organism that causes diphtheria) and those of *Clostridium tetani* (the causative agent of tetanus), with the altered form of the causative agent of pertussis, or whooping cough, has been an effective vaccine against three formerly lethal diseases of infancy and early childhood.

Generally, the only side effects are mild to moderate fevers for 24 to 48 hours after administration of the vaccine, although there may be tenderness at the site of the injection. In some cases, fevers have been severe enough to produce a febrile convulsion; however, this is rare.

After age 5 years, the diphtheria-tetanus (DT) vaccine (without pertussis) is administered. The dose and route are the same as for the DPT.

Dose: (IM) 0.5 cc at intervals of 4 to 8 weeks, followed by booster doses as outlined in the schedule in Table 30–1.

Diphtheria and Tetanus Toxoids and Pertussis Vaccine and Haemophilus B Conjugate Vaccine (Tetramune). This four-way vaccine will generally replace the old triple of DPT vaccine in the future. All four vaccines in one injection will minimize the number of injections for the infant.

Dose: 0.5 cc IM at 2, 4, 6, and 25 (or 18) months.

Poliovirus Vaccine, Inactivated, USP, BP, Poliovirus Vaccine Live Oral, USP, BP. The first polio vaccine was the injectable and inactivated form, commonly known as the Salk vaccine. It has generally been replaced by the more convenient live oral form, the Sabin vaccine, except in instances when the patient has a family member who is immunocompromised (i.e., receiving immunosuppressives after an organ transplant or on antineoplastic drugs). In these cases the immunosuppressed person would be at risk from the shedding of live oral poliovirus in the stool that occurs after the oral polio form, and the injectable form is given instead.

Dose: Inactivated: (IM, SC) Three doses at intervals of 4 to 6 weeks, with annual boosters. Live oral: Three doses at 6- to 8-week intervals over the first year of life, with booster doses as per the schedule in Table 30–1. It is not administered after age 18.

Measles, Mumps, and Rubella Virus Vaccine Live, USP, BP (MMR). Although all these virus vaccines are available as single vaccines, it has been shown that immunity is conferred just as effectively with the triple live virus vaccine. Immunity is less than optimum if administered before 15 months of age, and if it is administered early because of a community epidemic, the dose must be repeated at a later time.

Side effects are minimal with this vaccine; however, occasionally the patient may experience a low-grade fever and light pink rash 10 to 14 days after administration.

Dose: At 15 months or older: (SC) 0.5 mL.

Haemophilus B Vaccine (HIB). This vaccine is given to develop an immunity against *Haemophilus influenzae,* primarily for the prevention of meningitis from this organism. Three HIB vaccines are available. They have differing dosage schedules and should not be used interchangeably. All are given intramuscularly in 0.5-mL doses.

This vaccine will be replaced by the four-way Tetramune in the future.

Tetanus Toxoid, USP, Tetanus Vaccine, BP. Tetanus toxoid is a preparation of the formaldehyde-treated byproducts of the tetanus bacillus *Clostridium tetani*. Although combined with the DPT and DT series given routinely in childhood, the tetanus toxoid alone is often chosen for periodic boosters after childhood. An effective serum level is sustained for 10 years after the booster dose; however, boosters are given as often as every 5 years for extremely dirty lesions.

Dose: Adults: (IM) 0.5 mL.

Influenza Virus Vaccine, USP, BP. This vaccine contains virus material from several different strains of influenza A and B. It is given annually to high-risk groups but has limited effectiveness in influenza epidemics because of the new strains of the virus that develop periodically.

Dose: Adults: (IM) 0.5 mL in the autumn, annually.

Hepatitis B Vaccine (Heptavax-B). This vaccine developed from the surface antigen of hepatitis B, formerly called the Australia antigen, is recommended for administration to high-risk groups, particularly those in the medical and dental fields who are in contact with potentially infectious body fluids.

Dose: Adults: (IM) Three 1-mL injections, the second 1 month after the initial injection, the third 6 months after the initial injection.
Infants: 0.1 cc IM at birth, at 1 month, and at 6 months.

BCG Vaccine, USP, BP. The bacille Calmette-Guérin vaccine confers immunity against tuberculosis. It is generally recommended for high-risk groups, those who live in endemic areas, and medical personnel.

Dose: Adults: (Dermal) 0.1 mL administered by the multiple puncture technique.

Agents that Provide Passive Immunity

Various preparations of antibodies are available to provide a short-lived but immediately effective protection against disease. These include the following:

Diphtheria Antitoxin, USP, BP

Dose: Adults: (IM) Prophylactic: 10,000 U. (IM, IV) Therapeutic: 10,000 to 200,000 U.

Tetanus Antitoxin, USP, BP (Equine Antitoxin)

Dose: Adults: (IM, SC) Prophylactic: 3000 to 10,000 U. (IV) Therapeutic: 40,000 to 100,000 U.

Tetanus Immune Human Globulin, USP, BP

Dose: Adults: (IM) Prophylactic: 250 U. (IM) Therapeutic: 300 to 600 U.

Botulism Antitoxin, USP, BP

Dose: Adults: (IV) 1 mL (1000 U) in diluted solution 1:10 with 10% glucose solution injected slowly over 5 minutes. Subsequent dosage administration based on individual requirements.

Pertussis Immune Human Globulin, USP, BP

Dose: Adults: (IM) Prophylactic: 1.25 to 2.5 mL repeated in 1 to 2 weeks. (IM) Therapeutic: 1.25 mL every 24 to 48 hours.

Mumps Immune Human Globulin, USP, BP

Dose: Adults: (IM) Prophylactic: 3 to 4.5 mL. (IM) Therapeutic: 15 to 20 mL.

Immune Human Serum Globulin, USP, BP

Dose: Adults: (IM) 1.3 to 2 mL/kg for prophy-

laxis every 6 to 8 weeks. For dysgam-
maglobulinemia therapy may be 20
to 50 mL monthly.

Hepatitis B Immune Globulin

Dose: Adults: (IM) 0.06 mL/kg within 7 days
of exposure.

**Rho(D) Immune Human Globulin, USP
(RhoGAM).** This antibody preparation is used
to desensitize Rh-negative mothers after delivery of an Rh-positive infant. The sensitization
of the mother occurs when infant blood cells
enter the mother's blood stream, thus causing
antibody formation, which then causes erythro-
blastosis fetalis in subsequent Rh-positive infants that she may carry.

When administered within 72 hours of delivery, the immune globulin diminishes antibody
formation in the mother.

Slight temperature elevations and mild local
reactions at the site of injection may occur after
administration.

Dose: Adults: (IM) 2 mL.

IMMUNOSUPPRESSIVE AGENTS

The immune system has its origins in the
fetal thymus gland. A process occurs during intrauterine life whereby the infant recognizes
certain substances as its own and develops two
types of lymphoid cells, the T cells and the B
cells, which are activated to recognize and destroy foreign substances and tissues.

With the development of technology for organ
transplants, the rejection of foreign tissue had
to be altered. A great deal of refinement has
occurred in the matching of tissue samples. This
process, similar to but much more complex than
typing blood, has improved the outcome of organ transplants, but immunosuppressives are
also needed to prevent rejection by the recipient.

General complications of the immunosuppressives include increased susceptibility to infections and lethal effects when otherwise minor
illnesses such as chickenpox are contracted. Immunosuppressed patients may contract polio-

myelitis from the live virus shed by infants after
oral administration of polio vaccine. Family
members of immunocompromised patients are
generally administered the inactivated or Salk
vaccine for this reason. Central nervous system
toxicity may be observed, and symptoms include
dizziness, headache, confusion, slurred speech,
and paresthesias. Jaundice from liver damage
and symptoms of bone marrow suppression such
as sore throat, oral mucosal lesions, and excessive bruising may also occur.

The Corticosteroids. Primarily the synthetic corticosteroids prednisone, prednisolone,
and dexamethasone are used for immunosup-
pression. Side effects particular to this group
include salt and water retention, with the moon
face and fat distribution noted as the administration is prolonged.

Dose: Prednisone and Prednisolone: Adults:
(Oral) 10 to 100 mg daily in divided
doses.
Dexamethasone: Adults: (Oral) 0.75 to
9 mg daily in divided doses.
Children: (Oral) 0.3 mg/kg daily in divided doses.

Azathioprine, USP, BP (Imuran). Because
of its similarity to the naturally occurring purines, this agent acts as an antagonist to RNA
and DNA synthesis, thus interfering with cell
metabolism.

This agent is primarily used in the treatment
of renal transplant patients to prevent rejection.
It is occasionally used in the treatment of other
autoimmune disorders such as systemic lupus
erythematosus, hemolytic anemias, and idiopathic thrombocytopenia.

Liver damage, increased susceptibility to infection, and bone marrow depression are the
most common side effects of this agent.

Dose: Adults: (Oral) 3 to 5 mg/kg daily initially, then 1 to 2 mg/kg daily as a
maintenance dose.
Children: Same as that for adults.

Cyclophosphamide, USP, BP (Cytoxan).
By interfering with DNA and RNA activities,

this agent disrupts cellular function and destroys proliferating lymph cells.

It is used to treat autoimmune disorders, such as lupus erythematosus, rheumatoid arthritis, and the nephrotic syndrome and to prevent organ transplant rejection.

Dose: Adults: (Oral, IV) 1 to 5 mg/kg daily.
Children: Same as that for adults.

Cyclosporine. This agent acts primarily against the T lymphocytes and inhibits the factors that stimulate T lymphocyte growth. For this reason it is used to prevent rejection of organ and bone marrow transplants.

Dose: Adults: (Oral) 10 to 25 mg/kg daily.
Children: Same as that for adults.

Antilymphocytic Globulin (ALG). This antibody preparation is obtained from large animals, usually horses, after inoculation with human lymphoid cells. The antibody thus produced destroys circulating lymphocytes, particularly T cells, and thereby aids in the survival of organ transplants.

Dose: No standard dose, administered individually.

Implications for the Student

1. The nurse should be familiar with the childhood diseases now prevented by the routine immunizations.

2. The nurse has an effective role in promoting adherence to routine infant immunization.

3. When administering immunizations, the nurse should shake the vial carefully before withdrawing the required dose.

4. All biological agents have an expiration date; this should be checked before administration of the vaccine.

5. Immunizations are often withheld when the patient is receiving corticosteroids or antineoplastic agents. In some cases immunization is deferred when close family members are immunologically compromised.

6. Before administration of a biological vaccine from an animal source, the patient should be closely questioned for allergic reactions.

7. The patient should be counseled about expected side effects of the vaccines (i.e., pain, erythema, and swelling at the site of injection and a fever that may last for 24 to 48 hours).

8. When patients are receiving immunosuppressive medications, they should be observed for side effects, such as fever, sore throat, bone marrow depression, and bleeding disorders.

9. Oral hygiene should be maintained when a patient is receiving immunosuppressives. Lemon-glycerin swabs may be used in lieu of vigorous tooth brushing to prevent gingival bleeding.

10. Signs of renal toxicity in a patient receiving immunosuppressives should be observed; these include dark urine, decreased urine output, and peripheral edema.

11. Liver damage as a side effect of the immunosuppressives is manifested by jaundice, dark urine, clay-colored stools, and abdominal pain or swelling.

12. The patient should be observed for signs of skin rashes or petechiae when receiving immunosuppressives.

CASE STUDIES

1. Your neighbor, who is the proud parent of a 1-month-old daughter, is confused by what she hears of the dangerous effects of the "baby shots." She wants your honest opinion as to whether these are really necessary. How would you respond?

2. Susan F., age 18, is alarmed and dismayed at the fat face she now has after her kidney transplant. She is being treated with Imuran and Prednisolone. How would you discuss this problem with her?

3. John F., age 56, has never had a tetanus injection or any other childhood immunizations. He has just sustained deep lacerations after a fall off his tractor. How do you think tetanus immunity would be best attained?

Review Questions

1. Briefly outline the diseases prevented by the standard childhood immunizations. Become familiar with the possible sequelae of each disease.

2. In addition to the basic childhood immunizations, which immunizations may further benefit someone working in the health field?

3. Which drugs may be used to avoid rejection of a kidney transplant?

4. What is lupus erythematosus, and what are its complications? What drugs are helpful in lupus erythematosus?

5. Give the general side effects of the immunosuppressives and explain why each occurs.

APPLYING PHARMACOLOGICAL KNOWLEDGE

CHAPTER 31

Geriatric Medication

Objectives for the Student

BE

ABLE

TO

- 1. Define specific health problems seen in the elderly.
- 2. Become aware of the differences in drug metabolism in the elderly.
- 3. Become aware of nutritional problems in the elderly and their solutions.
- 4. Recognize health problems in the elderly, such as hypothyroidism, that may be confused with senility.
- 5. Recognize structural changes in the aging body, particularly those of the bone and connective tissue.
- 6. Recognize and assist in the solution of social problems when elderly are cared for in the home or a nursing center.

Currently, more than 30 million Americans are 65 years of age or older. By the year 2030, older people will represent approximately 22 percent of the population. As a result, geriatric medicine has emerged as a vital and necessary medical discipline. The American Geriatrics Society has been formed to increase the number of health professionals trained in geriatrics and to expand and implement geriatric education and training for physicians, nurses, allied health personnel, and the general public.

One of the most important conceptual advances in the last few years has been the greater attention paid to what distinguishes aging per se from other influences that may be modified or helped in some way. For example, disease conditions that some people acquire and some do not, environmental changes, lifestyle factors such as diet, use of alcohol or drugs, smoking, and exercise all impact on the personal environment.

A great deal of interest lies in the areas of health promotion, disease prevention, and maintenance of good health and maximum independence as long as possible throughout the lifespan. Interactions of the elderly with society should be productive, satisfying, and rewarding for all involved.

This chapter is designed to promote some specific thoughts on the treatment of the elderly and to address some specific problems seen in the geriatric patient.

NUTRITION IN THE ELDERLY

The elderly patient who is still in his or her home often becomes malnourished out of inattention or inability to obtain a sufficient supply of fresh food for a balanced diet. Depression and isolation are common problems that seem to increase as the patient ages, and they are accompanied by a decreased ability and interest in self-care and nutrition.

Social programs, such as Meals-on-Wheels, have improved the lives of these patients because it addresses both their isolation and their nutrition inadequacies.

Poorly fitting dentures or missing teeth create mechanical problems in chewing food. Dental needs may have to be addressed before nutrition deficits can be improved.

Many patients are on modified diets (e.g., a bland diet for ulcers, a low-fat or low-sodium diet, or a low-purine diet for the prevention of gout). Often the elderly patient did not comprehend the instructions or simply does not know what he or she can eat. Patients often restrict their diets so much that they lose weight and become malnourished. Vitamin and mineral supplements are very beneficial, but they do not provide additional calories. Dietary supplements are available that can enhance vitamin and mineral nutrition as well as provide additional calories.

> *Enrich* is a liquid nutrition with fiber. Eight ounces contains 260 cal and 3.4 gm of dietary fiber. It is low in sodium and cholesterol and contains a complement of vitamins and minerals.
>
> *Ensure* provides nutritional and caloric enrichment. There are 250 cal per 8-oz serving. Like Enrich, it is low in sodium and cholesterol.
>
> *Ensure Plus* is similar to Ensure but has 355 cal per 8-oz serving.

PREVENTIVE NUTRITION IN THE PATIENT WITH A CHRONIC DISEASE

Many factors have been recognized as affecting the course of many diseases of aging, such as coronary heart disease, hypertension, cancer, glucose intolerance, and osteoporosis.

Coronary Artery Disease. A diet including reduced fats, increased soluble fiber, vitamins with the trace elements copper and chromium, and a supplement of fish oil capsules has been found helpful. Fish oil capsules reduce serum lipids, and the prostaglandins reducing inflammation seem to be increased. Fish consumption could be increased to three to four times a week instead of taking the supplement capsules.

Hypertension. Hypertensive patients should decrease sodium intake and, particularly if diuretic medications are prescribed, should increase potassium intake. Potassium supplements can be given, or intake of foods high in potassium, such as oranges, bananas, and raisins, should be increased. Calcium and magnesium supplements or increases in dairy products and beans, brown rice, broccoli, and fish may be in order.

Cancer. A diet high in fiber appears to be protective against colon and breast cancers. Fiber is provided naturally in fruits, vegetables, beans, and whole grains, or it can be given as a supplement in wheat bran or commercial fiber supplements. The antioxidant vitamins A, C, E, and the trace mineral selenium are being studied as protective against cancer. Antioxidants probably function as scavengers of "free radicals," products of tissue oxidation that cause cellular damage. Oranges and dark green vegetables provide B-carotene as well as many dietary supplements.

Diabetes. A diet with complex carbohydrates and 25 to 30 gm of dietary fiber daily has been shown to increase diabetic control. A diet deficient in chromium has been shown to increase the incidence of type II diabetes; thus, chromium supplements should be given. Food sources of chromium include brewer's yeast and nuts.

Vision Problems. Macular degeneration and cataracts may be slowed by administration of zinc supplements. Food sources of zinc include wheat germ, wheat bran, and oysters. Vitamin E and C supplements have been beneficial in lowering the incidence of cataracts.

Osteoporosis. Calcium, vitamin D supplements, and trace minerals such as magnesium and manganese have been used in the treatment of osteoporosis.

ARTHRITIS AND THE ELDERLY

There have been many improvements made in the treatment of osteoarthritis, which is no longer looked on as a simple "wear and tear" disease. The articular cartilage has been found to be a dynamic tissue rather than the static or inert substance it was once thought to be.

Articular cartilage serves a number of important functions. It minimizes friction between joint surfaces, thereby minimizing wear; it increases the contact area between bones within the joint, thus decreasing contact stress; and it helps dissipate energy and absorb shock.

One of the earliest changes seen in osteoarthritis is an increase in the water content of cartilage. This is clinically important because this change increases the porosity of the cartilage and thus decreases the strength and load-carrying capacity of the tissue.

The nonsteroidal anti-inflammatory drugs (NSAIDs) have been shown to interrupt this inflammatory process and the subsequent degeneration of cartilage. Some NSAIDs have more effect on the cartilage metabolism than others. Aspirin, ibuprofen (Motrin), and fenoprofen (Nalfon) have been shown to be the most beneficial in treating osteoarthritis. These agents are discussed in Chapter 24 (see Prostaglandin Inhibitors).

OSTEOPOROSIS IN THE ELDERLY

As the lifespan increases, so do the long-term problems seen with osteoporosis in the elderly female. The morbidity and mortality resulting from vertebral compression and fractures are very significant.

The most rapid bone loss in the female occurs in the first 5 years after menopause, or cessation of menses. It has been demonstrated that calcium supplements and exercise will somewhat retard this process, but research has shown definitively that the only true "treat-

ment" is prevention in the form of supplemental hormone therapy. The vasomotor symptoms or "hot flashes" are reduced or eliminated as well with hormone therapy.

Annual physicals are necessary when hormone therapy is given to detect the early presence of hormone-dependent cancers such as breast or gynecological cancer.

Many of the estrogens commercially available can be given to prevent osteoporosis (see their discussion in Chapter 27). Conjugated estrogen (Premarin) is the most commonly prescribed.

THE AGING THYROID AND HOW IT AFFECTS THE ELDERLY

Changes in thyroid function occur as a natural consequence of aging. These are associated with a lowered rate of thyroid hormone secretion and clearance from the body or, less commonly, hyperthyroidism or carcinoma of the thyroid.

Hypothyroidism occurs commonly in the elderly person. It has been found that the pituitary secretion of thyroid-stimulating hormone (TSH) does not change with aging. When elevated levels of TSH are found in the blood, even if there are no recognizable signs of hypothyroidism, it is believed that the patient has subclinical hypothyroidism and should be given replacement therapy.

When hypothyroidism occurs in the elderly, it may differ greatly from the disorder in a younger person. The following clinical signs should increase the suspicion of hypothyroidism in the elderly:

- Unexplained elevations in plasma cholesterol or triglycerides
- Congestive heart failure
- Fecal impaction
- Macrocytic anemia
- Vague arthritic complaints
- Mild psychiatric disturbances
- The presence of a thyroidectomy scar
- A history of treatment with thyroid hormone
- Previous treatment with radioactive iodine
- Goiter

The treatment of hypothyroidism is replacement therapy with thyroid hormone. This can be given in the form of the natural gland, or Armour Thyroid, or in the form of the synthetic thyroxine Synthroid. In most cases the need for thyroid hormone replacement is permanent. The doses are individualized according to the patient's needs and responses. These agents are discussed in Chapter 27.

When hyperthyroidism, or Graves' disease, occurs in the elderly, the signs may be muted or masked. Congestive heart failure is the most common presenting symptom of hyperthyroidism. Weight loss, muscle weakness, palpitations, eyelid tremor, eyelid lag, exophthalmos, and nervousness are also seen.

The principal treatment for hyperthyroidism in the elderly is radioactive iodine. The antithyroid drugs propylthiouracil and methimazole are used in the younger patient, but they are less satisfactory in the elderly.

Thyroid cancer, or papillary carcinoma, is a more aggressive malignancy in the elderly. The aggressiveness includes a more rapid rate of growth, metastases to distant sites, and recurrence after surgery. Surgery remains the treatment of choice, followed by antineoplastic drug therapy.

HYPERTENSION IN THE ELDERLY

Hypertension in the elderly must be treated more carefully than in the younger patient. The elderly have sluggish sympathetic responsiveness and impaired autoregulation; thus, therapy should be slow and gradual, avoiding drugs that cause postural hypotension or exacerbate other medical problems that patients may have. The goal of therapy should be about 160/90, not a strictly "normal" pressure. Postural hypotension, dizziness, and falls, which commonly result in serious fractures, have often been caused in part by medications that lower blood pressure.

Diuretics may be used, even though they are no longer the primary drug of choice for the younger patient. Beta blockers should be used with caution; calcium channel blockers are a good choice as are angiotensin-converting enzyme inhibitors in certain patients. Long-acting dosage forms should be chosen whenever possible to keep the number of medication doses at a minimum.

ANTI-INFECTIVE THERAPY IN THE ELDERLY

The elderly experience a higher incidence of vascular, metabolic, degenerative, and neoplastic disorders. They are also very susceptible to infectious complications of all their disorders. Antibiotic therapy can be challenging because the infection is often well advanced before they seek therapy, and, when treatment is begun, drug penetration into infected tissues is inadequate because arteriosclerosis limits access.

In addition, physiological changes associated with aging result in alteration of drug metabolism. Renal plasma flow declines with age; thus, drugs dependent on the "average" renal function or excretion may build up in the body to toxic levels. Congestive heart failure may slow circulation further.

Some drug categories that must be monitored are as follows:

Aminoglycoside Antibiotics. Kanamycin, gentamicin, tobramycin, amikacin, and netilmicin are used in the elderly for infections caused by *Enterobacter* and *Pseudomonas* strains. Excretion of these agents is often delayed, however. Thus, blood levels must be monitored carefully. Nephrotoxicity and ototoxicity are common toxic effects.

Penicillins. Patients with impaired renal function may have acute renal failure or hemolytic anemia when large doses of penicillin are given parenterally. Neurotoxic symptoms of muscle twitching, myoclonic jerking, and seizures have been reported as well. Large parenteral doses may be necessary for life-threatening, severe infections; thus, choices may be limited.

Cephalosporins. Life-threatening hemorrhage may result from wound sites or the gastrointestinal tract. The risk of hemorrhage is greatest in the poorly nourished patient who has cancer and who has undergone a surgical procedure. It has been theorized that the cephalosporins interfere with intestinal microorganism production of vitamin K.

Nitrofurantoin. Elderly patients who have been administered this agent for urinary tract infections have been reported to have increased risk of agranulocytosis, hepatitis, and chronic pulmonary fibrosis. It is believed that this agent should be used with caution in the elderly if at all.

The Quinolones. This new class of antimicrobial agents has been shown to be highly favorable for use in the elderly. These agents (norfloxacin, ciprofloxacin, and ofloxacin) have a broad spectrum of activity, are active orally in twice-daily doses, and can be prescribed for penicillin-sensitive patients. They are contraindicated in patients with seizure disorders and are inactivated by the concurrent use of liquid antacids containing aluminum or magnesium.

ANXIETY IN THE ELDERLY

Anxiety is a prominent problem in the elderly. The older patient is likely to suffer from a wide array of medical illnesses that can produce symptoms that either mimic or trigger anxiety. These illnesses include cardiovascular disease; drug-related problems; endocrine, hematological, immunological, neurological, or pulmonary problems; and some form of cancer. In addition, the elderly are often engaged in less productive activities and, therefore, have more time to worry than do younger people.

There has been a great impetus toward the development and implementation of anxiolytic pharmacotherapeutic agents that do not carry the increased risks associated with the use of benzodiazepines in the elderly. The benzodiazepines are alprazolam (Xanax), chlorazepate (Tranxene), chlordiazepoxide (Librium), diazepam (Valium), flurazepam (Dalmane), halazepam (Paxipam), lorazepam (Ativan), midazolam (Versed), oxazepam (Serax), prazepam (Centrax), temazepam (Restoril), and trazolam (Halcion). Many of these agents are discussed in Chapter 23.

As a class, these are useful agents for the relief of anxiety and the treatment of insomnia. They have a mild sedative effect on the younger adult patient. In the elderly, however, owing to a decreased ability to detoxify these agents, there is often inadvertent overdosage and cumulative toxicity. Impaired motor function with frequent falls, a decrease in cognitive function, and extrapyramidal effects or tremors are frequently seen when these agents are used in the elderly.

Buspirone (Buspar) has been shown to be the drug of choice in many studies for the treatment of anxiety in the elderly. It is also discussed in Chapter 23.

PRESCRIPTION DRUG IMPAIRMENT IN THE ELDERLY

The elderly suffer a disproportionate number of adverse drug reactions. A significant factor in this problem is that older patients are more likely to have chronic diseases requiring long-term treatment. Eighty percent of those older than 65 years have one or more chronic illnesses.

Drug toxicity is likely to affect the central nervous system, and these symptoms may be attributed to underlying causes such as sepsis, neurological disease, and metabolic derangements. Adding to this difficulty is poor drug compliance in the elderly. Compliance has been estimated to be about 45 percent in most drug regimens.

Complex regimens, when different medications must be taken at different times, before or after meals, or on an empty stomach, are even more likely to confuse geriatric patients. Those with underlying cognitive impairment are even more susceptible to confusion.

Inadvertent drug overdoses are often prescribed. Owing to slowing of drug detoxification processes, the elderly can often obtain the desired pharmacological effect on a dose 25 to 50 percent lower than the average adult dose. This is particularly true of psychotropic medications.

When many drugs are prescribed for the patient, and this is particularly true when the patient is seeing more than one physician, there is the potential for adverse drug-drug reactions as well.

Drug absorption is altered by delays in gastric emptying, decreased gastrointestinal motility, decreased efficacy of cellular transport systems, and decreased gastrointestinal blood flow.

Drug distribution changes found in the aging include a smaller body size and decreased muscle mass, resulting in a lowered ratio of lean body tissue to fat. There is also decreased body water content. These phenomena have significant pharmacological effects, including a greater concentration of drugs distributed in body fluids, decreased storage of water-soluble drugs, prolonged storage of fat-soluble drugs, and decreased drug binding to albumin with correspondingly increased levels of free drug.

Drug metabolism is reduced owing to decreased blood flow to the liver, decreased liver size, and decreased enzyme activity. This increases the risk for accumulation of drugs in the elderly.

Drug excretion is reduced owing to a decline in renal function. Slower drug clearance by the kidneys increases the drug half-life in the body.

All these factors combined contribute to the effects of overdosage in the elderly. The doses of many agents should be lowered when administered to the elderly.

FAMILY CARE OF THE ELDERLY AND CAREGIVER STRESS

When the elderly patient is living at home, a caregiver is usually required. Meeting the needs of the elderly causes increased stress in the caregiver. There is often a sense of ambivalence because the son, daughter, or spouse who is the caregiver would otherwise be at a stage of life when most responsibilities are fulfilled, and this is the long-awaited free time for travel or other interests.

Concerns about the seemingly increasing incidence of elder abuse reflect a decompensation in the caregiver. Health personnel can play an important role in screening for elder abuse and offering appropriate support, education, advice, and intervention for the elderly person and his or her caregiver.

Parental care is different from child care. Child care is naturally expected to lessen as time goes on. The reverse is true with elder care. Adult children begin with grocery shopping and transportation, then add housecleaning and meal preparation, bathing and dressing, and, finally, feeding and coping with incontinence.

Caregiver stress can present as vague symptoms of fatigue, anxiety, depression, back strain, anger, guilt, frustration, social isolation, and a perception of poor health. Elements to screen for when interviewing the caregiver include a history of drug or alcohol abuse in the elderly person or the caregiver, a family history of violence, a mention of "punishment" of the elderly person by the caregiver, or a recent life stress for the caregiver.

Caregivers need specific advice. They must be encouraged to set realistic limitations on the amount of care they can give. Other family members should be encouraged to become involved and give relief to the primary caregiver. The use of day care centers for the elderly and temporary nursing home placement for time off should be encouraged.

Self-help or support groups for caregivers are available in many communities. In addition, there are support groups for those dealing with Alzheimer's disease in the elderly.

The health care worker should become familiar with support groups and services for the elderly in his or her community so that support and intervention can be given whenever necessary.

Implications for the Student

1. The metabolism of the geriatric patient differs significantly from that of the younger adult. The patient should be observed for signs of drug overdose.

2. Aging patients should not merely be considered as senile when behavior and abili-

ties begin to change. A look at the possibility of underlying diseases is always in order.

3. The geriatric patient should be counseled thoroughly on the choices in his or her special diet. Careful attention should be given to nutrition with the recommendation of supplemental vitamins and minerals and dietary supplements.

4. Drug compliance is a problem in the elderly. They should be counseled regarding the importance of taking the medications as prescribed.

5. Falling, confusion, and decreased cognitive abilities may be signs of overdosage of a sedative medication.

6. The use of over-the-counter medications such as aspirin and ibuprofen can alleviate many of the symptoms of osteoarthritis.

7. Congestive heart failure may point to thyroid abnormalities as well as specific problems with the myocardium of the heart.

8. The health care worker should be aware of problems with the elderly patient's caregiver. Skilled counseling is possible only if the social problems are recognized.

9. Anxiety is a common problem of the elderly. The use of anxiolytic agents can significantly relieve many of these symptoms.

10. Chronological aging does not in itself mean a loss of function or a poor quality of life. Good medical care and the proper use of community services can provide many improvements for the elderly.

11. Preventive nutrition may prevent or minimize some chronic illnesses in the elderly.

12. Hypertension must be treated with mild drugs; the goal of treatment is not as stringent as in the younger person.

13. When infections become more numerous and severe, the tolerance to many antibiotics is decreased.

CASE STUDIES

1. Minnie A., 72, came to the heart clinic today for her 6-month checkup. The chart shows a slow but steady weight loss for the past year. Minnie says that she is so tired it is hard to get to the grocery store, and mostly she just has toast and tea for lunch and a sandwich for dinner. What may be some of her additional problems? How may they be improved?

2. Harold P., 82, is admitted to the hospital for a broken hip. The physician ordered blood studies because of the large bruises over his shoulder and upper back. The blood studies are normal. His daughter says he "just falls a lot." Should further investigation and studies be made?

3. Sarah R., 68, has become more and more confused when she is seen in follow-up for her hypertension. Her medications include digoxin, Lasix, Slow-K, Valium, and Dalmane. Should any of the medications be considered part of her problem?

4. Sharon P., 50, came to her physician for "burnout." She works full time, has two teenage children, an elderly father with

Alzheimer's disease, and a married daughter with a new baby. With no time for herself, her marriage is suffering, and she complains of sleep problems and anxiety. What suggestions may be made to improve her situation?

Review Questions

1. Name five health problems commonly found in the elderly.

2. What is senility? Why should all elderly persons not be assumed to be senile when changes in behavior are observed?

3. What sort of interview may be made of a homebound elderly person to assess his or her diet and nutrition? What recommendations may be made to improve the diet?

4. List the symptoms of hypothyroidism in the elderly. How may these differ from the symptoms of hypothyroidism in the young child or younger adult?

5. What are the symptoms of hyperthyroidism in the elderly person? How may these differ from those seen in the younger adult?

6. Why is anxiety such a problem in the elderly? Describe various ways of improving anxiety in addition to medication.

7. How does the elderly person's metabolism differ from that of the younger person? How does this affect drug metabolism?

8. How would you interview the caregiver of an elderly person? What services are available in your community to assist the caregiver?

9. Should all bruises and injuries in the elderly be simply attributed to clumsiness and falling? Why or why not? What further steps may be taken to assess the cause of the injuries?

10. What general recommendations may be given to an elderly person to improve the quality of life?

11. What dietary improvements may help in the management of the following?
    a. Hypertension
    b. Cancer
    c. Coronary artery disease
    d. Diabetes
    e. Osteoporosis

12. What common debility of the aged patient may interfere with drug therapy, particularly antibiotics?

32

Drug Therapy in Home Health Care

Objectives for the Student

B E

A B L E

T O

■ 1. Understand the necessity for and objectives of home health care.
■ 2. Become aware of the different medications given in the home setting.
■ 3. Appreciate the expanded role of the nurse and allied health professional in the home health field.
■ 4. Assess the homebound patient, and evaluate the environmental factors that affect the quality of the treatment.
■ 5. Recognize side effects of medications administered.
■ 6. Recognize factors that change the goals of drug therapy for the terminally ill patient.

Home health care has grown rapidly, and with it has grown the opportunities for nurses and allied health care workers.

Home care offers an acceptable, effective alternative to extended hospitalization. Cost-containment efforts by payers, newer techniques, and the increasingly sophisticated home health care providers have made all in the health care field believe that this trend will only increase in the future.

The home health care professional is a part of a collaborative team of nurse, physician, and other health care providers. Usually the home health worker is the only one seeing the patient on a regular basis; thus, he or she must be responsible for the assessment of the patient and keep sufficiently detailed records so that changes in the patient's condition, mental state, blood pressure, and so on may be noted and reported in a timely fashion.

The health care worker must be acutely aware of the medications that each patient is taking and be knowledgeable of the effects, side effects, and potential toxic effect of each medication so that untoward effects may be avoided. Appropriate corrective actions may be taken by other members of the team only if problems are reported.

A new assessment of nursing theories and responsibilities must be made. The new role of providing home care places more emphasis on responsibility and decision-making skills for the nurse or health professional.

Some aspects of home health care are covered in this chapter, but it cannot be all inclusive.

HOME INFUSION THERAPY

Home infusion can shorten or prevent hospitalization for selected patients needing intravenous antibiotics, chemotherapy, hydration, pain management, immunoglobulins, transfusions, and parenteral nutrition.

The main advantage of home infusion is that it offers the patient a more normal lifestyle with reduced medical costs. Home infusion is generally safe and effective. The following list includes many of the home infusion therapies now considered standard:

- Short- and long-term antibiotics
- Antifungal and antiviral therapy
- Blood transfusions
- Total parenteral nutrition
- Pain management
- Chemotherapy
- Anticoagulation with heparin
- Suppression of premature labor with terbutaline

Patients who are referred for home infusion often have no previous experience in this type of therapy. They must be screened for intellectual, psychological, social, and environmental factors before home infusion is offered.

The patient should be medically stable after discharge, with the exception of the need for intravenous therapy. Patients with hypotension, unexplained fevers, respiratory distress, active bleeding, recent emboli, or other conditions that render them medically unstable are poor risks for home health care.

Medications that may cause allergic or severe adverse reactions should not be started in the home and should merely be continued by home therapy after initial doses are administered in a hospital setting.

Long-term central catheters are commonly used for home infusions. Occluded catheters may sometimes be reopened by infusing small amounts of acid or base solution, and clotted catheters may be opened by the infusion of urokinase. Pumps that can be programmed offer new alternatives for the administration of various medications at different times.

Pediatric Home Infusion

Home infusion therapy for the pediatric populations presents another set of obstacles and opportunities.

Hospitalization is a stressful and expensive event for a child and the family. The trend toward moving even high-technology care into the home is very beneficial. Particular problems occur with the pediatric patient, however. Fear and its associated lack of cooperation and the limited intellectual ability and maturity of the child will cause problems. Maturity and cooperation of the parent or caregiver cannot be ensured either. Parents may be of limited intelligence and may be visually or physically handicapped as well, and they may not be dependable as allies in the care of the child.

Hematology and oncology patients are often candidates for home care. Blood and blood product administration, intravenous medication administration, and total parenteral nutrition are often done in the home.

Families should be encouraged to discuss the procedures with the home health caregiver, and the child's questions should be answered truthfully; the child should be given as much explanation as the situation warrants. Much of the anxiety and fear experienced by the child and the family is associated with a lack of comfort in their roles as regards the infusion. Effective communication here is essential.

Cancer Pain Management

Pain is a major symptom of cancer patients. In many cases, the pain is poorly controlled, and it has been estimated that 25 to 35 percent of cancer patients die without adequate pain relief. It is difficult to understand why patients have uncontrolled pain when all experts acknowledge that almost all cancer patients will respond to appropriate doses of analgesic medication.

There are many oral, topical, and parenteral

medications for pain relief. Two of the most common reasons for poor pain control are as follows:

1. Underprescribing and underdosing of the analgesic medication, or failure to use appropriate drugs
2. Inappropriate fears and attitudes on the part of the health care provider that cancer pain is inevitable and untreatable and that drug addiction and tolerance must be continuously considered and avoided

To improve the quality of pain control, some issues must be kept in mind:

- Pain is what the patient says it is. Nurses should not place their feelings, impressions, or evaluations on patient reports.
- Narcotic medications should be given orally when appropriate, giving the patient more control over self-administration. Cancer does not cease at night; thus, pain medication should be prescribed in sufficient amounts for around-the-clock dosing.
- The fear of drug addiction is not an issue in the terminal patient. If tolerance to the drug occurs, the dose should be increased . . . period. The dose should be sufficient to manage the pain.

Pain control should begin with the least potent of the analgesics; even Tylenol and aspirin products may be effective in the beginning. Progression proceeds through the nonsteroidal anti-inflammatory drugs, to the nonopiate analgesics such as propoxyphene napsylate–acetaminophen (Darvocet) and aspirin-caffeine-butalbital (Fiorinal), then finally to the oral meperidines or hydromorphone (Dilaudid). Topical application of fentanyl (Duragesic) has been shown to be surprisingly effective in the management of chronic pain and may be used to further delay the time when parenteral analgesics must be given.

Pain control at all stages should be appropriate and sufficient.

Home Therapy for the Bone Marrow Transplant Patient

With the new ability to treat malignant and nonmalignant diseases with bone marrow transplants, there comes the attendant problems of long-term therapy for these patients, often in a home setting.

The patient first has bone marrow destroyed by myelosuppressive therapy of one sort or another and then receives a compatible marrow by infusion.

Prophylactic therapy is aimed at preventing infections in the immunocompromised state following transplantation. Antibiotics and antifungal and antiviral agents are used. Anemia is treated with whole blood transfusions or with packed cells after the blood products are irradiated.

There is often general denuding of the mouth and the entire gastrointestinal tract. Pain control, oral hygiene, adequate nutrition, and fluid intake must be managed. Hepatic, renal, and pulmonary dysfunction occur and must be managed appropriately.

Pain associated with all the attendant malfunctions must be managed within the guidelines of chronic pain management.

Diabetics in the Home Care Setting

The severe diabetic with secondary problems resulting from disease often becomes a candidate for home health services.

Diabetic retinopathy often leaves the patient severely visually compromised or even totally blind. The patient cannot then self-administer insulin injections or attend to personal hygiene, foot care, or skin care properly.

Syringes prefilled by a home health worker may facilitate the visually impaired to continue partial self-sufficiency. Continual observation of the patient for skin breakdown or infections and monitoring of blood glucose levels are necessary. Detailed inquiries about any diet management and assessment of the patient's level of skill in taking any other medications must be made.

Psychiatric Home Care

The move to decentralize health care and provide more services in the home has extended to psychiatric patients as well. To some patients discharge from the hospital may mean that "there is no more hope for me" rather than the improvement generally believed by other patients. To the other extreme, the "I'm cured" way of thinking may prompt the patient to stop taking medications altogether.

The home health care worker must be skilled in the assessment of the patient's medication needs and compliance in taking them. An understanding of adverse side effects of the psychotropic drugs and recognition that the dose may be too small or large are important factors to assess.

Food imbalances, imbalances of activity and rest, an inability to make appropriate food choices, poor self-care, and a deteriorating environment may be early signs that the mental status is declining.

Home health care workers who care for clients being treated for mental illness must be trained to collaborate with psychiatrists to provide adequate care.

When assessing a patient whose behavior indicates a mental illness, the nurse must evaluate four things:

- Whether the aberrant behavior reflects a new primary disorder or is secondary to another disease or a medication side effect
- Whether the behavior is precipitated by stress or is a sign that medication effects are different than predicted
- The level of aberrant behavior and whether it constitutes a threat to the patient or others
- The behavior with relation to the culture and environment

Assessing psychiatric issues requires that the nurse be trained to listen; most assessment involves interviews and observation.

Implications for the Student

1. The role of the home health provider places new responsibilities on the nurse or other health care provider.

2. Often the nurse is the only professional who sees the patient on a regular basis. It is important to remain alert for any changes in the patient's status.

3. Detailed records must be kept with regard to the patient's mental condition and personal hygiene or affect as well as the medical signs of blood pressure, pulse, and so on.

4. If there are signs that the patient is not medically stable, the medical provider should be notified immediately.

5. Pediatric patients may have excessive fears that interfere with therapy.

6. The abilities of the patient's home caregiver should be also assessed.

7. Effective communication skills with the patient, family, and others on the health team are essential.

8. New skills may need to be learned for infusions at the home site.

9. Pain management for the terminally ill patient has different goals than that for the acutely ill patient.

10. Fears of narcotic tolerance and habituation are not applicable when treating a terminally ill patient.

11. Skills in assessing patient compliance with medication are particularly important when visiting the psychiatric patient.

12. Clues from the home environment are often helpful when assessing the patient.

CASE STUDIES

1. Mrs. E., 76, has been an insulin-dependent diabetic for many years. Her blood sugar levels have been unstable lately with several high or low readings. After visiting with her, she asks you to set her oven because she is having trouble with the numbers. Would you have any recommendations for her care?

2. John P., 27, previously diagnosed as a schizophrenic, was sent home stable on his psychiatric medication. On your recent visit, you notice he is eating only bread, his appearance is becoming more disheveled, and he is obviously delusional. What would be your procedure?

3. Mr. P., 67, who is on intravenous medication for his colon cancer, reports more sores in his mouth today. What would you advise?

Review Questions

1. What would you look for when visiting a recently discharged psychiatric patient? What questions would you ask the patient?

2. Outline objectives for pain management for the following:
   a. An athlete recovering from a fractured pelvis
   b. A child undergoing prolonged treatment for osteomyelitis
   c. A mother of your homebound patient who complains of low back pain
   d. A terminally ill cancer patient

3. What drugs may be given to a cancer patient by home infusion? Look up the side effects of each, and list the ones that may cause the drug to be stopped.

4. Look up the antifungal and antiviral drugs that may be given to the bone marrow transplant patient, and list the effects and untoward reactions of each.

5. Discuss the nursing implications of the diabetic homebound patient.

33

Drug and Alcohol Abuse

Objectives for the Student

B E

A B L E

T O

- ■ 1. Identify the risk factors that predispose to drug abuse.
- ■ 2. Identify particular risk factors in the teenager.
- ■ 3. Have an understanding of drug addiction and its symptoms.
- ■ 4. Recognize withdrawal symptoms in drug dependence.
- ■ 5. Recognize the symptoms shown by a patient under the influence of drugs.
- ■ 6. Become familiar with the short- and long-term effects of alcohol abuse.
- ■ 7. Recognize drugs that are potentiated in their effects when taken with alcohol.
- ■ 8. Identify the physical symptoms and dangerous sequelae of a drug overdose.

Substance abuse has become a national and international problem of gigantic proportions and in some way affects all of us. The use of psychoactive drugs by children and adolescents is a fact no longer questioned. The most reasonable preventive effort is now focused on education. Rehabilitation programs have limited success but are increasing in numbers as the national problem persists.

According to a publication of the U.S. Department of Health and Human Services, more than 90 percent of adolescents in the United States will have used alcohol before graduating from high school, 50 percent will have used marijuana, 17 percent have used cocaine, and 12 percent will have used hallucinogens. Of the 25,000 accidental deaths among youths annually, approximately 40 percent are alcohol related.

Studies have been made of the risk factors that predispose to substance abuse. The studies have shown that vulnerability to drug use is increased in children who have low self-esteem, a feeling of not belonging, a high need for social approval, inadequate bonding to family and society, inadequate communication and coping skills, inability to defer gratification, and an inability to accept the consequences of their actions. A family history of alcoholism or drug abuse greatly increases the risk.

The drug-abusing teenager may first come to medical attention as a result of trauma related to intoxication or secondary to an acute drug overdose. The health care team should be responsible not only for treating the trauma but also for recognizing and assessing the substance abuse problem and, it is hoped, initiating some sort of remedial program. Most adolescents have three spheres of interaction: school, family, and peers. Adolescents who are having difficulty in any one of these spheres probably need referral for drug treatment. Convincing a patient and family members that a referral is needed may not be easy because there may be denial, a minimizing of the problem as a one-time occurrence, or a rejection of the values of society altogether.

During acute crises or overdoses in drug abusers, the health care worker has the responsibility of assessing the type of drug taken, the method of administration, the time the drug was taken, and the previous pattern of drug abuse. This information can be obtained from the abuser, if responsive, or the family or friends.

In the treatment and rehabilitation of the drug abuser, the health care worker is involved at many levels, assisting the patient through the withdrawal period, observing the patient for other problems, and observing the effects of therapy and the patient's level of cooperation.

SEVEN SIGNS OF POSSIBLE DRUG INVOLVEMENT

1. Change in school or work attendance or performance (e.g., the student whose grades begin to fall or whose absentee rate is a matter of concern)
2. Alteration of personal appearance (e.g., the student who was once neat now appears disheveled and disorderly)
3. Mood swings or attitude changes
4. Withdrawal from family contacts
5. Association with drug-using friends
6. Unusual patterns of behavior or mannerisms
7. Defensive attitude concerning drugs

DEPENDENCE ON NARCOTICS

Heroin is the drug of choice for most addicts in the United States. Although this drug is outlawed in this country, illicit drug channels keep the addicts supplied. Paregoric, morphine, and hydramorphine (Dilaudid) are often abused also.

The desired sensation is a euphoria after administration, usually intravenous. With continued use a tolerance to the drug occurs and higher doses are required for the euphoria. After a period of time, the addiction is so intense that the drug is taken for homeostasis and to prevent withdrawal symptoms. Accidental overdoses and death may occur inadvertently or in an attempt to obtain euphoria again.

The withdrawal symptoms from narcotics are severe and may be life threatening. The first abstinence symptoms are malaise and weakness about 6 to 12 hours after the last dose. After 12 hours, yawning and perspiration occur, and the patient becomes anxious. After 24 hours muscular contractions, chills, muscular pains, increased rate and depth of respiration, blood pressure elevation, pupil dilation, and extreme agitation occur. The withdrawal symptoms peak in 48 hours and begin to subside in 72 hours. General symptoms of weakness and malaise may be present for several weeks.

Methadone maintenance programs have been developed to sustain narcotic addicts after withdrawal. Although methadone is in itself an addicting narcotic, it produces little euphoria and allows the patient to function normally in society. Even with methadone, the percentage of permanent cessation of the addiction is small.

SEDATIVE-HYPNOTIC ABUSE

Although these agents can be obtained through illicit channels, they are often abused via the patient's prescription medications, often from many physicians simultaneously. These drugs become dangerous, particularly when combined with alcohol or other depressive drugs.

Withdrawal is not as severe as with the narcotic agents and is primarily characterized by insomnia, irritability, and anxiety-related symptoms.

MARIJUANA ABUSE

Marijuana is an intoxicant derived from the leaves and flowering tops of the *Cannabis* plant. It is generally smoked in cigarette form and produces a feeling of euphoria and a dreamy state. The length of the effect lasts 3 to 12 hours. Physical dependence most certainly occurs, although the question of true addiction is not settled.

Disorders have been attributed to long-term or chronic use of marijuana. These include chromosome breaks, personality and mental changes, anxiety, and irritation when the drug is not available.

One of its more notable disadvantages is that it leads the dependent person to try other and more addicting substances for a greater euphoric effect.

COCAINE ABUSE

Although cocaine was once thought to be a relatively "safe" recreational drug, it is now considered one of the most serious of all addictive drugs.

In 1984 the highly potent, highly addictive "crack" was introduced, and its availability, along with its relatively inexpensive price, has greatly increased the number of addicts. It is believed that even one use makes an addict, because the powerful urge for another "high" is so intense, even after the first experience with this drug.

Cocaine is a central nervous system stimulant with effects that are similar to those of amphetamine. It produces a strong stimulant and euphoric effect and increases pulse rate, blood pressure, and respiratory rate. The user feels a heightened sense of self-confidence, clarity of thought, alertness, and increased energy and well-being. Reductions in the need for sleep and food are common. The intoxicated individual has tremulousness, dysphoria, delirium, delusional thinking, and assaultive behavior.

Withdrawal symptoms include deep depression and profound exhaustion. Suicidal behavior is common in withdrawal.

Medications are now used to treat the cocaine addict and to assist in the withdrawal and replacement process. These include the antidepressants such as desipramine, imipramine, protriptyline, and trazodone. Lithium, usually prescribed for manic-depressive disorders, has been effective, especially if combined with an antidepressant. Supplements of the amino acids tyrosine and tryptophan, when combined with an antidepressant, seem to block the cocaine high.

ALCOHOL ABUSE

The most common "street drug" today, alcohol is losing much of its social acceptability as the effects of its abuse become recognized.

Unlike the other abused agents, alcohol does have some beneficial effects in moderation. It has been shown to raise the level of high-density lipoproteins (the "good" type of cholesterol) and thus reduce the risk of coronary disease. Its effect on behavior is well known, from a

Table 33-1. PRESCRIPTION DRUGS AFFECTED BY ALCOHOL

Alcohol Combined with	May Cause
Sleeping medication	Rapid intoxication with
Tranquilizers	small amounts of alcohol
Antidepressants	Excessive drowsiness
Motion sickness medication	Mental confusion
Pain relievers	
Muscle relaxants	
Antihistamines	
Allergy medicine	
Antiangina medication	Dizziness, fainting
Antihypertensives	Lack of muscle coordination, falling
Aspirin	Increase in gastric irritation
Nonsteroidal anti-inflammatory drugs	and bleeding
Potassium tablets	
Anticoagulants	
Metronidazole (Flagyl)	Severe reaction, similar to
Oral hypoglycemic agents	that of disulfiram
Certain antibiotics	(Antabuse); nausea, vomiting, flushing, tachycardia, dyspnea
Anticoagulants	Changes in the effectiveness
Oral hypoglycemic agents	of the drug controlling the
Seizure medications	condition

Table 33-2. COMPARATIVE SYMPTOMS OF DRUG USE

Drug	Physical Symptoms	Signs to Look for	Dangerous Effects
Inhalants (gas, aerosols)	Nausea, dizziness, headaches, lack of coordination	Odor of the substance on breath, intoxication symptoms	Unconsciousness, brain damage, sudden death
Heroin, narcotics	Euphoria, drowsiness, nausea, vomiting	Pinpoint pupils, needle tracks on arms	Death from overdose, AIDS, hepatitis from needles
Cocaine, amphetamine	Talkativeness, hyperalert state, increased blood pressure	History of weight loss, hyperactivity, ulcers in nasal mucosa	Sudden death, hallucinations, paranoia
Barbiturates, alcohol, tranquilizers	Intoxication, slowed heart and respiratory rate	Capsules and pills, history of seeing more than one physician, slurred speech	Death in overdose, especially in combinations with alcohol
Hallucinogens, LSD, PCP	Altered mood, panic, focus on detail	Capsules, blotter squares	Unpredictable and violent behavior
Marijuana	Altered perceptions, euphoria, laughing, red eyes, dry mouth	Cigarette papers, odor of burnt rope	Panic reaction, impaired memory

LSD = lysergic acid diethylamide; PCP = phencyclidine hydrochloride.

sense of relaxation in small doses to behavior aberrations, a loss of sensorimotor control, and coma in overdose.

As chronic intake progresses, the abuser loses the ability to perform fine motor movements, memory and discrimination become dulled, and nausea and vomiting result. It is believed that the cumulative effects on the central nervous system and liver progress with each dose.

Infants born to alcohol abusers have a cluster of birth defects known as the fetal alcohol syndrome. This is typified by a typical "elfin" facies and mental retardation. There is some feeling that even small doses of alcohol during pregnancy may harm the fetus.

Many prescription drugs are potentiated by even small amounts of alcohol. These generally are agents that have sedation as a side effect. They include antihistamines, tranquilizers, some antidepressants, sleeping medications, and many muscle relaxants. As a general rule, alcohol should be avoided when taking any prescription medication (Table 33–1).

Table 33–2 presents a general idea of the agent taken when a patient presents with aberrant or drug-induced behavior. It should always be remembered that drug abusers often do not take a single substance. Drugs are often taken in combination, and they are often combined with alcohol.

Implications for the Student

1. Drug abuse among adolescents is very common. An assessment of the patient should include some questions about drug and alcohol abuse.

2. A vigorous denial of drug use should not be accepted at face value if the adolescent has risk factors for substance abuse.

3. The withdrawal symptoms from drug usage are severe and life threatening. Many nursing interventions can be made to ease some of the discomfort.

4. After acute drug withdrawal the addiction problem remains. Subsequent follow-up is vitally important and must be reinforced and encouraged.

5. Substance abuse can occur using only prescription medications. Questioning for

drug compliance and the use of several physicians as drug sources can uncover this problem.

6. There is no "safe" recreational drug.

7. The most commonly abused substance is alcohol. Society provides many situations in which alcohol abuse is approved or tolerated. Societal norms are now found to be detrimental when attempting to control alcohol abuse.

8. Cocaine is a dangerous and extremely addicting drug, particularly in the "crack" form.

9. Many drugs are useful in the treatment of cocaine and heroin addiction. These agents both reduce the craving for the drug and prevent recurrence of the addictive pattern.

10. The symptoms of drug use, although not explicit in many cases, can enable the nurse to identify patients who may be under the influence of drugs.

CASE STUDIES

1. Patsy S., 17, has been brought to the emergency room after a car accident. She has a broken wrist and multiple bruises. Although it is expected that she would be worried and in pain, she is bright, cheerful, talkative, and alert. What other assessment may be made on this patient?

2. Mark M., 14, is brought in for psychological testing by his parents. While in grade school Mark was an excellent student. He seems to have adjustment problems in high school, however. His grades are barely passing, he seems to have no friends, and his clothes seem disheveled and dirty. What line of questioning may be appropriate here?

3. Mrs. Q., 47, calls the clinic to say she needs a new prescription for Valium. Her entire bottle of tablets somehow was flushed down the toilet. You notice on her chart that her purse was stolen, necessitating a new prescription just 2 weeks ago. She also has headaches that require numerous pain medications, often called in just before the office closes. What additional problems may need to be pursued?

Review Questions

1. List several symptoms of drug withdrawal from heroin.

2. What are the symptoms that may appear when a person has been drinking excessive amounts of alcohol?

3. What symptoms or social factors may identify an adolescent as being at risk for drug abuse?

4. How would you approach the subject of drug abuse with an adolescent?

5. What are the symptoms of cocaine use? What are the dangers of overdose?

6. Why does an individual become a heroin addict? Are treatment and rehabilitation effective?

7. What drug is used to treat former heroin addicts?

8. What drugs may help in the treatment of cocaine addiction?

9. Name seven signs of possible drug involvement.

10. What may be the signs that a person has been using the following?
    a. Freon as an inhalant
    b. Crack cocaine
    c. Alcohol
    d. Heroin

11. How can you tell the difference between "normal" aberrant teenage behavior and the behavior often associated with drug abuse?

GLOSSARY

Achlorhydria: the absence of hydrochloric acid in the stomach.

Acidosis: a decrease in the alkali reserve of the blood, notably in the bicarbonates, with lowering of the blood pH.

Addiction: the state in which the use of drugs is compulsive; withdrawal symptoms occur if the drug is withdrawn, owing to cellular dependence.

Addison's disease: adrenal insufficiency, fatal if not treated with corticosteroid hormones. Symptoms include bronzing of the skin, emaciation, and anemia.

Adrenergic: an agent that produces stimulating effects on the sympathetic nervous system (Adrenalin-like effects).

Adrenergic-blocking agent: a drug that interferes with the adrenergic, or sympathetic nervous system, actions.

Agranulocytosis: a toxic condition often caused by reactions to drug therapy in which a certain type of white blood cells—those with very small granules in the cell body—is deficient or absent.

Alkaloid: an organic substance, basic in reaction, often the active ingredient of plant medicinals.

Alkalosis: an increase in the bicarbonate content of the blood with subsequent raising of the blood pH.

Allergen: a substance capable of producing an allergic reaction.

Analgesic: a substance used to relieve pain.

Analog: a substance structurally or chemically similar to another related drug or chemical.

Anaphylaxis: a severe, life-threatening allergic reaction accompanied by vasodilation, lowered blood pressure, and shock.

Anemia: a reduction in the hemoglobin content or number of red blood cells.

Anesthetic, general: an agent that induces analgesia, then unconsciousness.

Anesthetic, local: an agent, usually injected, that interferes with local nerve transmission and produces deadening or anesthesia of a small area of the body.

Angina pectoris: severe chest pain resulting from ischemia of the cardiac muscle that may radiate to other locations, notably the left shoulder or arm.

Anorexia: a loss of appetite.

Antagonist: a drug that opposes a bodily system or expected effect.

Antibiotic: an agent that kills or inhibits microorganisms.

Antibody: a substance produced by the body as a reaction to the intrusion of a foreign compound, the substance being designed to counteract or neutralize the offending antigen.

Anticoagulant: a substance used to delay blood clotting.

Anticonvulsant: a substance used to prevent or treat seizures.

Antidepressant: a drug used to produce mood elevation or mild central nervous system stimulation.

Antiemetic: an agent that prevents vomiting.

Antigen: any substance that stimulates the production of antibodies in the body or any substance that reacts with previously formed antibodies.

Antihistamine: an agent that prevents or diminishes the pharmacological effects of histamine, hence used in the treatment of allergic-type syndromes.

Antihypertensive: an agent used in the treatment of high blood pressure.

Antineoplastic: an agent used in the treatment of cancer.

Antipyretic: a substance used to lower body temperature.

Antiseptic: a substance that inhibits the growth of microorganisms.

Antispasmodic: an agent used to decrease peristaltic activity of the gastrointestinal tract.

Aplastic anemia: dysfunction of the bone marrow, often occurring as a reaction of drug therapy, in which there is a severe decrease in the production of erythrocytes and white blood cells.

Ascites: the presence of large amounts of fluid in the abdominal cavity.

Asphyxia: suffocation.

Asthma: a condition in which there is constriction of the lung bronchioles in response to allergic or emotional phenomena, producing symptoms of dyspnea, constriction in the chest, coughing, and expiratory wheezing.

Ataxia: muscular incoordination with staggering gait.

Atherosclerosis: the deposition of fatty material in the walls of the blood vessels.

Athetosis: recurrent, slow, and continual body movements, usually the result of a brain lesion.

Atrium (pl. atria): the upper chambers of the heart.

Bacteremia: the presence of microorganisms in the blood stream.

Bactericide: a substance that kills bacteria.

Bacteriostatic: a substance that inhibits the growth of bacteria.

Beriberi: a condition caused by a nutritional deficiency of thiamine (vitamin B_1), with symptoms and neurological involvement such as weakness, paralysis, edema, and mental deterioration.

Bladder: the membranous sac that collects urine produced by the kidneys.

BNDD: Bureau of Narcotics and Dangerous Drugs.

Bowman's capsule: the renal glomerular capsule.

Bradycardia: slowing of the heartbeat.

Bronchiole: the tiny, thin-walled lung tubules near the alveoli.

Bronchodilator: an agent that causes relaxation and enlargement of the bronchi.

Cancer: a tumor or unnatural growth in the body.

Candidiasis: a superinfection with the fungus *Candida albicans.* May be in the form of diaper rash, oral mucous membrane involvement (thrush), vaginitis, or infection of the skin or nails. If superinfection occurs in the gastrointestinal tract, diarrhea commonly results.

Carcinogen: an agent that produces cancer.

Carminative: an agent used to expel gas from the gastrointestinal tract.

Catalyst: a substance that increases the speed of a chemical reaction but is not used up nor permanently changed in any way by the reaction.

Cathartic: a strong laxative that produces frequent, watery stools.

Cerebral palsy: a nonspecific term for motor, speech, and mental dysfunctions resulting from brain damage, usually at birth.

Chancroid: venereal infection with lesions involving the genitalia and enlarged, painful inguinal lymph nodes.

Cholinergic: an agent that produces the effects of stimulation of the parasympathetic nervous system (acetylcholine-like effects).

Cholinergic-blocking agent: an agent that interferes with the cholinergic, or parasympathetic nervous system, functions.

Colitis: inflammation of the colon with accompanying diarrhea, often associated with mucus or blood.

Contraceptive: an agent that prevents ovulation and, hence, conception.

Convulsion (seizure): involuntary muscle contractions either focal or generalized, usually occurring as a result of brain dysfunction.

Coryza: engorgement of the nasal mucous membranes accompanied by increased nasal discharge and often sneezing.

Cretin: mentally retarded dwarf with congenital hypothyroidism.

Crystalluria: crystals in the urine.

Cushing's disease (or syndrome): a condition caused by overactivity of the adrenal gland causing florid facies, edema, striae, demineralization of bone, and other effects.

Cyanosis: bluish tinge of the skin and mucous membranes, usually caused by excessive amounts of deoxygenated hemoglobin in the blood.

Cystitis: inflammation of the urinary bladder.

Dependence: a severe attachment to a drug or agent; an addiction.

Depressant: a reduction in activity of a bodily system.

Depression: an unnatural state of lethargy, inactivity, and sadness.

Dermatitis: an inflammatory condition of the skin.

Diabetes insipidus: a disease caused by a decrease in the hormone vasopressin, permitting large amounts of very dilute urine to be passed regardless of the body fluid status. The condition is accompanied by extreme thirst and dehydration.

Diabetes mellitus: a condition brought about by a deficiency of functional insulin from the pancreas, thus interfering with the body's ability to metabolize glucose. Hyperglycemia, glycosuria, atherosclerosis, decreased resistance to infection, retinal hemorrhages, and kidney damage are among the manifestations of the disease.

Disinfectant (germicide): a substance that destroys microorganisms on objects. Usually too irritating to be used on human tissue.

Diuretic: a substance used to increase the output of urine.

DNA: the component of chromosomes that carries information and determines the organism's appearance and function.

Dyscrasia: an abnormal state. **Blood dyscrasia:** any abnormal condition in the type or number of the formed elements (cells) of the blood.

Dysmenorrhea: painful menstruation.

Edema: the excessive accumulation of fluid in the tissue spaces.

Embolus: a blood clot, or portion of a clot, that has broken away from its site of formation and traveled via the blood stream to another site within the body.

Emetic: a substance used to induce vomiting.

Enzyme: a substance formed by living cells that promotes or enhances a particular chemical reaction in the body by functioning as a catalyst.

Epilepsy: a brain dysfunction in which abnormal electrical discharges occur at intervals, causing motor seizures or psychic phenomena.

Erythema: reddening of the skin.

Erythrocyte: red blood cell; contains hemoglobin, which is responsible for carrying oxygen to body tissues.

Fibrillation: quivering of cardiac muscle fibers, rendering the heart unable to contract with sufficient force to circulate blood effectively.

Ganglion: a group of nerve cell bodies.

Glaucoma: a serious eye disorder in which normal drainage of intraocular fluid is impaired, causing increased intraocular pressure. Blindness results if treatment is delayed.

Glomerulus: the tuft of capillaries projecting into the glomerular capsule. The capillaries allow filtration of water, salt, and impurities from the blood and thus are responsible for the first stage in urine formation.

Glycosuria or glucosuria: sugar in the urine.

Goiter: enlargement of the thyroid gland; may occur with either hypothyroidism or hyperthyroidism.

Habit formation: the condition whereby drugs are routinely taken as a matter of course, not as a matter of necessity. Withdrawal symptoms are not seen on cessation of the habit.

Hematinic: an agent that enhances the diet, tending to increase the hemoglobin content of the blood; usually contains iron.

Hemoglobin: the red pigment in erythrocytes that reversibly combines with oxygen, thus transporting it to tissues.

Hemosiderosis: a condition in which there is an excessive deposition of iron in the tissues, particularly in the liver, causing cirrhosis, and in the pancreas, causing diabetes mellitus.

Hepatitis: inflammation of the liver.

Hirsutism: excessive growth of facial or body hair.

Histamine: an amino acid that, when released in the body, produces the symptoms of allergic reactions; nasal secretions are increased, engorgement of capillary beds occurs, visceral muscles are stimulated, and lung bronchioles are constricted.

Hodgkin's disease: a form of lymphoma characterized by enlargement and malignant degeneration of the lymph nodes, eventually spreading to involve the liver, spleen, and other internal organs.

Hormone: an agent secreted by the endocrine glands into the blood stream that produces or alters bodily functions.

Hypertension: elevated blood pressure.

Hypertensive: an agent used to elevate blood pressure therapeutically.

Hyperthyroidism: a condition caused by excessive activity of the thyroid gland with accompanying hypertension, nervousness, tachycardia, and exophthalmos.

Hyperuricemia: increased uric acid levels in the blood, often associated with gout or gouty arthritis.

Hypnotic: an agent used to induce sleep.

Hypochlorhydria: a decrease in the amount of gastric hydrochloric acid.

Hypotension: lowered blood pressure.

Hypotensive: an agent used to decrease blood pressure therapeutically.

Hypothyroidism: decreased functioning of the thyroid gland with subsequent slowing down of mental and motor functions.

Immunity: the state whereby the individual is not susceptible to a certain disease.

Immunizing agent: a biological preparation injected to produce immunity to disease.

Immunosuppressive: an agent that interferes with the body systems that resist infection and foreign materials.

Intrinsic factor: a substance in the gastric wall that is necessary for vitamin B_{12} absorption.

Jaundice: yellow pigmentation noticeable in the skin and mucous membranes and caused by an increase in the amount of serum bilirubin, usually as a result of a liver disorder.

Leukemia: a condition characterized by uncontrolled proliferation of the leukocytes, or white cells, of the blood.

Leukocyte: a white blood cell; responsible for antibody production and defense against infectious agents in the body.

Leukopenia: a decrease in the number of white cells in the blood.

Lymphocyte: a white blood cell, formed in the lymph tissues of the body such as the spleen, lymph nodes, and tonsils. Cells are active in antibody formation to counteract infection.

Lymphoma: any of a group of malignant conditions involving lymphoid tissue.

Lymphosarcoma: a tumor of the lymph nodes in which the nodes contain masses of rounded malignant cells that resemble lymphocytes.

Malaise: generalized, nonspecific discomfort or unease.

Meningitis: infection of the meninges, the lining of the brain, and the spinal cord.

Menopause: the time at which female fertility ceases.

Menorrhagia: excessive menstrual flow.

Metabolism: the chemical changes in living organisms whereby energy is produced and tissue repairs are effected.

Migraine: paroxysmal, intensely painful headache caused by vasomotor disturbances in a scalp artery, often accompanied by psychic phenomena, nausea, and vomiting.

Mineral: a naturally occurring, inorganic substance necessary to body function.

Miosis: pupil constriction.

Moniliasis: superinfection with the fungus *Candida albicans*. See *Candidiasis*.

Multiple myeloma: a malignant disease characterized by bony destruction, often with pathological fractures, anemia, hyperglobulinemia, hypercalcemia, and increased numbers of immature cells in the bone marrow.

Mycosis fungoides: a form of lymphoma that has numerous cutaneous manifestations, such as eczema, nodules, tumors, infiltrations, and ulcerations.

Mydriasis: dilation of the pupil.

Myxedema: hypothyroidism with onset usually in late childhood or adulthood, characterized by puffiness of the skin and a slowing of mental and motor functions.

Neoplasm: an unnatural growth or tumor in the body; a cancer.

Nephritis: inflammation of the kidney.

Nephron: the functional unit of the kidney, consisting of the glomerulus, the glomerular capsule, and the collecting tubules.

Neurosis: an emotional disorder characterized by anxiety or depressive reaction but in which the patient has not lost contact with reality.

Neutropenia: a decrease in the number of neutrophils (a type of white cell) in the blood.

Nocardiosis: a systemic fungus infection, often with granuloma formation in various organs.

Opisthotonos: a tetanic muscle spasm characterized by arching of the back, inability to speak, and loss of muscle control. The patient is usually conscious; occurs as a rare drug hypersensitivity reaction.

Osmosis: the process in which water travels through a semipermeable membrane to equalize concentrations of fluid on either side of the membrane.

Osteomalacia: softening of the bones resulting from interference with calcium deposits in bony tissue.

Osteoporosis: thinning and increased porosity of the bone with resultant deformities or fractures. Common in postmenopausal women.

Oxytocic: a drug used to produce effects similar to those of oxytocin, especially stimulation of uterine contractions.

Palliative: an agent that lessens the effect of a microorganism or cancer in the body; improves the condition of the patient but does not cure.

Pancytopenia: a condition in which there are decreased numbers of all blood cells.

Paralysis: an inability to move an affected body part.

Parasympatholytic: an agent that counteracts the effects of the parasympathetic nervous system.

Parasympathomimetic: an agent that produces stimulating effects on the parasympathetic nervous system.

Paresis: weakness of an affected body part.

Paresthesia: the abnormal skin sensation of crawling, burning, or tingling, not caused by surface stimuli.

Parkinson's disease: a progressive condition resulting primarily from deterioration of certain brain nuclei; characterized by rigidity, tremors, akinesia, and loss of spontaneous or automatic movement.

Parkinsonism: usually refers to a short-term reversible syndrome, resembling Parkinson's disease but occurring instead as a side effect of certain drugs, notably the tranquilizers, and reversible following withdrawal of the drug.

Peristalsis: automatic contractions of the gastrointestinal tract.

Pheochromocytoma: a tumor of the sympathetic nervous system, usually located in the adrenal medulla, that may cause severe, intermittent, or persistent hypertension.

Polycythemia vera: a condition characterized by increased numbers of red blood cells in the blood. Occasionally occurs as a premalignant disorder before the onset of leukemia. Common in individuals living in high altitudes for prolonged periods of time.

Prostaglandins: short-acting hormones that perform many functions in the body and exert their effect close to the site of production.

Prostaglandin inhibitors: agents that interfere with the effects of prostaglandins.

Prothrombin: a protein produced by the liver necessary for normal blood clotting.

Prothrombin time: a measurement of the prothrombin level in the blood. Measurement performed routinely to assess the effectiveness of anticoagulant therapy.

Pruritus: an itching sensation of the skin.

Psychosis: a severe mental disease in which the patient's contact with reality is diminished or lost.

Purpura: multiple small hemorrhagic areas in the skin or mucous membranes.

Pyelitis: inflammation of the pelvis of the kidney.

Pyelonephritis: inflammation of the pelvis and glomerular tissues of the kidney.

Rickets: a condition caused by a deficiency of vitamin D. Calcium and phosphorus imbalances cause softening of the bones and characteristic deformations, such as bowed legs, rachitic "rosary" on the costochondral junctions, and so on.

Ringworm: a topical fungus infection of the skin, hair, or nails, often circular in appearance and spreading peripherally.

RNA: the component of the nucleus that carries information and aids in the correct assembly of DNA.

Schizophrenia: a type of psychosis in which the patient typically withdraws from reality, exhibiting unpredictable moods, disturbances in the stream of thought, and regressive tendencies to the point of deterioration, often with hallucinations and delusions.

Scurvy: a vitamin C deficiency characterized by weakness, gum hemorrhages, loosening of the teeth, and subcutaneous hemorrhages.

Sedative: an agent used to quiet the patient without inducing sleep.

Seizure: see *Convulsion.*

Shock: a sudden drop in blood pressure as a result of an injury or blood loss.

Status asthmaticus: a prolonged attack of asthma, poorly responsive to drug therapy and lasting as long as several days.

Status epilepticus: a rapid succession of epileptic seizures in which the patient does not regain consciousness between seizures.

Stevens-Johnson syndrome: a severe, life-threatening allergic drug reaction. Excoriations of the skin, mucous membranes, and cornea and inflammation of the internal organs occur. Decreased blood pressure may bring about shock and death.

Stimulant: an agent that promotes or enhances the activity of a body organ or tissue.

Sympatholytic: an agent that counteracts the effects of the sympathetic nervous system.

Sympathomimetic: an agent that produces stimulating effects on the sympathetic nervous system.

Synapse: the connection between two or more neurons.

Tachycardia: increased heart rate.

Tetany: a condition caused by a decreased concentration of ionized calcium in the blood, leading to increased irritability of muscles and painful tonic muscle spasms.

Thrombophlebitis: inflammation of the walls of a vein with resultant clotting of blood at the site.

Thrombus: a blood clot in the heart or blood vessels that remains attached at the site of formation.

Thrush: *Candida albicans* infection of the oral mucous membranes, typically in the form of small, white macular spots.

Toxin: the poisonous substance released by microorganisms.

Toxoid: an altered form of toxin that may be injected to produce immunity to a specific disease or microorganism.

Toxoplasmosis: a disease caused by infection with the protozoan *Toxoplasma*. May take the form of a respiratory infection, encephalomyelitis, or a dermatitis.

Trachoma: an inflammatory disease of the eye involving the conjunctiva and cornea, producing photophobia, pain, and excessive lacrimation. May lead to blindness through vascularization of the cornea if not treated.

Tranquilizer: a substance used as a calming agent during waking hours.

Tumor: an unnatural growth in the body.

Ureter: the tube that carries urine from the kidney to the bladder.

Urethra: the tube that carries urine from the bladder to the exterior of the body.

Urticaria (hives): a condition in which pruritic wheals or welts appear on the skin, usually as a response to an allergic phenomenon.

Vaccine: an agent injected to produce immunity to disease.

Ventricle: one of the lower chambers of the heart.

Vertigo: dizziness.

Vitamin: an organic compound that cannot be synthesized in the human body, but is present in minute amounts in foodstuffs. It is required for normal growth, development, and well-being.

Canadian Drug Information

Alfred J. Rémillard, Pharm.D.

INTERNATIONAL SYSTEM OF UNITS

In an attempt to standardize the large number of different units used worldwide and thus improve communication, the *Système International d'Unités* (International System of Units, SI) was recommended in 1954. In 1971, the mole (mol) was adopted as the standard for designating the amount of substance present, and the liter (L) was adopted as the standard for designating volume. The World Health Organization recommended the adoption of SI units in 1977. However, Canada had already implemented an equivalent system in 1971.

In therapeutics, the major change caused by adopting the SI was to express drug concentrations present in body fluids in molar units (e.g., μmol/L) rather than in mass units (e.g., mg/L). This allows us to better compare the pharmacological and pharmacodynamic effects of different drugs, since these effects are now related to the number of molecules (e.g., μmol) of drug present rather than to the number of mass units (e.g., mg).

DRUG SERUM CONCENTRATIONS

Many drugs have known therapeutic or toxic levels that are monitored in patients to ensure safety and efficacy. In Canada, clinical laboratories report these levels in SI units. Levels traditionally reported as μg/mL can be converted to μmol/L once the conversion factor (CF) is calculated:

$$CF = \frac{1000}{\text{molecular weight of the drug}}$$

To convert from μg/mL to SI units:

$$\mu g/mL \times CF = \mu mol/L$$

To convert from SI units to μg/mL:

$$\frac{\mu mol/L}{CF} = \mu g/mL$$

Table A–1 lists some important drugs for which therapeutic or toxic levels have been established. For most of these drugs, the levels presented are *trough* (minimum) values, which are measured in blood samples drawn just prior to the next dose. For the aminoglycosides and vancomycin, two levels are listed: a *trough* level and a *peak* (maximum) level. Levels must remain between the peak and trough to maintain efficacy of these drugs and to minimize toxicity.

From Lehne RA: Pharmacology for Nursing Care, 2nd ed. Philadelphia, W.B. Saunders, 1994.

Table A-1. THERAPEUTIC SERUM DRUG CONCENTRATIONS

Drugs	SI Reference Interval	SI Unit	Conversion Factor	Traditional Reference Interval	Traditional Reference Unit
Acetaminophen	13–40	μmol/L	66.16	0.2–0.6	mg/dl
Acetylsalicylic acid	7.2–21.7	μmol/L	0.0724	100–300	mg/dl
Amikacin*	—	—	—	15–25†; <8‡	μg/ml
Amitriptyline	430–900§	nmol/L	3.605	120–250§	ng/ml
Carbamazepine	17–42	μmol/L	4.233	4–10	μg/ml
Desipramine	430–750	nmol/L	3.754	115–200	ng/ml
Digoxin	0.6–2.8	nmol/L	1.282	0.5–2.2	ng/ml
Disopyramide	6–18	μmol/L	2.946	2–6	μg/ml
Gentamicin*	—	—	—	6–10‡; <2‡	μg/ml
Imipramine	640–1070§	nmol/L	3.566	180–300§	ng/ml
Lidocaine	4.5–21.5	μmol/L	4.267	1–5	μg/ml
Lithium	0.4–1.2	mmol/L	1.0	0.4–1.2	mEq/L
Netilmicin*	—	—	—	6–10†; <2‡	μg/ml
Nortriptyline	190—570	nmol/L	3.797	50–150	ng/ml
Phenobarbital	65–170	μmol/L	4.306	15–40	μg/ml
Phenytoin	40–80	μmol/L	3.964	10–20	μg/ml
Primidone	25–46	μmol/L	4.582	6–10	μg/ml
Procainamide	17–34§	μmol/L	4.249	4–8§	μg/ml
Quinidine	4.6–9.2	μmol/L	3.082	1.5–3	μg/ml
Theophylline	55–110	μmol/L	5.55	10–20	μg/ml
Tobramycin*	—	—	—	6–10†; <2‡	μg/ml
Valproic acid	300–700	μmol/L	6.934	50–100	μg/ml
Vancomycin*	—	—	—	25–40†; <10‡	μg/ml

*Aminoglycosides (amikacin, gentamicin, netilmicin, tobramycin) and vancomycin are not reported in SI units because of the variability of their molecular weights.
†Peak drug level.
‡Trough drug level.
§Drug level reported as the total of the parent drug and its active metabolite.

REFERENCES

1. SI Manual in Health Care, 2nd ed. Subcommittee of Metric Commission Canada, Sector 9.10, Health and Welfare, Ottawa, Canada, June 1, 1982.
2. McLeod DC: SI units in drug therapeutics. Drug Intell Clin Pharm 22:990–993, 1988.
3. Evans WE, Schentag JJ, Jusko WJ (eds): Applied Pharmacokinetics: Principles of Therapeutic Drug Monitoring. Applied Therapeutics, Inc., Spokane, WA, 1992.

CANADIAN DRUG LEGISLATION

In Canada, two acts form the basis of drug laws. The Food and Drug Act, which was amended in 1953, controls the manufacture, distribution, and sale of all drugs except narcotics. The Narcotic Control Act (1961) controls the manufacture, distribution, and sale of narcotic drugs. The responsibility for administering these acts rests with the Health Protection Branch, Department of National Health and Welfare. Both acts contain general statements relating to the safety and efficacy of drugs. Detailed requirements are outlined in the Regulations.

Prescription Drugs (Schedule F)

The Food and Drug Regulations separate drugs sold in Canada into several categories, referred to as Schedules. Schedule F lists all prescription drugs and includes a wide diversity of classes, such as antihypertensives, hormonal preparations, and psychotropic medications. These drugs are available to the general public only with a prescription from a medical practitioner. Prescriptions for Schedule F medications may be written or verbal (i.e., telephone order to the pharmacist) and can be refilled as often as indicated by the physician. More than 350 drugs are listed in Schedule F, which is subject to frequent changes. The symbol Pr must appear on all manufacturing labels. Although some drugs may be classified *federally* as nonprescription, the *provinces* may nonetheless require a prescription, as occurs with digoxin, for example.

Controlled Drugs (Schedule G)

Controlled drugs, listed in Schedule G of the Food and Drug Act, have a moderate potential for abuse. Accordingly, these agents require greater control than Schedule F drugs (prescription drugs), which have essentially no potential for abuse. Schedule G contains about 14 drugs, including potent analgesics (nalbuphine, butorphanol), amphetamine and its congeners, and the barbiturates (phenobarbital, amobarbital, secobarbital). The distribution of controlled substances is more restricted than the distribution of Schedule F drugs. Schedule G drugs can be obtained by a written or verbal prescription, but refills are only allowed on a written order. The symbol © must appear on the labels of these drugs. Schedule G is similar to Schedule III of the Controlled Substances Act in the United States.

Restricted Drugs (Schedule H)

These agents are hallucinogenic, potentially dangerous, and have no recognized medicinal use. Examples include LSD, peyote, and mescaline. These chemicals are available legally only to medical institutions involved in specialized research. This category is similar to Schedule I of the Controlled Substances Act in the United States.

Narcotic Drugs

Narcotic drugs are controlled by the Narcotic Control Act and Regulations. Examples include coca leaves (cocaine), opium, codeine, morphine, phencyclidine, and Cannabis (marijuana). The major clinical use for these drugs is strong analgesia. However, they all have potent psychotropic effects and addictive potential. As a result, their availability must be strictly controlled. Narcotic agents can be dispensed only with a written prescription. No refills are allowed. The letter **N** must appear on all labels and professional advertisements.

An exception to the narcotic drug regulations is low-dose codeine (8-mg tablets and 20 mg/30 mL liquid), which can be purchased without a prescription. The codeine must be in a preparation that contains at least two additional medicinal ingredients (acetylsalicylic acid and caffeine) and can be sold only by a pharmacist.

Nonprescription Drugs

Nonprescription drugs, also known as over-the-counter (OTC) medications, can be purchased without a prescription. These drugs represent an interesting class of compounds, as several prescription drugs shown to have a proven safety record are, in low-dose formulations, gradually being transferred to the OTC category. Examples include ibuprofen (Motrin) in 200-mg tablets and hydrocortisone in 0.5% topical preparations.

Although the Food and Drug Act and Regulations place no restrictions on how OTC drugs are sold, most provinces have drug schedules—administered by their respective Pharmacy Acts—to determine the conditions and place of sale. As a result, there are three categories of nonprescription medications in Canada. These are described below.

The first category represents general proprietary (GP) medicines and can be purchased at any retail outlet. These products are intended for the symptomatic treatment of self-limiting minor illness, injury, or discomfort. Proprietary medications have adequate information on the packages so that they can be administered without the assistance of a health professional. Examples include medicated shampoos, minor analgesics, and cough drops.

Agents in the second category are generally available only in pharmacies. Although these drugs are intended for treating minor self-limiting conditions, it is recommended that the advice of a health professional be obtained concerning their proper use. Examples of this category include laxatives, cough and cold preparations, disinfectants, and many vitamins.

The third category consists of medicines that should be taken only on the recommendation of a physician. These drugs, which are available in pharmacies, include insulin, nitroglycerin, muscle relaxants, and antispasmodics. Also in this category are medications that are not accessible to the public but may be purchased after consultation with the pharmacist. These include ibuprofen, hydrocortisone, and low-dose preparations of codeine.

Schedule Harmonization

The Health Protection Branch (HPB) has expressed concern about the proliferation of differing provincial schedules that regulate the sale of nonprescription drugs. In an attempt to address the problems of the current regulatory system at both the federal and provincial levels, the HPB has proposed to harmonize drug schedules throughout the country, using a three-Schedule system. Schedule I would include all prescription drugs (Schedules F and G, and Narcotics); Schedule II would consist of pharmacist-monitored nonprescription drugs; and Schedule III would consist of nonprescription drugs that are not appropriate for inclusion in Schedule I or II. For Schedule III drugs, there would be no restrictions on the place of sale.

The first step toward harmonization is to develop scientific criteria to determine the degree of professional involvement required for the sale and judicious use of drug products. Criteria for determining which drugs will be assigned to Schedule II will be the greatest challenge. Creation of Schedule II represents a very progressive step in drug regulation, as it is anticipated that many prescription drugs with a proven safety profile, such as cimetidine, may be transferred to this Schedule. The HPB is currently reviewing comments received and is expected to publish its proposals soon in the form of draft regulations.

REFERENCES

1. Health Protection and Drug Laws. Health and Welfare Canada, Canadian Publishing Center, Ottawa, Canada, 1988.
2. Johnson GE, Hannah KJ, Zerr SR: Pharmacology and the Nursing Process, 3rd ed. WB Saunders, Philadelphia, 1992.
3. Health Protection Branch, Information Newsletter. Issue No. 798, September 9, 1991.

NEW DRUG DEVELOPMENT IN CANADA

The process for approving a new drug in Canada is very similar, if not identical, to the process in the United States. The same drug data that are required for approval by the Food and Drug Administration in the United States are required by the Health Protection Branch (HPB) in Canada. The principal difference between Canada and the United States is one of nomenclature: once preclinical testing is completed, the manufacturer in Canada applies for a *Preclinical New Drug Submission,* versus an Investigational New Drug in the United States; at the end of clinical testing, the manufacturer in Canada seeks a *New Drug Submission* (NDS), versus a New Drug Application in the United States.

After all the information on a new drug has been submitted—including results of preclinical and clinical testing, method of manufacturing, packaging, labeling, and results of stability testing—the pharmaceutical company receives a *Notice of Compliance* (NOC) from the HPB, and the drug enters the market.

Although data collection for a new drug is thorough, there is no guarantee that all adverse reactions are known, especially when the drug is used concurrently with other drugs. Also, long-term effects are not fully appreciated. For these reasons, postmarketing surveillance plays a major role in monitoring these drugs. The manufacturer must immediately report any new clinical findings, unexpected adverse effects, or therapeutic failures to the HPB.

Patent Laws

In 1969, changes were made to the Patent Act, and Compulsory Licensing was introduced. The license allowed generic drug companies to manufacture and distribute patented drugs in Canada, provided that a minimal 4 percent royalty fee was paid to the patent holder. This system was introduced to help control drug prices. Unfortunately, the system caused a decline in revenue to "innovative" pharmaceutical companies, with a resultant decline in research on new drug development. After much debate, and retroactive to June 1987, the Patent Act was amended to allow market exclusivity for either (1) 7 to 10 years, or (2) until the 17-year patent (from date of filing) expires, whichever comes first. A Price Review Board was created to monitor the prices of new drugs and those under Compulsory Licensing.

Anticipated Patent Law Changes

Further changes in the Patent Act are expected. As a result of extensive lobbying from representatives of the pharmaceutical industry, provisions were included in the North American Free Trade Agreement (1992) and the General Agreement on Tariffs and Trade (1991) that require Canada to repeal its patent laws and bring them into agreement with international rules on the protection of intellectual property. At the time of this writing, the Canadian Parliament approved Bill C-91, which will extend patent protection by 3 years, thereby providing 20 years of exclusivity for companies that develop new drugs. This would be consistent with patent laws in the United States and other industrialized nations.

REFERENCES

1. Health Protection and Drug Laws. Health and Welfare Canada, Canadian Publishing Center, Ottawa, Canada, 1988.
2. Mailhot R: The Canadian drug regulatory process. J Clin Pharmacol 26:232–239, 1986.
3. Sullivan P: CMA to support increased patent protection for drugs but will attach strong qualifications. Can Med Assoc J 147:1669–1701, 1992.

INDEX

Note: Page numbers followed by t refer to tables.